Pain Management - From Acute to Chronic and Beyond

Edited by Theodoros Aslanidis and Christos Nouris

Published in London, United Kingdom

Pain Management - From Acute to Chronic and Beyond
http://dx.doi.org/10.5772/intechopen.107760
Edited by Theodoros Aslanidis and Christos Nouris

Contributors
Tej Prakash Sinha, Sakshi Yadav, Anuj Ajayababu, Sanjeev Bhoi, Björn Gerdle, Marcelo Rivano Fischer, Åsa Ringqvist, Denberu Eshetie Adane, Kristina Ryliškienė, Mantas Jokubaitis, Mamta Latwal, Ganesh Pandey, Maria I. Trapali, Ahmed Adebayo Ishola, Lucia Merlino, Luca Titi, Alba Crognale, Maria Grazia Piccioni, Maria Grazia Porpora, Carlo Della Rocca, Roberto Senatori, Stephen Sciberras, Theodoros Aslanidis, Christos Nouris, Juliet Lee, Gustavo Rodriguez, Emma Whiting, Boris Hait, Agnès Mazic De Sonis, James A. Tolley, Dimitar Tonev, Yoram Braw, Itay Goor-Aryeh, Motti Ratmansky, Dong Ha Lee, Jung Wook Huh

First published in London, United Kingdom, 2024 by IntechOpen
IntechOpen is the global imprint of INTECHOPEN LIMITED, registered in England and Wales, registration number: 11086078, 5 Princes Gate Court, London, SW7 2QJ, United Kingdom
Printed in Croatia

British Library Cataloguing-in-Publication Data
A catalogue record for this book is available from the British Library

Additional hard and PDF copies can be obtained from orders@intechopen.com

Pain Management - From Acute to Chronic and Beyond
Edited by Theodoros Aslanidis and Christos Nouris
p. cm.

This title is part of the Pharmaceutical Science Book Series, Volume 1
Topic: Pharmacology
Series Editor: Rosario Pignatello
Topic Editor: Cristina Manuela Drăgoi
Associate Topic Editor: Alina Crenguţa Nicolae

Print ISBN 978-1-83768-797-8
Online ISBN 978-1-83768-816-6
eBook (PDF) ISBN 978-1-83768-817-3
ISSN 3033-3318

For EU product safety concerns:
IN TECH d.o.o., Prolaz Marije Krucifikse Kozulić 3, 51000 Rijeka, Croatia,
info@intechopen.com or visit our website at intechopen.com.

IntechOpen Book Series
Pharmaceutical Science
Volume 1

Aims and Scope of the Series

Pharmaceutical science focuses on the design, synthesis, formulation, targeting, distribution, safety, and efficacy of active compounds as potential therapeutics. It is a large interdisciplinary discipline that aims to integrate the basic principles of physical and organic chemistry, biochemistry, biology, and engineering to discover, develop, and characterize active compounds and to optimize the formulation and delivery of drugs in the body for offering new and improved safe and efficacious therapies against human diseases. The research areas covered by the pharmaceutical sciences range from medicinal chemistry and pharmaceutical technology to pharmacology and toxicology, which represent the preliminary phases of drug development. Medicinal chemistry involves the design and synthesis of pharmaceuticals as well as the isolation of active agents from natural sources. Computer-aided strategies are increasingly involved in this drug discovery process. Pharmaceutics is a multidisciplinary science that examines the relationships between drug formulation, delivery, distribution, and clinical outcomes. Modern clinical approaches are increasingly relying on controlled release strategies and drug delivery and targeting systems, including nanotechnological platforms (nanomedicine). Pharmacology is the science of drug action in biological systems. Pharmacologists also make drugs as tools to explore aspects of cell and tissue functions. Toxicology is the study of the adverse effects of active agents on living organisms and the ecosystem, including the prevention and amelioration of such adverse effects. This book series includes volumes on Drug Discovery, Delivery, and Pharmacology. Their overall aim is to present the latest research in the whole path of drug discovery and development from different points of view of this multidisciplinary and dynamic field.

Meet the Series Editor

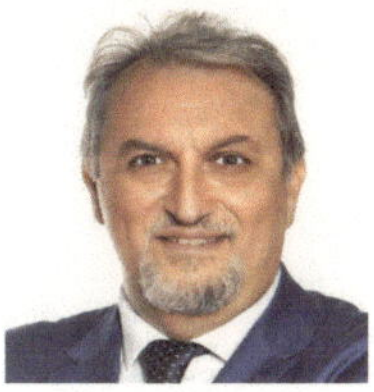

Prof. Rosario Pignatello is a Full Professor of Pharmaceutical Technology and Legislation at the University of Catania, Italy. He is the Director of the Department of Drug and Health Sciences. He has nearly 30 years of experience in the research and development of innovative formulations for the controlled release and targeting of bioactive molecules, through chemical approaches as well as nanotechnological carriers, aimed at treating different disorders. Prof. Pignatello has coauthored about 180 papers and edited a series of textbooks on biomaterials and their application in medicine. The main areas of his research are polymeric and lipid-based micro- and nanoparticles as modified drug delivery systems; vesicular nanocarriers (liposomes, micelles); lipophilic prodrugs and conjugates; synthesis and evaluation of new polymeric biomaterials for drug delivery and tissue regeneration. In particular, Prof. Pignatello works actively in the field of ocular drug delivery, leading the Research Centre for Ocular Nanotechnology, within the NANOMED Centre (Centre for Nanomedicine and Pharmaceutical Nanotechnology) at the University of Catania.

Meet the Volume Editors

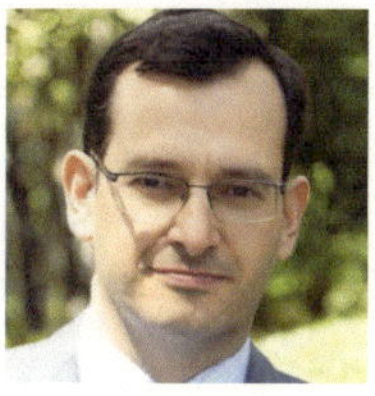

Dr. Theodoros K. Aslanidis received his MG from Plovdiv Medical University, Bulgaria and his Ph.D. from Aristotle University of Thessaloniki, Greece. After serving as a medical doctor in the Hellenic Army Force and as a rural physician at Outhealth Centre, Iraklia and Serres' General Hospital, Greece, he completed anesthesiology specialty training at "Hippokratio" Thessaloniki's General Hospital, critical care subspecialty training at AHEPA University Hospital, and a prehospital emergency medicine postgraduate program at the Hellenic National Centre for Emergency Care. He served as an EMS physician and emergency communication center medic before moving to his current post as a consultant-researcher at the Intensive Care Unit and Anesthesia Department of Agios Pavlos General Hospital of Thessaloniki, Greece. He also serves as Head of Postgraduate Studies, College of Offshore and Remote Medicine, Pretty Bay, Malta.

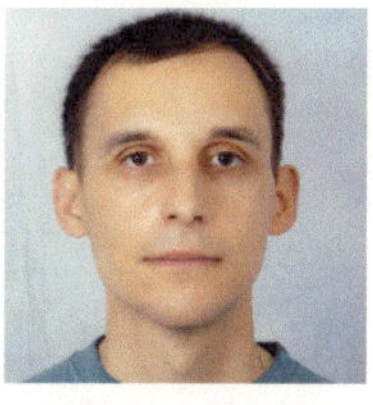

Dr. Christos Nouris received his MD from the School of Medicine, Aristotle University of Thessaloniki, Greece. He also obtained an MSc in Medical Research Methodology from the same university. After completing his residency in anesthesiology at AHEPA University Hospital, Greece, he worked as a consultant anesthesiologist at the District General Hospital of Veria, Greece. Later, he completed his fellowship in intensive care at "G. Papageorgiou" General Hospital, Greece, where he is currently an ICU consultant. From 2017 he worked as a consultant at AHEPA University Hospital, Greece, as well as taught medical students at the School of Medicine, Aristotle University of Thessaloniki; in the Postgraduate Nursing Specialties Program, AHEPA University Hospital; and the Committee for the European Education in Anesthesiology (CEEA) teaching programs.

Contents

Preface

The 2020 revised definition of the International Association for the Study of Pain states that pain is "An unpleasant sensory and emotional experience associated with, or resembling that associated with, actual or potential tissue damage". The definition is expanded by other keynotes for further valuable context. Such notes are, for example, that pain is a personal experience, and that pain differs from nociception. Yet, pain management has always been a quest for humankind. In fact, the world's oldest recorded list of medical prescriptions from a Sumerian clay tablet dating to about 2100 BC is about pain.

Medicine has made tremendous progress in the field of algology. However, the personal and societal burden of pain, either acute or chronic, remains extremely high. The incorporation of genetic testing and artificial intelligence in daily practice is expected to change our understanding about the pathophysiology of pain, facilitating assessment and monitoring and boosting the development of innovative models of personalized care.

Within this framework, this book provides an overview of pain in two areas. The first section of the book is dedicated to pain management in different conditions and various populations, including in the emergency department and the intensive care unit. It also discusses multimodal analgesia and enhanced recovery after surgery (ERAS) protocols for vestibular migraine, nociplastic pain in gynecology, interdisciplinary rehabilitation programs to palliative, and end-of-life care. The second section highlights the pharmacology of analgesics, with a focus on aspirin, as well as discusses topics in pain research and genetics.

The diversity of the subjects presented makes this book a valuable resource, opening pathways for future researchers.

Theodoros Aslanidis
Intensive Care Unit and Anesthesia Department,
"Agios Pavlos" General Hospital,
Thessaloniki, Greece

Christos Nouris
Intensive Care Unit,
"G. Papageorgiou" General Hospital,
Thessaloniki, Greece

Section 1

Management

Chapter 1

Introductory Chapter: Pain in ICU

Theodoros Aslanidis and Christos Nouris

1. Introduction

According to the International Association for the Study of Pain (IASP), pain is defined as "an unpleasant sensory and emotional experience associated with actual or potential tissue damage or described in terms of such damage" [1]. This "pain distress" is usually augmented in the ICU where patients suffer the additional psychological distress of hospitalization, communication difficulty, and self-control loss [2]; and it is considered the main source of anxiety, agitation and sleep deprivation, and delirium in the ICU [3].

Apart from that, sustained pain leads to a state of persistent adrenergic activation and systemic inflammatory response syndrome encapsulating which are related to tachycardia, hypertension, increased myocardial oxygen consumption, and myocardial ischemia [4]; atelectasis, diaphragmatic dysfunction, respiratory impairment, increased catabolism, hyperglycemia, immunosuppression impaired wound healing and hypercoagulation [5–8].

The former result not only in a higher ICU length-of-stay, ICU morbidity, and mortality but also long-term consequences even after ICU discharge. The incidence of chronic pain (duration of more >3 months) after ICU varies from 28 to 77% and risk factors for chronification of pain involve pre-existing chronic pain, the intensity of acute pain, and the presence of acute pain at discharge from ICU [9, 10]. Chronic pain is a key element of Post Intensive Care Syndrome, a physical, cognitive, and psychological entity that may persist for years after ICU discharge [2].

Despite these facts, pain continues to be a commonly reported experience among ICU patients. More than half of critically ill patients report moderate to severe pain at rest and 80% experience pain during procedures with fewer than 25% receiving analgesics before painful procedures [11–15].

The rates of pain do not defer between medical and surgical ICUs [16]. Patients in ICU experience pain due to their illness or the diagnostic and therapeutic procedures carried out by medical and nursing staff. ICU-related procedures characterized as uncomfortable are repositioning, physiotherapy and mobilization, wound and burn dressing changes, tracheal suctioning, and mechanical ventilation but the care-related procedures described as most painful are arterial line insertion, chest tube removal, and wound drain removal [14].

2. Assessment of pain in ICU

Diagnosing and quantifying pain in ICU is a complex matter and a systematic and thoughtful approach is needed. It is essential to differentiate pain from other causes of distress, like delirium, hypoxemia, hypotension or withdrawal of alcohol and drugs, and address the issue accordingly [1]. The approach should be systematic and protocolized. However, surveys have shown that only 50% of ICU professionals assess pain and they only do it infrequently [17]. Clinicians should assess critically ill patients for their level of pain regularly, that is every 2–3 hours and every time before a painful procedure or mobilization, using validated scales [3]. Vital signs associated with pain (hypertension, tachycardia, tachypnea) are poor indicators of pain because physiological parameters related to pain can be augmented or inhibited by several other factors in the ICU setting [1].

When patients in ICU can interact and communicate, either verbally or not, commonly used pain scales are very useful in the assessment of pain. The most valid and feasible among several pain intensity rating scales is a visually enlarged numeric rating scale (NRS) from 0 to 10, where 0 represents no pain and 10 represents severe pain [18]. Intubated patients can report their level of pain either by pointing on a large board that includes the numeric rating scale or by nodding as a provider holds up the board with the scale and points at the specific rating of their pain.

When patients in ICU are unable to communicate, scales that rest upon patient's behavior are implemented. Behavioral Pain Scale (BPS) and Critical-Care Pain Observation Tool (CPOT) are the most effective. Behavioral Pain Scale relies on the observation of the patient's expressions, upper limp movements, and synchrony with mechanical ventilation. It ranges between 3 and 12 and any value over 6 necessitates treatment of pain [19]. Critical-Care Pain Observation Tool is similar. It includes four components: facial expressions, body movements, muscle tension, and compliance with the ventilator for intubated or vocalization for extubated patients. This scale scores from 0 to 8 and a score over 2 indicates high levels of pain that need to be addressed [20]. Behavioral scales have been validated in critically ill patients [21, 22], but their correlation with self-reported scales is poor [23].

Despite the high availability of assessment tools for the diagnosis of pain in the ICU, existing literature suggests that as little as 19% of intensive care personnel adhere to the actual implementation of standardized diagnostic protocols [24]. Even then, adequate assessment must be partnered with an appropriate and adequate analgesic strategy to alleviate pain.

3. Treatment of pain in ICU

The pain must be treated before the administration of sedation, which should be initiated only if needed. It should rely on an algorithm-based approach using evidence-based protocols in response to pain scores [3, 16] and must be multimodal and holistic based on a variety of combined interventions to achieve the best analgesic effect with minimal side effects [15]. Furthermore, pain should, whenever possible, be treated preemptively, before the initiation of potentially painful procedures. Lastly, the specific analgesic pharmacological agents chosen to treat pain and the administrated dosage must be tailored to each patient concerning the patient's specific needs.

Non-pharmacologic methods include massage therapy [25–27], cold therapy [28, 29], music and sound [30, 31], and relaxation therapy [32, 33]. They have been shown to decrease patient-reported and behavioral pain scores and the need for pharmacologic interventions [3] but are time-consuming requiring the engagement of the patient's family and should always be used in conjunction with pharmacologic therapy [16].

Pharmacologic therapy is based on the administration of numerous different classes of drugs that are often simultaneously used to block the various receptors and pathways of pain. Intravenous is the main route of administration but other options exist too. Regional analgesia, for example, and the use of local anesthetics can play a fundamental role in postoperative and post-trauma pain control in ICU. Central and peripheral neuraxial blocks have been shown to ensure adequate pain control with less opioid consumption and reduced stress response to surgery or trauma [34].

3.1 Opioids

Opioids are the mainstay for the treatment of acute non-neuropathic pain in the ICU. They are mostly administered intravenously by infusion following an initial bolus dose but can also be given by other routes like enteral (oxycodone, diamorphine, tramadol, codeine, morphine) or transcutaneous (fentanyl). Even when opioids are titrated to effect, prolonged use has been associated with several side effects: hemodynamic instability (bradycardia, hypotension), respiratory depression, gastrointestinal dysfunction (constipation, ileus, nausea, and vomiting), delirium and muscle rigidity, tolerance, dependency and iatrogenic withdrawal syndrome [35].

All opioids have the same analgesic efficacy, respecting the equianalgesic table. Except for meperidine which should be avoided in ICU, there is no evidence to favor the use of one opioid over another. Fentanyl is a highly lipid soluble short-acting potent drug with low impact on the hemodynamic status of the patient with safe renal and hepatic profile [36]. However, it accumulates displaying a prolonged duration of action, when given in high doses for long periods. Remifentanil has quick onset and offset of action, and it is metabolized to inactive metabolites through hydrolysis by plasma esterase. Alfentanil also has quick onset and offset of action, but its clearance is prolonged in liver failure. Morphine still has a place in ICU pain management. Caution is warranted because morphine is metabolized by the liver to morphine-3-glucoronide and morphine-6-glucoronide which are cleared by the kidneys. The former metabolite can cause delirium and the latter is more potent than morphine itself. Thus, accumulation and toxicity are possible in hepatic and renal failure. Other opioids like oxycodone, diamorphine, codeine, and tramadol are less commonly used in ICU.

3.2 Non-opioids

Paracetamol can be given through many routes (oral, intravenous, and rectal). It is effective in the treatment of mild to moderate pain and can be used in combination with opioids for the management of severe pain [18]. It should be given with caution in patients with reduced glutathione stores (malnutrition, co-morbidity) because of the potential risk of liver injury [18, 36, 37].

Non-steroidal anti-inflammatory drugs (NSAIDs) inhibit the regulation of cyclooxygenase enzymes COX-1 and/or COX-2. Their analgesic properties in critically ill patients have not been studied elaborately [36]. Their use can cause kidney injury and gastrointestinal bleeding and are to be used with great caution in patients with renal dysfunction, congestive heart failure, and coagulopathy [38]. Thus, they are generally avoided in critically ill patients.

Alpha (a_2)-adrenergic receptors agonists, clonidine and dexmedetomidine, are also implemented for the management of pain in the ICU. The latter has eight times more affinity for a_2-receptors than the former. They are both used in the ICU mostly for sedation. Even though they can have opioid-sparing properties they are not routinely used for reducing opioid administration in the ICU [18, 35–38]. They are mainly used to treat opioid, benzodiazepine, and alcohol withdrawal syndrome or improve analgesia quality in opioid-tolerant individuals. They can cause hypotension and bradycardia or, in case of abrupt cessation, rebound hypertension.

Ketamine is a sedative and analgesic agent that is reserved for special circumstances in ICU. It has an opioid-sparing effect for opioid-tolerant and dependent patients and has been shown to be effective in the management of pain in sickle cell crisis and after major abdominal surgery [39]. It reduces cough and stress response during tracheal suctioning attenuating intracranial pressure increase in head-injured and neurosurgical patients. It is also indicated in refractory status epilepticus and status asthmaticus.

Neuropathic pain is a disturbing condition resilient to the usual treatment regimens which call for special measures. Gabapentinoids are useful in the treatment of neuropathic pain. Gabapentin and pregabalin are brought into play for the management of pain in conditions like multiple sclerosis, spinal cord injuries [40], and demyelinating polyradiculoneuropathies such as Guillain-Barré syndrome [41] by reducing the central sensitization and hyperalgesia developed in these situations. They are only available in the enteral formulation and are excreted unchanged in the urine, so their dosage needs to be adjusted for renal impairment. Finally, useful adjuvants are tricyclic antidepressants (TCAs) with amitriptyline being the main representative.

4. Conclusion

Pain is a common issue in critically ill patients and remains poorly assessed and treated, despite its detrimental effects. Recognition of pain among ICU patients, whether they are communicative or not, is essential and is based on the regular assessment of pain with the use of validated tools. Effective treatment relies on a multimodal protocol-based analgesic strategy tailored to each patient that incorporates numerous pharmacologic agents.

Author details

Theodoros Aslanidis[1]* and Christos Nouris[2]

1 Intensive Care Unit/Anesthesiology Department, St. Paul General Hospital of Thessaloniki, Greece

2 Intensive Care Unit, G. Papageorgiou General Hospital of Thessaloniki, Greece

*Address all correspondence to: thaslan@hotmail.com

References

[1] Barr J, Fraser GL, Puntillo K, et al. Clinical practice guidelines for the management of pain, agitation, and delirium in adult patients in the intensive care unit. Critical Care Medicine. 2013;**41**(1):263-306

[2] Nordness MF, Hayhurst CJ, Pandharipande P. Current perspectives on the assessment and Management of Pain in the intensive care unit. Journal of Pain Research. 2021;**14**:1733-1744

[3] Devlin JW, Skrobik Y, Gelinas C, et al. Clinical practice guidelines for the prevention and management of pain, agitation/sedation, delirium, immobility, and sleep disruption in adult patients in the ICU. Critical Care Medicine. 2018;**46**(9):825-873

[4] Burton AR, Fazalbhoy A, Macefield VG. Sympathetic responses to noxious stimulation of muscle and skin. Frontiers in Neurology. 2016;7:109

[5] Narayanan M, Venkataraju A, Jennings J. Analgesia in intensive care: Part 1. BJA Education. 2016;**16**(2): 72-78

[6] Swinamer DL, Phang PT, Jones RL, Grace M, King EG. Effect of routine administration of analgesia on energy expenditure in critically ill patients. Chest. 1988;**93**(1):4-10

[7] Reade MC, Finfer S. Sedation and delirium in the intensive care unit. The New England Journal of Medicine. 2014;**370**(5):444-454

[8] Colacchio TA, Yeager MP, Hildebrandt LW. Perioperative immunomodulation in cancer surgery. American Journal of Surgery. 1994;**167**(1):174-179

[9] Makinen JO, Backlund ME, Liisanantti J, Peltomaa M, Karlsson S. Kalliomaki ML persistent pain in intensive care survivors: A systematic review. British Journal of Anaesthesia. 2020;**125**(2):149-158

[10] Lavan d'H P. The progression from acute to chronic pain. Current Opinion in Anaesthesiology. 2011;**24**:545-550

[11] Fink RM, Makic MB, Poteet AW, Oman KS. The ventilated patient's experience. Dimensions of Critical Care Nursing. 2015;**34**(5):301-308

[12] Damico V, Macchi G, Murano L, Forastieri MA. Incidence of pain at rest and during nursing procedures in ICU patients: A longitudinal observational study. Annali di Igiene. 2020;**32**(4):407-418

[13] Alasad JA, Abu Tabar N, Ahmad MM. Patients' experience of being in intensive care units. Journal of Critical Care. 2015;**30**(4):859

[14] Puntillo KA, Max A, Timsit JF, et al. Determinants of procedural pain intensity in the intensive care unit. The Europain(R) study. American Journal of Respiratory and Critical Care Medicine. 2014;**189**(1):39-47

[15] Chanques G, Sebbane M, Barbotte E, Viel E, Eledjam JJ, Jaber S. A prospective study of pain at rest: Incidence and characteristics symptom in surgical and trauma versus intensive care patients. Anesthesiology. 2007;**107**(5):858-860

[16] Puntillo KA, White C, Morris AB, Perdue ST, Stanik-Hutt J, Thompson CL, et al. Patients' perceptions and responses to procedural pain: Results from thunder

project II. American Journal of Critical Care. 2001;**10**(4):238-251

[17] Payen JF, Chanques G, Mantz J, et al. Current practices in sedation and analgesia for mechanically ventilated critically ill patients: A prospective multicenter patient-based study. Anesthesiology. 2007;**106**:687-695

[18] Joffe AM, Hallman M, Gélinas C, Herr DL, Puntillo K. Evaluation and treatment of pain in critically ill adults. Seminars in Respiratory and Critical Care Medicine. 2013;**34**(2):189-200

[19] Payen JF, Bru O, Bosson JL, et al. Assessing pain in critically ill sedated patients by using a behavioral pain scale. Critical Care Medicine. 2001;**29**(12):2258-2263

[20] Gélinas C, Johnston C. Pain assessment in the critically ill ventilated adult: Validation of the critical-care pain observation tool and physiologic indicators. The Clinical Journal of Pain. 2007;**23**(6):497-505

[21] Severgnini P, Pelosi P, Contino E, Serafinelli E, Novario R, Chiaranda M. Accuracy of critical care pain observation tool and behavioral pain scale to assess pain in critically ill conscious and unconscious patients: Prospective, observational study. Journal of Intensive Care. 2016;**4**:68

[22] Kanji S, MacPhee H, Singh A, et al. Validation of the critical care pain observation tool in critically ill patients with delirium: A prospective cohort study. Critical Care Medicine. 2016;**44**(5):943-947

[23] Bouajram RH, Sebat CM, Love D, Louie EL, Wilson MD, Duby JJ. Comparison of self-reported and behavioral pain assessment tools in critically ill patients. Journal of Intensive Care Medicine. 2018;**35**(5):453-460

[24] Burry LD, Williamson DR, Perreault MM, et al. Analgesic, sedative, antipsychotic, and neuromuscular blocker use in Canadian intensive care units: A prospective, multicentre, observational study. Canadian Journal of Anaesthesia. 2014;**61**(7):619-630

[25] Boitor M, Gélinas C, Richard-Lalonde M, Thombs BD. The effect of massage on acute postoperative pain in critically and acutely ill adults' post-thoracic surgery: Systematic review and meta-analysis of randomized controlled trials. Heart & Lung. 2017;**46**(5):339-346

[26] Boitor M, Martorella G, Maheu C, Laizner AM, Gélinas C. Effects of massage in reducing the pain and anxiety of the cardiac surgery critically ill-a randomized controlled trial. Pain Medicine. 2018;**19**(12):2556-2569

[27] Jagan S, Park T, Papathanassoglou E. Effects of massage on outcomes of adult intensive care unit patients: A systematic review. Nursing in Critical Care. 2019;**24**(6):414-429

[28] Gorji HM, Nesami BM, Ayyasi M, Ghafari R, Yazdani J. Comparison of ice packs application and relaxation therapy in pain reduction during chest tube removal following cardiac surgery. North American Journal of Medical Sciences. 2014;**6**(1):19-24

[29] Aktaş YY, Karabulut N. The use of cold therapy, music therapy and lidocaine spray for reducing pain and anxiety following chest tube removal. Complementary Therapies in Clinical Practice. 2019;**34**:179-184

[30] Saadatmand V, Rejeh N, Heravi-Karimooi M, Tadrisi SD, Vaismoradi M, Jordan S. Effects of natural sounds on pain: A randomized controlled trial with patients receiving mechanical ventilation

support. Pain Management Nursing. 2015;**16**(4):483-492

[31] Richard-Lalonde M, Gélinas C, Boitor M, et al. The effect of music on pain in the adult intensive care unit: A systematic review of randomized controlled trials. Journal of Pain and Symptom Management. 2020;**59**(6):1304-1319

[32] Rose L, Haslam L, Dale C, Knechtel L, McGillion M. Behavioral pain assessment tool for critically ill adults unable to self-report pain. American Journal of Critical Care. 2013;**22**(3):246-255

[33] Williams TA, Martin S, Leslie G, et al. Duration of mechanical ventilation in an adult intensive care unit after introduction of sedation and pain scales. American Journal of Critical Care. 2008;**17**(4):349-356

[34] De Pinto M, Dagal A, O'Donnell B, Stogicza A, Chiu S, Edwards WT. Regional anesthesia for management of acute pain in the intensive care unit. International Journal of Critical Illness and Injury Science. 2015;**5**(3):138-143

[35] Karamchandani K, Carr JZ, Bonavia A, Tung A. Critical care pain Management in Patients Affected by the opioid epidemic: A review. Annals of the American Thoracic Society. 2018;**15**(9):1016-1023

[36] Pota V, Coppolino F, Barbarisi A, Passavanti M, Aurilio C, Sansone P, et al. Pain in intensive care: A narrative review. Pain and Therapy. 2022;**11**:359-367

[37] Jefferies S, Saxena M, Young P. Paracetamol in critical illness: A review. Critical Care and Resuscitation. 2012;**14**(1):74-80

[38] Candiotti KA, Bergese SD, Viscusi ER, Singla SK, Royal MA, Singla NK. Safety of multiple-dose intravenous acetaminophen in adult inpatients. Pain Medicine. 2010;**11**(12):1841-1848

[39] Guillou N, Tanguy M, Seguin P, et al. The effects of small-dose ketamine on morphine consumption in surgical intensive care unit patients after major abdominal surgery. Anesthesia and Analgesia. 2003;**97**:843-847

[40] Mehta S, McIntyre A, Dijkers M, et al. Gabapentinoids are effective in decreasing neuropathic pain and other secondary outcomes after spinal cord injury: A meta-analysis. Archives of Physical Medicine and Rehabilitation. 2014;**95**:2180-2186

[41] Moulin DE, Hagen N, Feasby TE, Amireh R, Hahn A. Pain in Guillain-Barré syndrome. Neurology. 1997;**48**:328-331

Chapter 2

Postoperative Analgesia

Denberu Eshetie Adane

Abstract

A failure to maintain adequate pain control is a substandard and unethical practice. Pain has disastrous effects in which poorly controlled acute postoperative pain is associated with increased morbidity and mortality, impaired quality of life, delayed recovery time, prolonged opioid usage, and higher healthcare costs. Inadequate knowledge about analgesia and pain management leads the healthcare profession to ineffective postoperative pain management. The main goal of postoperative analgesia is to reduce or eliminate pain and discomfort with a minimum of side effects. Assessment of pain severity is vital before managing it. There are many analgesic options that can be used to manage acute and chronic postoperative pain. Recently, non-opioid analgesia methods are encouraged for acute postoperative pain control due to the side effect of opioids and the advancement of recent technologies for peripheral nerve block.

Keywords: postoperative pain, pain management, analgesia, postoperative analgesia, pain assessment scale

1. Introduction

Pain after surgery is a common phenomenon, especially in patients who underwent general anesthesia, around half of the patients experience moderate to severe acute pain [1, 2]. The immediate experience of pain may be associated with the patient's attitude, belief, and their personality [3].

Appropriate postoperative analgesia administration is associated with lower cardiopulmonary complications, lower mortality and morbidity, reduced hospital costs, and increased patient satisfaction [4, 5]. Standardizing multimodal analgesia combined with enhanced recovery after surgery (ERAS) are considered a quality improvement initiative in healthcare [6]. The American Pain Society introduced pain as the fifth vital sign. A failure to maintain adequate pain control is a substandard and unethical practice. The World Health Organization and the International Association for the Study of Pain have recognized pain relief as a human right [7, 8].

Unmanaged or poorly managed acute pain can lead to complications and prolonged rehabilitation. Poorly managed postoperative is associated with the development of chronic pain with a reduction in quality of life [9, 10].

Even though there are different modalities of pain management, the anesthesia type plays a great role in the decrement of postoperative pain scores. Regional anesthesia is more beneficial to control postoperative pain than general anesthesia [11]; from general anesthesia, a single controlled trial concluded that propofol anesthesia has a better analgesia outcome compared with sevoflurane anesthesia after open gastrectomy procedure in the early postoperative period [12], but a meta-analysis study concluded that there is no significant difference between propofol and inhalational anesthetics regarding postoperative pain, even though there was heterogeneity between the studies [13].

Pain management is one of the major components of ERAS protocol, and it is recommended that early and effective multimodal analgesia while decreasing opioids improves postoperative complications for colorectal surgeries [14]. Regional anesthetic techniques are the most effective methods to treat postoperative pain. A meta-analysis study suggests that epidural analgesia can no longer be considered the "gold-standard," and another RCT study also outweighs transversus abdominis plane (TAP) block combined with opioid-sparing analgesia for laparoscopic colorectal surgery, than epidural analgesia [15, 16].

2. Pain pathophysiology acute pain

Acute pain is caused due to a response to tissue injury; during surgery, there is tissue damage and injury of small nerve fibers. The afferent nociceptors, A-delta, and C-sensory fibers (A mechano-thermal and C-polymodal) are peripheral nerve endings that normally have a high threshold for pain sensation/activation. So, noxious sensation produced by direct stimulation of A-delta and C-sensory fiber nerve endings and the inflammation due to a surgical incision will produce a peripheral sensitization enhancing the sensitivity of these nociceptors. Nociception follows four process: transduction, transmission, perception, and modulation [17]. From the damaged cells, mediators like substance P, prostaglandins, serotonin, histamine, bradykinins, and other mediators trigger the nociceptors (**transduction**) to send afferent impulses via the dorsal root ganglion to the spinal cord (**transmission**) [18]. Activation of substance P and other neurotransmitters carry the action potential to the dorsal horn of the spinal cord, from where it ascends the spinothalamic tract to the thalamus and the midbrain. From the thalamus, fibers send the nociceptive message to the somatosensory cortex, parietal lobe, frontal lobe, and the limbic system, where the third nociceptive process **perception** occurs [17, 19]. Finally, activation of the midbrain will result in the release of counter neuroinhibitory neurotransmitters like endorphins, serotonin, enkephalin, and dynorphin which descend to the lower central nervous system. The activation of these neurotransmitters triggers the release of endogenous opioids. Both centrally and peripherally opioid receptors are synthesized or upregulated in the sensory neurons. Binding of endogenous opioids to these receptors will reduce the excitability. From the periphery, immunocompetent cells seem to produce opioid peptides. Centrally, the opioid receptors will act as presynaptic receptors. In the dorsal horn, opioid peptides are released by the inter neurons, so the inhibition of pain transmission will occur (**modulation**) [20–22].

3. Pain assessment

Before an administration of analgesics, it is better to assess the pain to understand the severity of the pain. There are different options for pain assessment.

3.1 Numeric rating scale (NRS)

It is the most popular pain assessment scale which is simple to use and widely used for research purposes, and the patient is ordered to indicate the number that is ordered from 0 to 10 which best reflects the intensity of their pain. 0 indicates no pain and 10 indicates the worst pain [23].

It is further categorized for the sake of intervention 0 = no pain, 1–3 mild pain, 4–6 moderate pain, and 7–10 = severe pain. The numeric rating scale (NRS) can be administered verbally (therefore also by telephone) or graphically for self-completion.

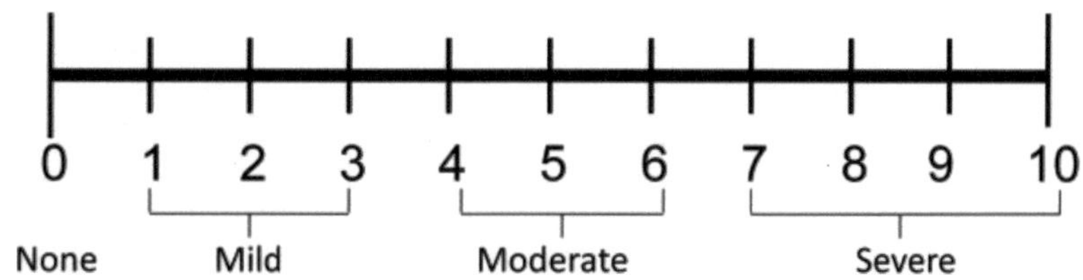

3.2 Visual analog scale (VAS)

Visual analog scale (VAS) has a sensory component and is considered a reliable measurement of pain [24]. It is subjective and measured by using a ruler, and the score is determined by measuring the distance (mm) on the 10-cm line between the "no pain" and the patient's mark, providing a range of scores from 0 to 100. As with the NRS, categories may be imposed on this (no pain 0–4 mm; mild pain 5–44 mm; moderate pain 45–74 mm; and severe pain 75–100 mm), but this is arbitrary and does not necessarily reflect patients' meanings.

0mm____**100mm**

There are also other types of pain assessment tools such as Defense and Veterans Pain Rating Scale (DVPRS), adult Non-Verbal Pain Scale (NVPS), pain, assessment in Advanced Dementia Scale (PAINAD), Behavioral Pain Scale (BPS), Critical Care Pain Observation Tool (CPOT), and the rater can use the convenient method of assessment and can categorize the pain intensity as mild, moderate, and severe for the sake of analgesia administration.

4. WHO analgesic ladder

The WHO analgesic ladder was primarily proposed for cancer pain and other chronic pain management, but it can be applied for postoperative pain management too. Analgesia administration is based on the severity of the pain from mild to severe pain, but the revised 2021 WHO analgesic ladder includes invasive and minimally invasive treatments for patients with no pain relief/persistent pain despite managing with strong opioids. The invasive or minimally invasive procedures include epidural analgesia, intrathecal administration of analgesic and local anesthetic drugs with or without pumps, neurosurgical procedures (e.g. lumbar percutaneous adhesiolysis and cordotomy), neuromodulation strategies (e.g. brain stimulators and spinal cord stimulation), nerve blocks, ablative procedures (e.g. alcoholization, radiofrequency, microwave, cryoablation ablations, laser-induced thermotherapy, irreversible electroporation and electrochemotherapy), cementoplasty, and palliation radiotherapy [25] (**Figure 1**).

5. Postoperative analgesia/postoperative pain management

Postoperative analgesia administration is depending on the severity of the pain, and it is a wastage and disastrous to administer strong opioids for mild pain and is wrong and unethical to not to manage pain while the patients are crying due to severe pain. Pain management after having surgery depends on many factors such as type of surgery, site of surgery severity of the pain, the impact of the pain on the life quality, the medical status of the patient, and the intake of other medications [8, 24, 26].

When we describe postoperative analgesia, primitive analgesia will be remembered. Primitive analgesia is a treatment that prevents the establishment of altered sensory processing that amplifies postoperative pain. The effective preemptive analgesic technique requires a multimodal approach of nociceptive input, increasing the threshold for nociception and decreasing nociceptor receptor activation. Primitive analgesics are safe and effective and have superior pain control with a decreased VAS score of pain [27].

5.1 Multimodal analgesia

Multimodal analgesia was developed for the management of postoperative pain, and the concept is clear and reasonable. It is an administration of two or more drugs that have a different mechanism of action that maximizes pain control and minimizes the side effects of a single drug [28]. Opioids, acetaminophen, nonsteroidal anti-inflammatory drugs (NSAIDs), local anesthetics, regional anesthesia, peripheral nerve block (PNB), local/wound site infiltration, N-methyl-d-aspartate receptor antagonists, anticonvulsants, alpha $_2$ agonists, etc., are commonly used multimodal analgesia drugs/techniques [29–32].

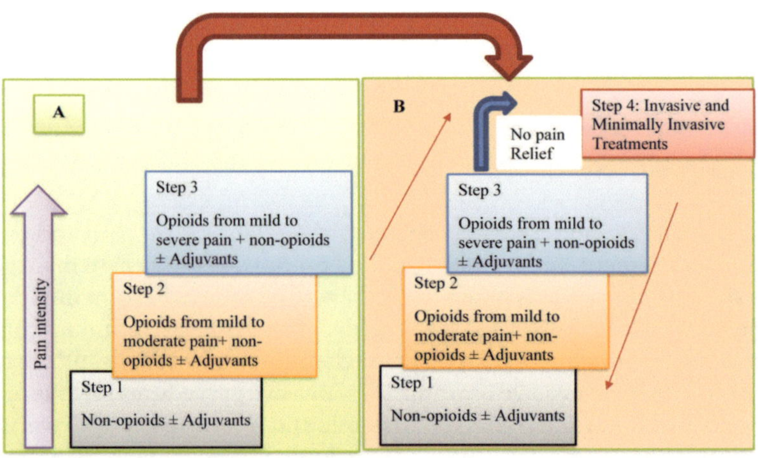

Figure 1.
Transition from the original three-step WHO analgesic ladder (A) to the revised four-step form [25].

MMA generally involves optimizing non-opioid pharmacologic and nonpharmacologic interventions and reserving opioid use to treat breakthrough pain. A review of articles regarding MMA generalizes the implementation of MMA that should involve different stakeholders. The article concluded that health system benefits can also be realized from the implementation of an effective MMA, as fewer opioid-related side effects can improve patient recovery and lead to faster discharge and improved utilization of resources [33].

5.2 Lidocaine infusion

Lidocaine is an amide local anesthetic agent which can be used for various pain management techniques; beyond this, it can be used for cardiac arrhythmia management. Infiltration of lidocaine is commonly known; but apart from infiltration, continuous perioperative lidocaine infusion has a clear advantage in patients undergoing abdominal surgery, provides significant pain relief, reduces postoperative opioid consumption, decreases opioid-induced side effects including postoperative nausea and vomiting, and promotes the faster return of bowel function, which decreases the length of hospital stay [34].

Lidocaine has a potent anti-inflammatory effect which is more potent than other known anti-inflammatory drugs and decreases circulating inflammatory cytokines. Lidocaine infusion is also used to treat chronic pain neuropathic pain by relieving the mechanical effect of allodynia and hyperalgesia, and it found to relieve pain caused by diabetic neuropathy [35, 36].

To achieve steady-state concentrations of 3 mg/mL, an infusion rate of 30 mg/kg/minute or 1.8 mg/kg/hour would be required. The weight-based lidocaine regimens used in the studies reviewed, which ranged from 1.33 to 3 mg/kg/hour, should have achieved adequate plasma concentrations in the range of 2–5 mg/ml. The optimum dose, timing, and duration of infusion of lidocaine also need to be established [34, 37].

5.3 Acetaminophen/Paracetamol

Paracetamol is a commonly used postoperative analgesic that can decrease opioid consumption by 20–30%. Its mechanism of action is not well known but believed that it may act through cyclooxygenase inhibition, serotonergic activation, and/or cannabinoid pathways, and it can easily cross the blood-brain barrier [38]. For postoperative pain management, it can be applied and effective for mild to moderate pain either combined with other analgesic techniques or alone. A systematic review and meta-analysis showed that an administration of prophylactic intravenous (IV) acetaminophen reduces postoperative nausea and vomiting through its direct effect of reduction in postsurgical pain but not due to decrement in opioid consumption [39].

Both oral and intravenous (IV) prophylactic acetaminophen before the surgical incision were found to be equally efficacious, and no superiority was found in the IV acetaminophen regarding immediate postoperative pain, postoperative nausea, vomiting reduction, and length of hospital stay according to a randomized placebo-controlled trial study [40]. A single dose of paracetamol is also effective to treat pain for about 50 % of patients for the first 4 hours with minimal side effects, but the use of postoperative IV acetaminophen does not affect the reduction of hypoxemia over 48 hours [41, 42].

The therapeutic window of acetaminophen is low, so administration beyond 4 g in a single day for a fit adult is not recommended, and a small amount of paracetamol overdose can result in liver damage. A single dose of 40–60 mg/kg rectal paracetamol is safe for children [43].

5.4 Nonsteroidal anti-inflammatory drugs (NSAIDs)

According to a review, NSAIDs have been shown to increase patient satisfaction, decrease opioid requirements, and decrease opioid-induced side effects. They have no increased incidence of adverse effects during the acute postoperative period. NSAIDs and COX-2 inhibitors, however, should use cautiously for colorectal surgical patients, and they were found to cause an anastomotic leak [44].

5.5 Regional analgesia/anesthesia

Regional anesthesia is a technique with an administration of a local anesthetic agent with or without adjuvants near the nerve roots so that the patient can get better analgesia. It includes both epidural and intrathecal analgesia/anesthesia and can be applied as a single injection or continuous catheter technique, and the latter is more advantageous than a single injection, because the analgesic agent can be added when the patients complain pain [45].

A level 1 evidence study showed that regional blocks have improved analgesia at rest and reduced incidence of postoperative ileus, pulmonary complications, surgical stress response, negative nitrogen balance, and other analgesic requirements [11]. Beyond analgesic purpose, malignant surgical procedures which underwent regional anesthesia are proposed to lower the recurrence of cancer after surgery compared with general anesthesia and opioid analgesia, and they are also used as a preventive measure for deep venous thrombosis [46, 47].

A meta-analysis of 141 RCTs where most of them were after major orthopedic surgery concluded that neuraxia blockade reduces the risk of deep venous thrombosis by 44%, pulmonary embolism by 55%, blood transfusion requirements by 50%, pneumonia by 39%, respiratory depression by 59%, and myocardial infarction by 30%. The mortality rate with a single dose of neuraxia also decreased by 30% [48].

5.6 Peripheral nerve blocks

Peripheral nerve blocks (PNBs) are a type of regional anesthesia. The local anesthetic is injected near a specific nerve or bundle of nerves that can block sensations of pain from a specific area of the body. PNBs usually last longer than local infiltration anesthesia. They are most commonly practiced for surgery on the arms and hands, the legs and feet, or the face. Beyond upper and lower extremity blocks, abdominal field/truncal blocks can be performed solely or as a part of multimodal analgesia [49, 50]. Peripheral nerve blocks are practiced with blind landmark technique, using a nerve stimulator, or ultrasound-guided technique either a single injection or continuous using a catheter. Technological advances, such as real-time ultrasonography, allow more accurate identification of plexuses and peripheral nerves, resulting in the improvement of block success [51, 52].

A meta-analysis of RCTs to determine the analgesic efficacy of postoperative peripheral catheter analgesia is compared with opioid-based analgesia. Catheter-based analgesia provided a statistically and clinically superior postoperative pain control compared with opioids with decreased side effects [53].

Although PNBs are overall safe when performed correctly, there are rare but serious risks associated with them. Risks include block failure, bleeding, infection, damage to surrounding structures, transient/permanent nerve injury, inadvertent intravascular injury, and intravascular uptake of local anesthetic resulting in systemic toxicity.

5.7 Wound site infiltration

Wound site infiltration has a good option for postoperative pain management as part of multimodal analgesia, and it has comparable result with ultrasound-guided transversus abdominis plane block for lower abdominal surgeries [54]. A systematic review regarding wound infiltration analgesia showed that it has better pain relief if it is used correctly, and in adequate doses, wound infiltration analgesia can be used in a multimodal analgesic regime without major complications, with low cost in a single injection [55, 56].

5.8 Miscellaneous

Other drugs and techniques are also used to treat postoperative pain regarding the severity of pain. Antidepressants, anticonvulsants, NMDA receptor blockers, alpha 2 agonists, corticosteroids, cannabinoids, GABA agonists, neuroimmunomodulators, etc., can be used to treat pain majorly as an adjuvant but can also use as a primary treatment for a specific type of pain [57].

Alpha 2 agonists (dexmedetomidine and clonidine): they were found to reduce postoperative opioid consumption and increase the duration of nerve block, but they cause hemodynamic instability (hypotension) and sedation [58, 59].

Dexamethasone: it is associated with a decrease in pain scores during mobilization postoperatively. As part of multimodal analgesia, high-dose dexamethasone (more than 0.2 mg/kg) was found to have an opioid-sparing effect. It has also been shown to delay the time to first postoperative analgesic intake when used in conjunction with peripheral nerve blocks [60, 61].

Ketamine: it is NMDA receptor blocker that decreases postoperative opioid consumption at 24 and 48 hr. Along with decreasing pain intensity, it reduces opioid consumption by decreasing central excitability and possibly modulates opioid receptors. It is also effective when used as a sole agent, or in conjunction with opioids, NSAIDs, and paracetamol; surprisingly, it has the potential to decrease pain scores from weeks to months [29, 62, 63].

Ketamine was found beneficial for painful procedures, including, upper abdominal, thoracic, and major orthopedic surgeries. Its analgesic effect was independent of the type of intraoperative opioid administered, timing of ketamine administration, and its dosage of administration [64].

5.9 Non-opioid analgesia

Non-opioid analgesics play an important role in treating postoperative pain as monotherapy or combined with weak/strong opioids. Non-opioid analgesics are usually indicated to treat mild to moderate pain with fewer side effects compared with opioids because opioids have many deleterious effects. But peripheral nerve blocks and regional blocks can be considered as non-opioid analgesics and can be used to treat severe pain. Short-term effects seen in the perioperative period include postoperative nausea and vomiting, and gastrointestinal dysfunctions like ileus, pruritus, urinary retention, somnolence, and respiratory depression [43, 65].

5.10 Nonpharmacological

During the postoperative period, nonpharmacologic methods of pain management can increase the effect of analgesics. They can be applied when there is no availability of analgesics and when the analgesic drugs are perceived to cause deleterious effects. Exercise, aromatherapy, therapeutic touch, positioning, music, reflexology, hypnosis, acupuncture, acupressure, transcutaneous electrical nerve stimulation (TENS), prayer, relaxation hot application, cold application, meditation, imagination, bio-feedback, distraction, massage, etc. [66].

6. Conclusion

Due to inadequate pain management having deleterious effects, optimal and multidisciplinary pain management protocol is recommended, especially to accomplish fast recovery after surgery. Recently, there are many choices for pain management that are used to decrease the side effects of opioids. Even though there are many options, the management of pain should be based on the pain severity.

Author details

Denberu Eshetie Adane
Department of Anesthesia, Debre Tabor University, Debre Tabor, Ethiopia

*Address all correspondence to: dinberueshetie@gmail.com

References

[1] Tiruneh A, Tamire T, Kibret S. The magnitude and associated factors of post-operative pain at Debre Tabor compressive specialized hospital, Debre Tabor Ethiopia, 2018. SAGE Open Medicine. 2021;**9**:205

[2] Gan TJ. Poorly controlled postoperative pain: Prevalence, consequences, and prevention. Journal of Pain Research. 2017;**10**:2287

[3] Carr DB, Goudas LC. Acute pain. The Lancet. 1999;**353**(9169):2051-2058

[4] Tsui SL, Law S, Fok M, Lo JR, Ho E, Yang J, et al. Postoperative analgesia reduces mortality and morbidity after esophagectomy. The American Journal of Surgery. 1997;**173**(6):472-478

[5] Kehlet H, Holte K. Effect of postoperative analgesia on surgical outcome. British Journal of Anaesthesia. 2001;**87**(1):62-72

[6] Kaplan JAFE, Auerbach AD. Impact of multimodality pain regimens on elective colorectal surgery outcomes. The American Surgeon. 2017;**83**(4):414-420

[7] Sullivan MD, Ballantyne JC. The Right to Pain Relief: Its origins in end-of-life care and extension to chronic pain care. The Clinical Journal of Pain. 2022;**38**(1):58-63

[8] Jukić M, Puljak L. Legal and ethical aspects of pain management. Acta Medica Academica. 2018;**47**:1

[9] Chapman CRVC. The transition of acute postoperative pain to chronic pain: An integrative overview of research on mechanisms. Journal of Pain. 2017;**18**:359

[10] R. S. Causes and consequences of inadequate management of acute pain. Pain Medicine. 2010;**11**:1859

[11] Nimmo SM, Harrington LS. What is the role of epidural analgesia in abdominal surgery? Continuing Education in Anaesthesia. Critical Care & Pain. 2014;**14**(5):224-229

[12] Ji F-h, Wang D, Zhang J, Liu H, Peng K. Effects of propofol anesthesia versus sevoflurane anesthesia on postoperative pain after radical gastrectomy: A randomized controlled trial. Journal of Pain Research. 2018;**11**:1247

[13] Peng K, Liu H-Y, Wu S-R, Liu H, Zhang Z-C, Ji F-H. Does propofol anesthesia lead to less postoperative pain compared with inhalational anesthesia?: A systematic review and meta-analysis. Anesthesia and Analgesia. 2016;**123**(4):846-858

[14] Simpson JC, Bao X, Agarwala A. Pain management in enhanced recovery after surgery (ERAS) protocols. Clinics in Colon and Rectal Surgery. 2019;**32**(02):121-128

[15] Rawal N. Current issues in postoperative pain management. European Journal of Anaesthesiology| EJA. 2016;**33**(3):160-171

[16] Pirrera B, Alagna V, Lucchi A, Berti P, Gabbianelli C, Martorelli G, et al. Transversus abdominis plane (TAP) block versus thoracic epidural analgesia (TEA) in laparoscopic colon surgery in the ERAS program. Surgical Endoscopy. 2018;**32**(1):376-382

[17] Summers S. Evidence-based practice part 1: Pain definitions, pathophysiologic mechanisms, and theories. Journal of Perianesthesia Nursing. 2000;**15**(5):357-365

[18] Cousins MJ. Acute pain and the injury response: Immediate and

prolonged effects. Regional Anesthesia and Pain Medicine. 1989;**14**(4):162-179

[19] Meyr AJ, Steinberg JS. The physiology of the acute pain pathway. Clinics in Podiatric Medicine and Surgery. 2008;**25**(3):305-326

[20] Stein C. Peripheral and non-neuronal opioid effects. Current Opinion in Anesthesiology. 1994;**7**(4):347-351

[21] Lambert DG. Opioid receptors. Current Opinion in Anesthesiology. 1995;**8**(4):317-322

[22] Arnstein P. Clinical Coach for Effective Pain Management. Philadelphia PA: FA Davis; 2010

[23] Hartrick CT, Kovan JP, Shapiro S. The numeric rating scale for clinical pain measurement: A ratio measure? Pain Practice. 2003;**3**(4):310-316

[24] Coll AM, Ameen JR, Mead D. Postoperative pain assessment tools in day surgery: Literature review. Journal of Advanced Nursing. 2004;**46**(2):124-133

[25] Anekar AACM. WHO Analgesic Ladder. Treasure Island (FL): StatPearls Publishing; 2021

[26] Hodgins MJ. Interpreting the meaning of pain severity scores. Pain Research & Management. 2002;**7**(4):192-198

[27] Zhang L-k, Li Q, Quan R-F, Liu J-S. Is preemptive analgesia a good choice for postoperative pain relief in lumbar spine surgeries?: A meta-analysis of randomized controlled trials. Medicine. 2021;**100**:13

[28] Buvanendran A, Kroin JS. Multimodal analgesia for controlling acute postoperative pain. Current opinion in Anesthesiology. 2009;**22**(5):588-593

[29] Young A, Buvanendran A. Recent advances in multimodal analgesia. Anesthesiology Clinics. 2012;**30**(1):91-100

[30] Bailey JG, Morgan CW, Christie R, Ke JXC, Kwofie MK, Uppal V. Continuous peripheral nerve blocks compared to thoracic epidurals or multimodal analgesia for midline laparotomy: A systematic review and meta-analysis. Korean Journal of Anesthesiology. 2021;**74**(5):394-408

[31] Rosero EB, Joshi GP. Preemptive, preventive, multimodal analgesia: What do they really mean? Plastic and Reconstructive Surgery. 2014;**134**(4S):85-93

[32] Tornero CT, Rodríguez LF, Valls JO. Multimodal analgesia and regional anaesthesia. Revista Española de Anestesiología y Reanimación (English Edition). 2017;**64**(7):401-405

[33] Bhatia A, Buvanendran A. Anesthesia and postoperative pain control—multimodal anesthesia protocol. Journal of Spine Surgery. 2019;**5**(Suppl 2):S160

[34] McCarthy GC, Megalla SA, Habib AS. Impact of intravenous lidocaine infusion on postoperative analgesia and recovery from surgery. Drugs. 2010;**70**(9):1149-1163

[35] Kastrup J, Petersen P, Dejgård A, Angelo HR, Hilsted J. Intravenous lidocaine infusion—a new treatment of chronic painful diabetic neuropathy? Pain. 1987;**28**(1):69-75

[36] Cassuto JSR, Bonderovic M. Anti-inflammatory properties of local anesthetics and their present and

potential clinical implications. Acta Anaesthesiologica Scandinavica. 2006;**50**:265-282

[37] Woosley RLSD. Pharmacokinetics of antiarrhythmic drugs. The American Journal of Cardiology. 1978;**41**:986-995

[38] Oscier CDMQ. Perioperative use of paracetamol. Anaesthesia. 2009;**65-72**:65-72

[39] Apfel CC, Turan A, Souza K, Pergolizzi J, Hornuss C. Intravenous acetaminophen reduces postoperative nausea and vomiting: A systematic review and meta-analysis. Pain®. 2013;**154**:677-689

[40] Hickman SR, Mathieson KM, Bradford LM, Garman CD, Gregg RW, Lukens DW. Randomized trial of oral versus intravenous acetaminophen for postoperative pain control. The Bulletin of the American Society of Hospital Pharmacists. 2018;**75**(6):367-375

[41] Toms L, McQuay HJ, Derry S, Moore RA. Single dose oral paracetamol (acetaminophen) for postoperative pain in adults. Cochrane Database of Systematic Reviews. 2008;**4**:1465-1858

[42] Turan A, Essber H, Saasouh W, Hovsepyan K, Makarova N, Ayad S, et al. Effect of intravenous acetaminophen on postoperative hypoxemia after abdominal surgery: The FACTOR randomized clinical trial. Journal of the American Medical Association. 2020;**324**(4):350-358

[43] Dahl V, Raeder J. Non-opioid postoperative analgesia. Acta Anaesthesiologica Scandinavica. 2000;**44**(10):1191-1203

[44] Gupta A, Bah M. NSAIDs in the treatment of postoperative pain. Current Pain and Headache Reports. 2016;**20**(11):1-14

[45] Maurice-Szamburski A, Grillo P, Cuvillon P, Gazeau T, Delaunay L, Auquier P, et al. Comparison of continuous with single-injection regional analgesia on patient experience after ambulatory orthopaedic surgery: A randomised multicentre trial. British Journal of Anaesthesia. 2022;**129**(3):435-444

[46] Mantilla CB, Horlocker TT, Schroeder DR, Berry DJ, Brown DL. Risk factors for clinically relevant pulmonary embolism and deep venous thrombosis in patients undergoing primary hip or knee arthroplasty. The Journal of the American Society of Anesthesiologists. 2003;**99**(3):552-560

[47] Sessler DI. Does regional analgesia reduce the risk of cancer recurrence? A hypothesis. European Journal of Cancer Prevention. 2008;**17**(3):269-272

[48] Rodgers AWN, Schug S, et al. Reduction of postoperative mortality and morbidity with epidural or spinal anaesthesia. Results from overview of randomised trials. British Medical Journal. 2000;**321**:1493-1497

[49] Chang A, Dua A, Singh K, White BA. Peripheral Nerve Blocks. Treasure Island (FL): StatPearls Publishing; 2017

[50] Finnerty O, Carney J, McDonnell J. Trunk blocks for abdominal surgery. Anaesthesia. 2010;**65**:76-83

[51] Marhofer PCV. Ultrasound-guided regional anesthesia: Current concepts and future trends. Anesthesia and Analgesia. 2007;**104**:1265-1269

[52] Alemnew EF, Lemma DT. Analgesic effectiveness of transversus abdominis plane block versus wound site infiltration

after cesarean delivery under spinal anesthesia at Debre Tabor General Hospital, Debre Tabor, Ethiopia: A prospective cohort study, 2019. International Journal of Surgery Open. 2020;**23**:17-22

[53] Richman JM, Liu SS, Courpas G, Wong R, Rowlingson AJ, McGready J, et al. Does continuous peripheral nerve block provide superior pain control to opioids? A meta-analysis. Anesthesia & Analgesia. 2006;**102**(1):248-257

[54] Pratheeba N, Remadevi R, Raajesh IJ, Bhavani V, Tripathy D, Bhat RR. Comparison of postoperative analgesic efficacy of wound site infiltration and ultrasound-guided transversus abdominis plane block with 0.5% ropivacaine in lower abdominal surgeries under spinal anesthesia. Anesthesia, Essays and Researches. 2018;**12**(1):80

[55] Gupta A. Wound infiltration with local anaesthetics in ambulatory surgery. Current Opinion in Anesthesiology. 2010;**23**(6):708-713

[56] Banerjee P, Rogers BA. Systematic review of high-volume multimodal wound infiltration in total knee arthroplasty. Orthopedics. 2014;**37**(6):403-412

[57] Knotkova H, Pappagallo M. Adjuvant analgesics. Anesthesiology Clinics. 2007;**25**(4):775-786

[58] Grape SKK, Frauenknecht J, Albrecht E. Intra-operative analgesia with remifentanil vs. dexmedetomidine: A systematic review and meta-analysis with trial sequential analysis. Anaesthesia. 2019;**74**:793-800

[59] Jessen Lundorf LKNH, Møller AM. Perioperative dexmedetomidine for acute pain after abdominal surgery in adults. Cochrane Database System Review. 2016;**2**:CD010

[60] De Oliveira GAM, Benzon H, et al. Perioperative single dose systemic dexamethasone for postoperative pain: A meta-analysis of randomized control trials. Anesthesiology. 2011;**115**:575-588

[61] Clement JCBG, Puyraveau M, et al. Clinical Effectiveness of single dose of intravenous dexamethasone on the duration of ropivacaine axillary brachial plexus block: The randomized placebo-controlled ADEXA trial. Regional Anesthesia and Pain Medicine. 2019;**44**:370-374

[62] Aroni FIN, Dontas I, Pourzitaki C, Xanthos T. Pharmacological aspects and potential new clinical applications of ketamine: Reevaluation of an old drug. Journal of Clinical Pharmacology. 2009;**49**:957-964

[63] Loftus RWYM, Clark JA, et al. Intraoperative ketamine reduces perioperative opiate consumption in opiate-dependent patients with chronic back pain undergoing back surgery. Anesthesiology. 2010;**113**:639-646

[64] Laskowski K, Stirling A, Mckay WP, Lim HJ. A systematic review of intravenous ketamine for postoperative analgesia. Canadian Journal of Anesthesia/Journal canadien d'anesthésie. 2011;**58**(10):911-923

[65] Dunn LK, Durieux ME, Nemergut EC. Non-opioid analgesics: Novel approaches to perioperative analgesia for major spine surgery. Best Practice & Research. Clinical Anaesthesiology. 2016;**30**(1):79-89

[66] Yaban ZS. Usage of non-pharmacologic methods on postoperative pain management by nurses: Sample of turkey. International Journal of Caring Sciences. 2019;**12**(1):529-541

Chapter 3

Pain Management in the Emergency Department – Newer Modalities and Current Perspective

Sakshi Yadav, Anuj Ajayababu, Tej Prakash Sinha and Sanjeev Bhoi

Abstract

Pain is one of the most common complaints and yet one of the most neglected aspects of management in the emergency department. Optimal pain management is a nuanced skill which focusses on reduction of pain to an acceptable level to allow for safe discharge and return to normal activities, in addition to improving patient satisfaction and comfort during their stay in hospital. Adequate analgesia also improves physiological parameters such as heart rate and blood pressure. The aim is improving rather than eradication of pain altogether while maintaining an acceptable level of adverse effects. This chapter will discuss assessment of pain in the emergency department along with various modalities of pain management with specific focus on newer modalities including ultrasound guided regional nerve blocks. Ultrasound guided nerve blocks are associated with better analgesia and have fewer chances of drug related adverse events, especially in older patients and those with comorbidities where large doses of systemic medications are associated with a significant risk of adverse effects.

Keywords: pain management, emergency department, pain score, nerve blocks, USG guided

1. Introduction

Pain is one of the most common complaint of patients presenting to the Emergency Department (ED), with the frequency of severe pain reported anywhere between 20% and 40% worldwide [1]. Regardless, pain management in ED is often delayed due to overcrowded emergency rooms (ER) [2, 3] or poorly treated (oligo-analgesia) due to improper analgesic dosing [4–6]. Pain management in the ED can be used as an indicator of quality care [7–11]. Studies have shown that patients want to be treated for their pain in less than half an hour, yet the normal duration of treatment is at least 78 minutes [12]. The primary goal of acute pain management is not complete relief from pain, but reduced pain to an acceptable level that will allow for safe discharge by returning to daily patient activities in addition to improving patient comfort while in hospital. Uncontrolled pain can contribute to the development of comorbidities such as depression, high blood pressure, and immune system deficiency [13]. The type of treatment should be chosen and managed in such a way that with the reduction of pain in the patient, the analgesia method should have as few side effects as possible. The most widely used analgesics, both in ED and during discharge are acetaminophen (alone or in combination with hydrocodone), ketorolac, and ibuprofen [14]. Neuraxial analgesia is increasingly becoming an integral part of emergency management of various clinical situations and emerging emergency physicians need behavioral training. As a practice, they provide better long-term analgesia with reduced side effects at the hands of trained emergency care physicians.

2. Pain assessment

The intensity of the patient's pain is not always obvious. Facial expressions and behavior may give some clues but they are unreliable. Number of dosages or tools available to patients to indicate the severity of their pain, response to analgesic agents, or both. Using a pain screening tool directs the selection of analgesic agents and provides an indication of the patient's pain response.

2.1 Verbal descriptor scale

These are quick and easily implemented and particularly appropriate for older patients. In descriptive scales, we simply ask the patient to estimate their pain [15]. Choose from (**Figure 1**).

2.2 Numerical and combined rating scales

They offer a wide range of choices and avoid vague descriptive words. They need more concentration and communication. Good visual acuity is required for the visual analogue scale [18]. These include:

a. Visual analog scales

b. Verbal numerical rating scale

c. Combined verbal and numerical rating scales

2.2.1 Visual analog scales

The visual dimensions of the analogue are 100 mm lines with verbal anchors. Patients may be asked to mark their pain or relief of pain in a horizontal line depending on how severe or how much relief occurs in treatment (**Figures 2** and **3**).

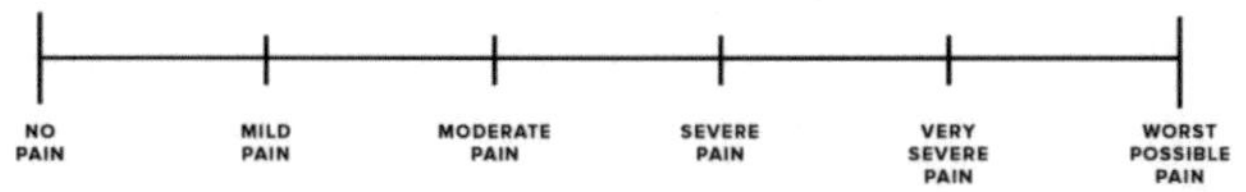

Figure 1.
Verbal descriptor scale. From references [16, 17].

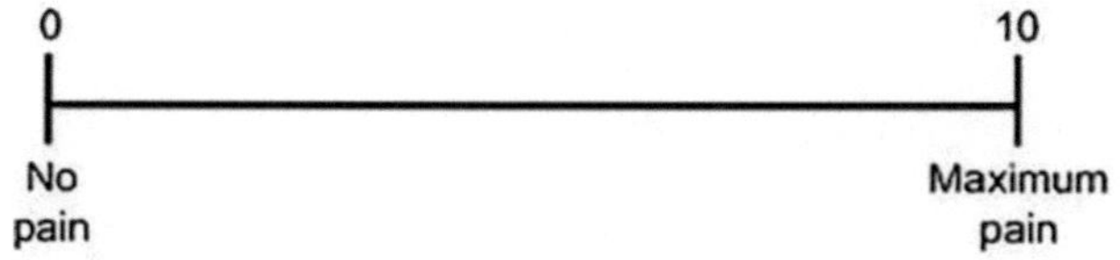

Figure 2.
Visual analogue scale for pain assessment.

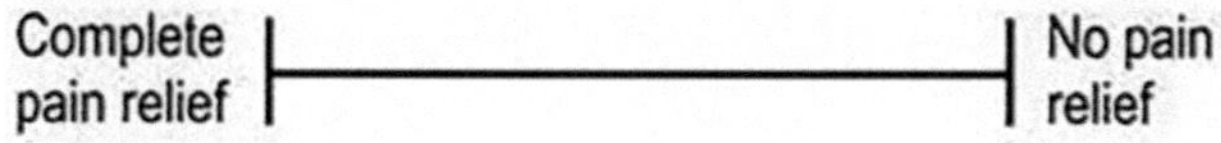

Figure 3.
Visual analogue scale for analgesia testing.

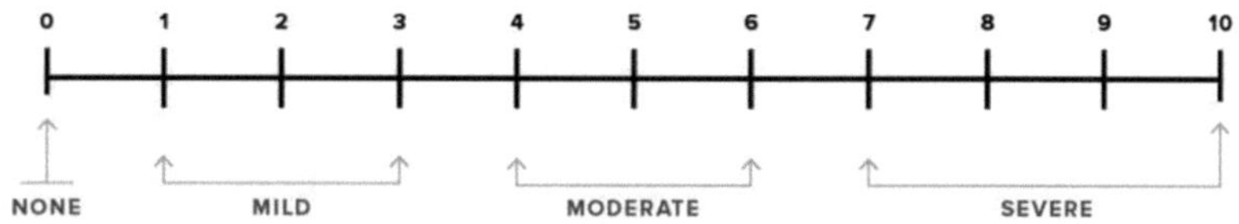

Figure 4.
Verbal numerical rating scale.

2.2.2 Verbal numerical rating scale

Patients should score their pain scores on a scale from 0 to 10, where 0 is painless and 10 is the most severe pain imaginable (**Figure 4**).

2.2.3 Combined verbal and numerical scale

Patients have further descriptive meanings in addition to numerical points to guide them in calculating pain (**Figure 5**).

One of the most commonly used standardized pain measurements is the Defense and Veterans Pain Rating Scale (DVPRS) (**Figure 6**) which has been validated in a variety of hospital and patient settings and is one of the most commonly used pain measurements in emergency departments. Uses improved numerical range of active word dictionaries, color coding, and graphic facial expressions matched by pain levels [16].

3. Principles of pain management

There are a number of pain management principles to keep in mind when choosing an analgesic agent. The WHO Analgesic Ladder has been the most frequently cited topic for decades and has five themes that guide our choices [19].

a. Oral administration is preferred whenever possible

b. Analgesics should be given regularly enough to maintain pain control

c. Agents should be selected based on the magnitude of the reported pain

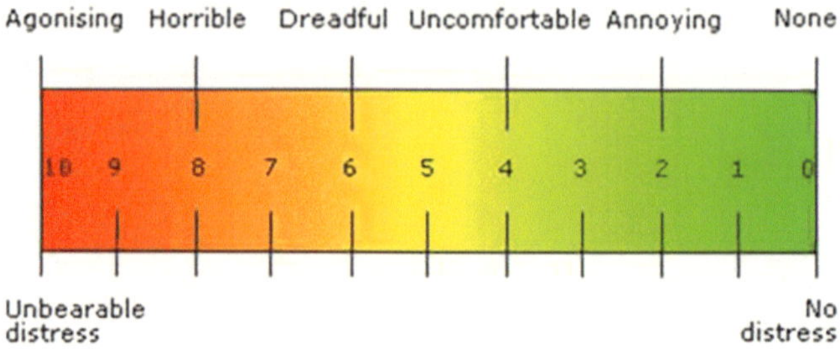

Figure 5.
Verbal and numerical measurements.

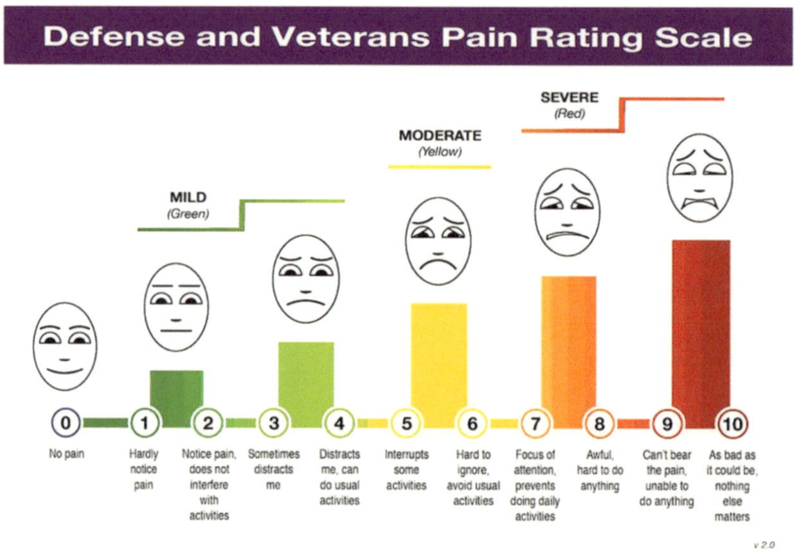

Figure 6.
DVPRS Defense and veteran pain rating scale.

d. The dose of agents should be appropriate for the patient

e. Patients should be given clear instructions on how/when to take their medication.

4. Common analgesics used in ED

Non-opioid analgesics include acetaminophen, non-steroidal anti-inflammatory drugs (NSAIDs), and cyclooxygenase 2 (COX-2) inhibitors. NSAIDs and COX 2 inhibitors have anti-inflammatory properties.

4.1 Acetaminophen

Acetaminophen is usually a first-line agent in ED for minor pain. This is due to the effective treatment of low grade pain and the little side effects that come with it. Its mechanism of action is inhibition of prostaglandin endoperoxide H2 synthase and cyclooxygenase activity [20]. Its central antipyretic effect is widely used when fever needs to be reduced. Unlike NSAIDs, Acetaminophen does not fight inflammation and therefore its use is limited to non-inflammatory conditions only. Studies have shown that injected acetaminophen can have similar analgesic effects to injectable NSAIDs in ED, as well as morphine in other painful processes [21–24]. It has also been shown that the addition of paracetamol to NSAIDs increases the effect of analgesia compared with NSAID use alone [25].

4.2 NSAIDs

NSAIDs reduce pain by preventing prostaglandin synthesis involved in both acute and chronic painful conditions [26]. The synergistic combination of 400 mg ibuprofen and 1000 mg paracetamol (acetaminophen) is an early example of moderate analgesia and has long been considered the first analgesic drug for mild to moderate pain [27, 28]. The reduction in pain by this compound has analgesic activity almost similar with oral opioid compounds (oxycodone/hydrocodone-acetaminophen) used in the treatment of acute musculoskeletal pain [29]. NSAIDs are best for inflammatory pain associated with prostaglandins such as renal colic and menstrual pain [30]. Lack of respiratory depression, lack of dependence, and long-term relief effect are some of the most important benefits of NSAIDs compared to injectable opioids. The main side effects of NSAIDs include intestinal obstruction, kidney failure, platelet obstruction, cardiovascular effects and anaphylaxis. Kidney failure is caused by decreased prostaglandin production, which contributes to afferent glomerular arteriole vasodilation. NSAIDs contribute to arteriolar vasoconstriction, leading to a decrease in renal pressure and a decrease in glomerular filtration levels [31]. This is made worse by dehydration. The most common side effect of NSAIDs is gastrointestinal injury, such as bleeding or dyspepsia and gastric ulcer. Patients at high risk for peptic ulcer or its complications, such as the elderly, those with bleeding diathesis, or patients taking glucocorticoids, have objections related to NSAID use. In addition, it has also been shown that certain COX 2 inhibitors may promote heart failure associated with kidney function by causing sodium retention. There is no guaranteed efficacy of one type of NSAID over another, including administration route [32–34].

4.3 Ketamine

For decades, ketamine has been used in the ED for procedural sedation but is now gaining attention as a potential alternative to opioids because of its unique analgesic effect. It is an effective N-methyl-d-aspartate (NMDA) receptor antagonist that provides safe and effective analgesia in subdissociative doses 0.1–0.3 mg/kg IV or less while maintaining respiratory and cardiopulmonary stability in an emergency [35, 36]. Side effects of ketamine include nausea, stomach upset, tremors, dizziness, and nystagmus (detected immediately after onset of action) [36]. These effects are increasingly evident among older patients where sub-dissociative doses should be used with caution. Infusing ketamine over 15 min (as opposed to IV push) reduces these side effects. Co-administration of prophylactic ondansetron and midazolam may be used to treat post-ketamine nausea and the onset of consecutive reactions [37].

4.4 Opioid medications

Opioids have been the gold standard for pain management in cancer patients for a long time. Its use has now been increased nearly 10 times in patients without cancer as well. They work on one of the three main opioid receptor systems (mu, kappa, delta). They can have analgesic and depressant effects on the central nervous system (CNS). Most opioids used in the clinic target μ-opioid (mu) receptors. These receptors mediate analgesia as well as common side effects such as nausea, constipation, and respiratory depression. Within the gastrointestinal system, opioids cause constipation [32]. However, Opioid prescription in ED serves as major factor for long term opioid usage and hence limiting its use. In 2019, an average of 38 people died each day from overdoses involving prescription opioids, totaling more than 14,000 deaths [38]. While prescription opioids were involved in over 28% of all opioid overdose deaths in 2019, there was a nearly 7% decrease in prescription opioid-involved death rates from 2018 to 2019 [39].

4.4.1 Morphine

It is one of the most widely used opioids in ED. Side effects ranges from hypotension, pruritus, nausea, vomiting, and respiratory depression. Respiratory depression is caused by medullary desensitization of carbon dioxide, with opioids binding to mu receptors. Cardiovascular effects are mediated directly through the sinoatrial node. A person should start with a recommended dose of 0.1 mg/kg if side effects are severe; However, rebolus with same dose can be given if the pain is not relieved in next 5–15 minutes. The study also found that obese patients do not need extra morphine and that, indeed, weight-based dosage is not really necessary [40, 41]. Widely used for dyspnea, especially in cancer patients and palliative care, nebulized morphine has also been found to be effective in cases of severe pain and difficult IV access (e.g., critical lung disease in sickle cell patients) [42].

4.4.2 Fentanyl

Fentanyl is 100 times more potent than morphine which allows for faster onset and shorter duration if needed in order to reduce titration faster in chronic severe pain compared to traditional analgesics. Its initial duration is 1–2 minutes and usually lasts about 30 minutes [20]. The initial IV dose is 1.5 μg/kg, and has the advantage of a short half-life. Fentanyl causes a slight release of histamine, making it ideal for patients with high blood pressure. It can also be given orally as a lollipop or intra-nasal or by nebulisation. Compared with morphine and hydromorphone, which is converted by the liver to active metabolites that require renal clearance, fentanyl is digested by the liver into inactive metabolites that are safer in patients with renal failure [43].

4.4.3 Tramadol

Tramadol is partial mu-opioid receptor agonist that doubles as a serotonin and norepinephrine reuptake inhibitor (SNRI) [44]. The analgesic effect showed that it was less than a combination of 500 mg acetaminophen and 5 mg hydrocodone for severe muscle and bone pain [45], no more than 1 mg/kg IV diclofenac for extremity injury limit [46], and no more than 5–10 mg IV morphine for organ pain [47]. Tramadol abuse has been shown to be a major component of ED visits [48]. It can cause nausea, tachycardia, convulsions, confusion, high blood pressure, hypoglycemia, and low consciousness [49].

5. Peripheral nerves

Peripheral nerve blocks prevent the need for process sedation and provide adequate anesthesia during painful procedures. This procedure can be performed in the emergency department with the help of ultrasound imaging to identify targeted sensors [50]. The ability to manage peripheral nerve blocks in ED has the potential to provide faster and more accurate analgesia with less systemic side effects compared to parent drugs. The effectiveness and duration of block time depends on the pharmacology of the analgesic/anesthetic agent used, dosage, and concentration. In peripheral nerve block, the purpose is to place a local anesthetic near the nerve because of which there is always a growing chance of nerve damage. However, most neurological injuries are temporary, with most patients recovering within 3 weeks. Ultrasound and nerve stimulator techniques have been shown to reduce complications from peripheral nerve blocks. Prior to the decision to perform a peripheral nerve block, a careful medical history should be obtained including allergies, anticoagulants use, pre-existing nerve damage, active site-specific diseases, and the ability to cooperate with procedures.

5.1 Femoral nerve block

Commonly used to anesthetize the hip, front thigh and knee. The femoral nerves exit the lumbar plexus and the subjects near the psoas muscle, before passing down the lateral inguinal muscle to the femoral artery within the femoral triangle. The fascia iliaca lies deep in the fascia lata, and separates the femoral nerve from the femoral artery [51, 52]. The patient is placed in supine position with the affected extremity in abduction and external rotation, as tolerated. The high-frequency linear probe is used to visualize the femoral nerve and artery by placing the probe in the inguinal crease, corresponding to the inguinal muscle, and the probe mark to the right of the patient (**Figure** 7). The nerve is hyperechoic, usually oval or triangular shape, and is located approximately 2–6 cm below the skin. Using a sterile method, insert a long needle into the plane at the edges of the probe, directing the space behind the sensor. One will often feel "the give away feel" as the tip of the needle exceeds the resistance of the iliac fascia. Once the tip of the needle is positioned, inject 1–2 mL of local anesthetic to ensure the placement of the tip of needle. Proper placement is confirmed by seeing a local anesthetic around the nerve, which improves its visibility on the ultrasound monitor. Once the correct placement has been confirmed, 10–20 ml of the selected anesthetic is injected. It may take 10–20 minutes to work [52, 53].

5.2 Fascia iliaca block

This block was originally used for hip and knee surgery and analgesia following hip or knee procedures is increasingly being used as part of pain management for fractures including hip and femoral neck and shaft fractures. In this process the femoral artery is first visualized by placing the transducer opposite to the inguinal crease, followed by a gradual lateral or medial movement. Tilt the probe to detect the hyperechoic fascia iliaca on the surface of the hypoechoic iliopsoas muscle. Medially, the femoral nerve appears deep in the fascia and lateral to artery. Laterally, the sartorius muscle is identified by its normal triangular shape when pressed by a transducer. The tip of the needle is placed under the fascia iliaca about one-third of the posterior

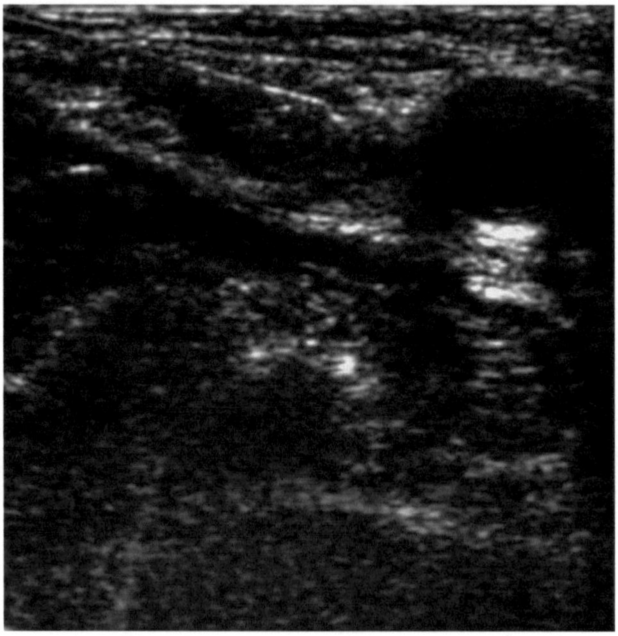

Figure 7.
Femoral nerve block.

line connecting the anterior iliac spine to the pubic tubercle (injection is performed several inches along the femoral artery). As the needle eventually pierces the fascia, one may feel loss of resistance, and the fascia may appear to "repeat" backwards in the US image. After negative aspirations, 1–2 mL of local anesthetic is injected to ensure proper injection plane between the fascia and iliopsoas muscle. A relatively large dose (20–40 mL) of local anesthesia is injected until it is spread along the iliac spine and femoral vein. Proper injection will result in splitting the fascia iliaca with a local anesthetic in the center from the injection site.

5.3 PENG block

Latest literature has described the nerve supply of the anterior capsule of the hip joint as the obturator nerve, accessory obturator nerve, and femoral nerve. These studies also examined the relationship between these nerves and other symptoms of soft or soft tissue that are detected by ultrasound guidance [54]. Studies have shown histologically that the anterior capsule has multiple nociceptive fibers, while the posterior capsule is primarily composed of mechanoreceptors [55]. The pericapsular nerve group (PENG) block is introduced to direct and block these articular branches that provide stability within the hip. This regional anesthetic was described in 2018 by Giron-Arango et al. [56]. In this case, the ultrasound probe is placed in a flexible plane over the anterior iliac crest (AIIS) and proceeds upwards to visualize the pubic ramus. The femoral artery and ilio-pubic eminence (IPE) are then visualized. Using in plane procedure the needle was developed from side to side, and 20–25 ml local anesthetic of 0.5% ropivacaine was inserted between the psoas tendon in the front and the pubic ramus in the back. As this blocks the accessory obturator nerve, theoretically provides better analgesia compared to the fascia iliaca block.

5.4 Brachial plexus block

It is used to help reduce fractures of the upper extremities and even reduce shoulder dislocations. There are two basic methods of Brachial plexus block - Interscalene and Supraclavicular. The Interscalene block is not used for the procedure below the elbow.

5.4.1 Interscalene block

The patient is placed on the supine, with the head turned away from the affected side. The probe is placed almost in the middle of the neck, in line with the clavicle. After identifying the common carotid artery and internal jugular vein, the probe slides sideways to detect the frontal and medial scalene muscles. The roots of the brachial plexus emerge between these two muscles as three different nerve bonds in this area. Next, aspiration is performed to rule out the vascular perforation, and the placement is confirmed by the anesthetic injection. Depending on the agent used, the local anesthetic dose can be 15–45 ml.

5.4.2 Supraclavicular block

The patient is placed supine and the head is turned away from the side of interest. The probe is placed at the base of the neck in the supraclavicular groove, which corresponds to the clavicle. The subclavian artery is identified and lateral to subclavian hypoechoic trunks of the brachial plexus can be seen. The 27 gauge needle is then used to inject into the skin with 1–2 ml of local anesthetic just along the canal. The block needle, 22-gauge, is then advanced in a plane toward the brachial plexus from laterally to medially.

Sometimes a person may experience "the give away feeling" when the brachial sheath is inserted. The person then wishes to confirm intravenous infusion and inject 1–2 ml of anesthetic to check the brachial plexus. Next, about 20–25 ml of anesthesia is injected, until a sufficient spread around the brachial plexus appears. Proximity of the artery and pleura carries a real risk of injury to these vital structures.

5.5 Erector spinae plane block (ESPB)

Pancreatitis is the most common gastrointestinal complaint that needs to be admitted to the emergency department (ED). The most common complaint of pancreatitis is severe abdominal pain. The T7 vertebrae is identified by counting from C7, the most prominent cervical vertebrae. Place the linear probe on the parasagittal plane, 3 cm lateral to T7 vertebral level to see the dynamic process. The erector spinae fascia appears just next to the flexible process. The needle is inserted between the flexible process and the erector spinae fascia and approximately 30 ml of local anesthetic is injected [57]. ESPB may be used for rib fractures, lumbar fractures, post herpetic neuralgia, back pain and renal colic (**Figure 8**) [58].

5.5.1 Injuries to the chest wall and nerve blocks

Broken ribs are common not only in patients with chest injuries but also common in patients with polytrauma. It is the cause of significant illness and death in such patients and adequate analgesia is very important in improving impaired ventilatory function, preventing atelectasis, and reducing the need for mechanical ventilation

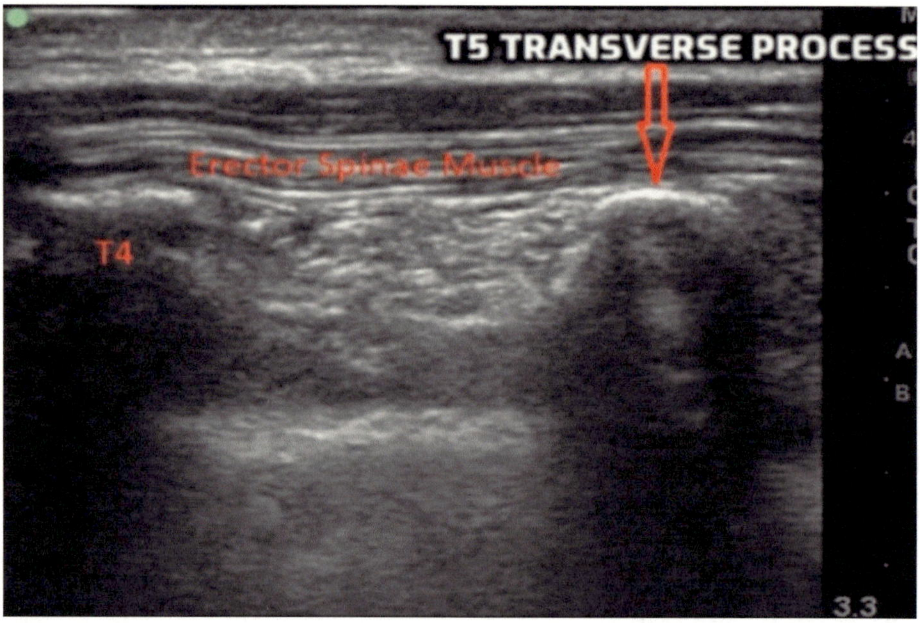

Figure 8.
Erector spinae block.

and associated diseases, in addition to improving patient outcomes and patient comfort. Opioids which are the mainstay of treatment in such patients have a variety of side effects including respiratory depression, coughing, and delirium. Nerve blocks develop into a critical component of emergency management of such injuries leading to better patient outcomes and patient satisfaction with analgesia. The Erector spinae block has already been shown to be effective in terms of analgesia for fractures of the posterior ribs and fractures of transverse processes of the vertebrae as shown by previous studies involving authors in this book [59].

5.6 Serratus anterior plane block

Serratus anterior plane block is increasingly becoming part of the clinical practice of treating patients with multiple rib fractures in the ED. Its efficacy, easy procedure and single-injection method in supine position with limited side effect has made it more popular in polytrauma patients with rib fractures. In a study published by the authors [60], a method within the serratus anterior plane block was used. In this case, the probe was placed in the sagittal plane, and the 5th rib in the medial axillary line appeared first. The Latissimus dorsi and the serratus anterior muscles are identified by over 5th ribs. The plane between the two muscles was further confirmed by identifying thoraco dorsal vein using color doppler. A small induration is made in the area marked with the injection of 1% lignocaine and adrenaline. A gap of 3–5 min is allowed to confirm the onset of skin anesthesia after which bupivacaine (0.5% at a dose of 1 mg/kg body weight and diluted with an equal volume of NS to make a solution of 0.25% while not exceeding the total volume 40 ml) injection using a 50 mm 18 g catheter needle using in plane method from superior anterior to posterior inferior for proper absorption. Once the plane between the serratus anterior and the latissimus dorsi is reached (**Figure** 7), rule out any vascular injury. Initially, 2–3 ml of LA is

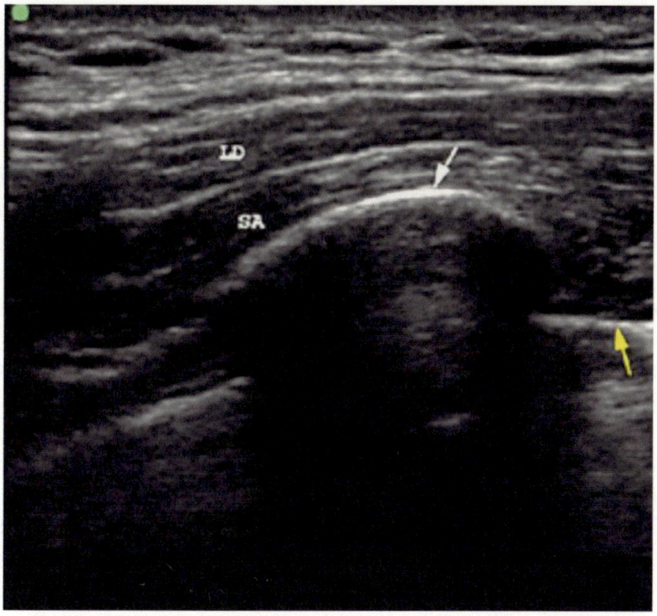

Figure 9.
Serratus anterior plane block. SA serratus anterior, LD latissimus dorsi.

injected to confirm hydro dissection between the latissimus dorsi and serratus muscle visible on ultrasound. The remaining solution is given gradually under continuous ultrasound guidance (**Figure 9**).

5.7 Pecs block

Both pecs I and Pec II block are widely used for fractures of the anterior ribs in patients with chest trauma. In pecs I nerve block, the plane between the major and minor pectoralis is hydrodissected to block the private and middle cutaneous nerves.

Pecs I nerve block involves the hydro separation of the plane between the pectoral muscles with local anesthetic to the lateral and the medial pectoral nerves. First, the major and minor pectoralis and pectoral branch of the thoraco-acromial artery are detected using ultrasound guidance. The lower border of the probe is rotated slightly to the side to visualize the pectoral branch of the thoraco-acromial artery and using the local anesthetic method is injected after initial confirmation using hydro-dissection of the space between the two pectoral muscles.

In the Pecs II nerve block, infiltrate the two fascial segments (pectoral and clavipectoral) by separating the local anesthetic volume between the pectoral nerves (pectoral fascia and clavipectoral fascia) and below the pectoralis minor muscle (middle) of the clavipectoral fascia and outer border. Serratus muscles). In the patient's supine position, the first injection is made in the form of pecs I block and the second is made in the anterior axillary line at a depth of 3-6 cm between the pectoralis minor and the anterior serratus muscle. In this block place the transducer is first in the midclavicular line and it is infero-laterally angle to identify the axillary vein, artery and second rib. The transducer is then moved sideways until the pectoralis minor and serratus anterior are visible. With continuous lateral movements, the third and fourth ribs appear. The local anesthetic is injected into two points: The first injection is usually made between the pectoralis major and pectoralis minor, and the second injection is made between the pectoralis minor muscles and the anterior serratus.

5.8 Adverse effects of nerve block

Although ultrasound guided nerve blocks have no side effects especially when performed by trained doctors, there are rare cases of traumatic events involving a vessel or temporary sensory injury that lead to sensory or motor impairment and infection at the injection site. In particular, Local Anesthetic Systemic Toxicity (LAST) is one of the complication that an emergency physician should pay attention to. It is a serious life-threatening event with incidence rate of approximately 0.04 [61]. While the LAST presentation is multifactorial, the most prominent neurological presentation [62] includes sensory and visual changes, decreased muscle function, and fainting. However, approximately one-fifth of all cases are characterized by cardiovascular manifestations including motor impairment, myocardial dysfunction, and decreased peripheral vascular tone. Prevention is the key to reducing the frequency and intensity of LAST. These include the use of ultrasound-guided blocks, reduction of the anesthetic dose, selective anesthesia with high levels of CC/CNS side effects (heart failure and central nervous system) [63] including ropivacaine and levobupivacaine, to avoid high-risk patients like patients with advanced age, kidney disease or those with mild heart disease.

6. Conclusion

In conclusion, although new pain management techniques are widely used by emergency physicians to improve patient outcomes both during their emergency stay and during their hospital stay, there are clinical settings where they should still be used but are not explicitly specified. Although neuraxial analgesia using ultrasound guided nerve blocks has been shown to be simpler and easier to perform by trained emergency physicians and provide better and more lasting analgesia, a good pain management protocol with specific step-by-step guidelines is not available in most emergency departments unlike other diseases. Future policy guidelines should address this aspect of emergency management.

Disclosures

None.

DOI: http://dx.doi.org/10.5772/intechopen.105952

Author details

Sakshi Yadav[1], Anuj Ajayababu[2], Tej Prakash Sinha[1*] and Sanjeev Bhoi[1]

1 Department of Emergency Medicine, All India Institute of Medical Sciences, New Delhi, India

2 Department of Medicine, All India Institute of Medical Sciences, New Delhi, India

*Address all correspondence to: drsinha123@gmail.com

References

[1] Chang HY, Daubresse M, Kruszewski SP, et al. Prevalence and treatment of pain in EDS in the United States, 2000 to 2010. The American Journal of Emergency Medicine. 2014;**32**:421-431

[2] Pines JM, Hollander JE. Emergency department crowding is associated with poor care for patients with severe pain. Annals of Emergency Medicine. 2008;**51**(1):1-5

[3] Mills AM, Shofer FS, Chen EH, et al. The association between emergency department crowding and analgesia administration in acute abdominal pain patients. Academic Emergency Medicine. 2009;**16**(7):603-608

[4] Gallagher RM. Physician variability in pain management: Are the JCAHO standards enough? Pain Medicine. 2003;**4**(1):1-3

[5] O'Connor AB, Zwemer FL, Hays DP, et al. Outcomes after intravenous opioids in emergency patients: A prospective cohort analysis. Academic Emergency Medicine. 2009;**16**(6):477-487

[6] Bijur PE, Latimer CT, Gallagher EJ. Validation of a verbally administered numerical rating scale of acute pain for use in the emergency department. Academic Emergency Medicine. 2003;**10**(4):390-392

[7] Schull MJ, Morrison LJ, Vermeulen M, Redelmeier DA. Emergency department overcrowding and ambulance transport delays for patients with chest pain. CMAJ. 2003;**168**(3):277-283

[8] Gordon DB, Dahl JL, Miaskowski C, McCarberg B, Todd KH, Paice JA, et al. American pain society recommendations for improving the quality of acute and cancer pain management: American pain society quality of care task force. Archives of Internal Medicine. 2005;**165**(14):1574-1580

[9] Hwang U, Richardson LD, Sonuyi TO, Morrison RS. The effect of emergency department crowding on the management of pain in older adults with hip fracture. Journal of the American Geriatrics Society. 2006;**54**(2):270-275

[10] Balbin JE, Nerenberg R, Baratloo A, Friedman BW. Intravenous fluids for migraine: A post hoc analysis of clinical trial data. The American Journal of Emergency Medicine. 2016;**34**(4):713-716

[11] Baratloo A, Negida A, El Ashal G, Behnaz N. Intravenous caffeine for the treatment of acute migraine: A pilot study. Journal of Caffeine Research. 2015;**5**(3):125-129

[12] Fosnocht D, Heaps N, Swanson E. Patient expectations for pain relief in the ED. The American Journal of Emergency Medicine. 2004;**22**:286-288

[13] Downey LVA, Zun LS. Pain management in the emergency department and its relationship to patient satisfaction. Journal of Emergencies, Trauma, and Shock. 2010;**3**(4):326-330

[14] Pitts S, Niska RW, Xu J, Burt C. National Hospital Ambulatory Medical Care Survey: 2006 emergency department summary. National Health Statistics Report. 2008;**7**:1-39

[15] Royal College of Physicians. British Geriatrics Society and British Pain Society, the Assessment of Pain in Older People: National Guidelines Concise Guidance to Good Practice Series, No 8. London, UK: RCP; 2007

[16] Rosemary C. Polomano, Kevin T. Galloway, Michael L. Kent, Hisani Brandon-Edwards, Kyung Nancy Kwon, Carlos Morales, Chester Trip Buckenmaier, III, Psychometric. Testing of the Defense and veterans pain rating scale (DVPRS): A new pain scale for military population, Pain Medicine. 2016;**17**(8):1505-1519

[17] Yanev N, Vlaskovska M. Treatment of pain in pediatric patients. Journal of IMAB. 2016;**22**(2):1175-1181

[18] Cleeland CS, Chapman CR, Loeser JD. Measurement of Pain by Subjective Report, Advances in Pain Research and Therapy Volume 12: Issues in Pain Measurement. New York: Raven Press; 1989. pp. 391-403

[19] Forbes K. Pain in patients with Cancer: The World Health Organization analgesic ladder and beyond. Clinical Oncology. 2011;**23**(6):379-380

[20] Miner JR, Burton J. Pain Management. In: Marx JA, Hockberger RS, Walls RM, Biros MH, editors. Rosen's Emergency Medicine 1. 8th ed. Philadelphia, PA: Elsevier Saunders; 2014. pp. 31-49

[21] Zhou TJ, Tang J, White PF. Propacetamol versus ketorolac for treatment of acute postoperative pain after total hip or knee replacement. Anesthesia and Analgesia. 2001;**92**(6):1569-1575

[22] Dejonckheere M, Desjeux L, DeneuS,EwalenkoP.Intravenoustramadol compared to paracetamol for postoperative analgesia following thyroidectomy. Acta Anaesthesiologica Belgica. 2001;**52**(1):29-33

[23] Hernandez-Palazon J, Tortosa JA, Martinez-Lage JF, Perez-FloresD.Intravenousadministration of propacetamol reduces morphine consumption after spinal fusion surgery. Anesthesia and Analgesia. 2001;**92**(6):14736

[24] Van Aken H, Thys L, Veekman L, Buerkle H. Assessing analgesia in single and repeated administrations of propacetamol for postoperative pain: Comparison with morphine after dental surgery. Anesthesia and Analgesia. 2004;**98**(1):159-165

[25] Hyllested M, Jones S, Pedersen J, Kehlet H. Comparative effect of paracetamol, NSAIDs or their combination in postoperative pain management: A qualitative review. British Journal of Anaesthesia. 2002;**88**(2):199-214

[26] Cashman JN. The mechanisms of action of NSAIDs in analgesia. Drugs. 1996;**52**(Suppl. 5):13-23

[27] Seymour RA, Ward-Booth P, Kelly PJ. Evaluation of different doses of soluble ibuprofen and ibuprofen tablets in postoperative dental pain. The British Journal of Oral & Maxillofacial Surgery. 1996;**34**(1):110-114

[28] Bailey E, Worthington H, Coulthard P. Ibuprofen and/or paracetamol (acetaminophen) for pain relief after surgical removal of lower wisdom teeth, a Cochrane systematic review. British Dental Journal. 2014;**216**(8):451-455

[29] Chang AK, Bijur PE, Esses D, et al. Effect of a single dose of oral opioid and nonopioid analgesics on acute extremity pain in the emergency department: A randomized clinical trial. Journal of the American Medical Association. 2017;**318**(17):1661-1667

[30] Shapiro AG. Emergency treatment of menstrual disorders in a nonpregnant woman. Emergency Medicine Clinics of

North America. 1987;**5**(3):559-568 PMID: 3653022

[31] Mernis D, Mehmet TI, Guksum K, Sezer A, Sut N. Intravenous paracetamol reduced the use of opioids, extubation time, and opioid-related adverse effects after major surgery in intensive care unit. Journal of Critical Care. 2010;**25**(3):458-462

[32] Thomas S. Management of Pain in the emergency department. ISRN Emergency Medicine. 2013;**2013**:19

[33] Turturro MA, Paris PM, Seaberg DC. Intramuscular ketorolac versus oral ibuprofen in acute musculoskeletal pain. Annals of Emergency Medicine. 1995;**26**(2):117-120

[34] Wright JM, Price SD, Watson WA. NSAID use and efficacy in the emergency department: Single doses oral ibuprofen versus intramuscular ketorolac. The Annals of Pharmacotherapy. 1994;**28**(3):309-312

[35] Yeaman F, Meek R, Egerton-Warburton D, et al. Sub-dissociative-dose intranasal ketamine for moderate to severe pain in adult emergency department patients. Emergency Medicine Australasia. 2014;**26**(3):237-242

[36] Motov S, Drapkin J, Likourezos A, et al. Continuous intravenous sub-dissociative dose ketamine infusion for managing pain in the emergency department. The Western Journal of Emergency Medicine. 2018;**19**(3): 559-566

[37] Motov S, Hossain R. Tarascon Pain Pocketbook. Burlington, MA: Jones and Bartlett Learning LLC; 2018

[38] Wide-Ranging Online Data for Epidemiologic Research (WONDER). Atlanta, GA: CDC, National Centre for Health Statistics; 2020

[39] https://www.cdc.gov/drugoverdose/deaths/prescription/maps.html

[40] Francis RC, Bubser F, Schmidbauer W, et al. Effects of a standard operating procedure on prehospital emergency care of patients presenting with symptoms of the acute coronary syndrome. European Journal of Emergency Medicine. 2014;**21**(3):236-239

[41] Patanwala AE, Edwards CJ, Stolz L, Amini R, Desai A, Stolz U. Should morphine dosing weight based for analgesia in the emergency department? Journal of Opioid Management. 2012;**8**:51-55

[42] Ballas SK, Viscusi ER, Epstein KR. Management of acute chest wall sickle cell pain with nebulized morphine. American Journal of Hematology. 2004;**76**(2):190-191

[43] Poklis A. Fentanyl: A review for clinical and analytical toxicologists. Journal of Toxicology. Clinical Toxicology. 1995;**33**(5):439-447

[44] Minami K, Sudo Y, Miyano K, et al. micro-opioid receptor activation by tramadol and O-desmethyltramadol (M1). Journal of Anesthesia. 2015;**29**(3):475-479

[45] Dezieck L, Hafez Z, Conicella A, et al. Resolution of cannabis hyperemesis syndrome with topical capsaicin in the emergency department: A case series. Clinical Toxicology. 2017;**55**(8):908-913

[46] Barden J, Edwards J, Moore A, et al. Single dose oral paracetamol (acetaminophen) for postoperative pain. Cochrane Database of Systematic Reviews. 2008;**2008**(4):CD004602

[47] Yeh YC, Reddy P. Clinical and economic evidence for intravenous acetaminophen. Pharmacotherapy. 2012;**32**(6):559-579

[48] Furyk J, Levas D, Close B, et al. Intravenous versus oral paracetamol for acute pain in adults in the emergency department setting: A prospective, double-blind, doubledummy, randomised controlled trial. Emergency Medicine Journal. 2018;**35**(3):179-184

[49] Ryan NM, Isbister GK. Tramadol overdose causes seizures and respiratory depression but serotonin toxicity appears unlikely. Clinical Toxicology. 2015;**53**(6):545-550

[50] Bhoi S, Chandra A, Galwankar S. Ultrasound guided nerve blocks in the emergency department. Journal of Emergencies, Trauma, and Shock. 2010;**3**(1):82-88

[51] Otterness K, Vermeulen M. Practical Tips: When and How to Use a Femoral Nerve Block. EM Resident Magazine [cited December 18, 2015]; 2014. Available from: emra.org

[52] Dewitz A, Jones RA, Goldsetin JG, Stone MB. Additional ultrasound guided procedures. In: Ma O, Mateer JR, Reardon RF, Joing SA, editors. Ma and Mateer's Emergency Ultrasound. 3rd ed. New York: McGraw-Hill; 2014

[53] Bunting LV, Calvello EJB. Femoral Nerve Block, 3-in-1 Block Variation. Ultrasound Guide for Emergency Physicians [cited December 18, 2008]; 2015. Web. Available from: http://www.acep.org/sonoguide

[54] Short AJ, Barnett JJG, Gofeld M, Baig E, Lam K, Agur AMR, et al. Anatomic study of innervation of the anterior hip capsule: Implication for image guided intervention. Regional Anesthesia and Pain Medicine. 2018;**43**:186-192

[55] Bugada D, Bellini V, Lorini L, Mariano ER. Update on selective regional analgesia for hip surgery patients. Anesthesiology Clinics. 2018;**36**:403-415

[56] Giron-Arango L, Peng PWH, Chin KJ, Brull R, Perlas A. Pericapsular nerve group (PENG) block for hip fracture. Regional Anesthesia and Pain Medicine. 2018;**43**:859-863

[57] Abdelhamid K, ElHawary H, Turner JP. The use of the erector spinae plane block to decrease pain and opioid consumption in the emergency department: A literature review. The Journal of Emergency Medicine. 2020;**58**:603-609

[58] Gopinath B, Mathew R, Bhoi S, Nayak R, Muvalia G. Erector spinae plane block for pain control in patients with pancreatitis in the emergency department. Turkish Journal of Emergency Medicine. 2021;**21**(3): 129-132

[59] Kumar G, Kumar Bhoi S, Sinha TP, Paul S. Erector spinae plane block for multiple rib fracture done by an emergency physician: A case series. Australasian Journal of Ultrasound in Medicine. 2020;**24**(1):58-62

[60] Paul S, Bhoi SK, Sinha TP, Kumar G. Ultrasound-guided serratus anterior plane block for rib fracture-associated pain Management in Emergency Department. Journal of Emergencies, Trauma, and Shock. 2020;**13**(3):208-212

[61] Liu SS, Ortolan S, Sandoval MV, et al. Cardiac arrest and seizures caused by local Anesthetic systemic toxicity after peripheral nerve blocks: Should we still fear the reaper? Regional Anesthesia and Pain Medicine. 2016;**41**:5

[62] El-Boghdadly K, Pawa A, Chin KJ. Local anesthetic systemic toxicity: Current perspectives. Local and Regional Anesthesia. 2018;**11**:35-44

[63] El-Boghdadly K, Chin KJ. Local anesthetic systemic toxicity: Continuing professional development. Canadian Journal of Anaesthesia. 2016;**63**(3):330-349

Chapter 4

ERAS Protocols and Multimodal Pain Management in Surgery

Gustavo Rodriguez, Emma Whiting and Juliet Lee

Abstract

Pain is inherent to trauma and surgery, either by direct tissue trauma or by the activation of a surgical stress response characterized by endocrine, metabolic, and immunologic responses. Most pain from trauma and surgery is nociceptive in nature, but patients may also experience inflammatory and neuropathic pain. Therefore, it is necessary to consider the clinical context, patient factors, the type of trauma injury and surgery, the extent and degree of tissue involvement, and the severity of the response when deciding on pain management choices. In the past, surgery was approached mostly in an open fashion and led to a greater stress response and pain. Over the last 30 years, the minimally invasive approach with laparoscopic and robotic surgery has improved the experience of patients with regard to peri-operative pain. In addition, the advent of enhanced recovery protocols have sought to minimize this surgical stress response through targeting of pain control and pain management regimens. This chapter will focus on enhanced recovery after surgery protocols and multimodal pain regimens and will consider trauma and cancer patients as examples of surgical patients who benefit from this type of approach.

Keywords: enhanced recovery after surgery, multimodal pain management, post-operative pain, surgical stress response, trauma, cancer

1. Introduction

Trauma is sometimes described as the transfer of external energy to the human body, causing tissue disruption. Therefore, surgery can be considered controlled and orderly penetrating trauma in which the act of an incision, dissection, and retraction also imposes tissue changes. Both trauma and surgery can lead to similar stress responses including endocrine, metabolic, and immunologic or inflammatory responses.

The endocrine response to surgery includes activation of the hypothalamus, pituitary gland and the sympathetic nervous system [1]. Multiple endocrine effects such as secretion of cortisol from the adrenal cortex and vasopressin from the pituitary gland lead to metabolic changes. These culminate in an overall systemic effect characterized by increased catabolism, water resorption, and mobilization of stored energy within fat, glucagon within the liver, and skeletal and visceral protein. The activation of thyroid hormone increases glucose absorption from the gastrointestinal tract and stimulates the central and peripheral nervous systems.

The immunologic stress response involves the elaboration of cytokines where neutrophils, fibroblasts, and endothelial cells are activated. These proteins play a role in the inflammatory response to surgery and tissue trauma and promote systemic changes. The most prominent cytokines released in the post-operative period are interleukin-1, interleukin-6, and tumor necrosis factor-α. As a result, the secretion from the pituitary gland is augmented through secretion of adrenocorticotropic hormone and increasing the release of cortisol. In turn, this additional stimulation of cortisol amplifies the endocrine and metabolic responses to trauma and surgery [2].

Pain is an expected part of trauma and surgery and the wound itself elicits inflammatory and metabolic responses [3]. Direct stimulation of the hypothalamic–pituitary–adrenal axis is transmitted through small myelinated A-delta fibers and unmyelinated C fibers [4]. These nociceptive signals are then transmitted via sympathetic pathways at the level of the spinal cord. As a result, pro-inflammatory cytokines are secreted via the spinal cord as well as systemically [5]. Also, the pain stimulus itself has been demonstrated to elaborate endocrine, metabolic, and inflammatory responses [6].

From a clinical perspective, acute pain after trauma and surgery is a reminder of the local tissue injury and that pain is a protective mechanism to move away from a painful stimulus or to limit behaviors that would cause further tissue damage. Patients experience pain in both a physical and cognitive manner. Whether the physical pain is nociceptive, inflammatory or pathologic, insults from an external source or internally from a disease process lead to a systemic response. The affective and cognitive aspect includes the way patients experience pain and the cortical processing that occurs when pain is experienced.

In order to treat acute pain resulting from trauma and surgery, strategies should address the physical and cognitive aspects of how patients experience pain. Surgical and anesthetic techniques that mute the body's endocrine, metabolic or immunologic responses may serve to reduce pain responses.

2. ERAS protocols

Enhanced Recovery After Surgery (ERAS) is a multimodal perioperative protocol focused on evidence-based interventions to improve patient outcomes and recovery. ERAS was developed from the foundational work of Professor Henrik Kehlet of the University of Copenhagen in the 1990s where he discussed the pathophysiology behind the "surgical stress response" and designed a multimodal perioperative approach that differed from existing traditional consensus guidelines [7]. Building off Kehlet's early work, Professor Ken Fearon of the University of Edinburgh and Professor Olle Ljungqvist of the Karolinska Institutet founded the ERAS Study Group in 2001. The ERAS Study Group later became the ERAS Society, a non-profit organization whose mission is "to develop perioperative care and to improve recovery through research education, audit and implementation of evidence-based practice" [8]. ERAS protocols are based on more than 20 principal interventions throughout the pre-, intra-, and post-operative periods that aim to minimize surgical trauma and adverse outcomes, preserve appropriate physiologic function, as well as enhance the rate of recovery. ERAS guidelines exist for a variety of surgical subspecialties and even specific surgical interventions. ERAS compliance has been repeatedly demonstrated to reduce length of admission and complication rates [9] as well as be financially beneficial [10, 11].

2.1 Pre-operative interventions for pain in ERAS

In the pre-operative period, a variety of interventions are used to optimize a patient's readiness for surgery. These interventions are targeted to address modifiable risk factors and stabilize pre-operative physiology. The components of ERAS in the pre-operative period include preadmission counseling, pre-operative medical optimization, pre-rehabilitation, pre-operative nutrition and carbohydrate loading, thromboprophylaxis, and antibiotic prophylaxis.

An important initial part of pain management in ERAS is appropriate preadmission counseling. Pre-operative counseling is designed to ready the patient for surgery and provide the patient with needed information and realistic expectations regarding the peri-operative period. Ideally, this pre-operative education will include a discussion of post-operative pain. Although there is little up to date research into benefits of pre-operative education, general consensus guidelines support the use of pre-operative counseling in the case of all non-emergent surgeries. Egbert et al. [12] demonstrated a statistically significant reduction in post-operative narcotic use in patients who received pre-operative education of pain including relaxation techniques and discussion of pharmacologic methods to control pain. This was despite noting no difference in subjective grading of pain severity in this group compared to patients who did not received education or counseling. Additional benefits of pre-operative pain discussions include reduced fear and anxiety and reduced distress due to pain [13, 14].

2.2 Intra-operative interventions for pain in ERAS

At the time of surgery, ERAS protocol items are targeted to maintaining physiologic function and minimizing surgical trauma. These interventions are designed to attenuate the surgical stress response and prevent adverse outcomes as a result. The components of ERAS in the intra-operative period include preventing intra-operative hypothermia, anesthetic management, opioid-sparing pain control, minimally-invasive surgery techniques, avoidance of prophylactic NG tubes and drains, nausea management, and peri-operative fluid management.

2.2.1 Surgical technique

Historically, procedures were performed in an open manner, where incisions allowed wide exposure of the involved structures. Newer developments in surgical technique such as minimally invasive surgery (MIS) require smaller surgical incisions and are designed to inflict less pain and trauma on the body. MIS encompasses both laparoscopic and robotic-assisted surgery techniques. Laparoscopy involves the use of a camera, also known as a laparoscope, and other elongated forms of surgical tools which are inserted through port sites at various locations on the abdomen or thorax. This allows surgeons to visualize structures and perform an operation entirely through multiple small surgical incisions. Robotic-assisted surgery is a newer approach where a surgeon controls laparoscopic tools from a console. This system uses instruments with an additional point of articulation as compared to laparoscopic instruments, which may allow for more precise, fine motor movements in the confined space of the abdomen, pelvis or thorax. The increased articulation of the robotic arms may further minimize tissue injury by decreasing the torque on the abdominal and chest wall and compensate for surgeon and patient characteristics that affect the ergonomics during the surgical intervention.

Open versus laparoscopic techniques have been extensively studied across a wide range of surgical procedures. In our review of the ERAS protocols for gastrectomy, bariatric surgery, and colorectal surgery, all protocols recommend the use of minimally-invasive surgery techniques whenever possible, appropriate, and within the expertise of the operating surgeon [15–17]. There is some variation in the grade of recommendation with colorectal and bariatric surgery giving a strong recommendation for MIS technique and gastrectomy recommendation varying based upon procedure and level of disease progression. In nine meta-analyses comparing open versus laparoscopic techniques in either distal gastrectomy [18–23] or total gastrectomy [24–26], the laparoscopic approach was consistently shown in all studies to have lower volume of blood loss. Laparoscopic surgery was associated with longer operating times and shorter hospital stays in 6 out of the 9 meta-analyses. In the studies that demonstrated shorter hospital stays with the minimally invasive approach, the hospital stay was 4–5 days less on average. A laparoscopic approach to gastric bypass was associated with shorter length of stay (LOS), earlier recovery, reduced rate of hernia and infection [27–30]. In multiple controlled trials in colorectal surgery, laparoscopic technique was associated with improved recovery, reduced length of stay, reduced blood loss, and complications [31–37]. Research comparing outcomes between laparoscopic and robotic-assisted surgery for colonic and rectal resection did not demonstrate significant differences in primary outcome measurements aside from reduced conversion rate associated with robotic technique and reduced operating time associated with laparoscopic method. Robotic-assisted surgery was associated with significantly increased cost despite not conferring major additional advantages [38, 39].

The LAFA-study, a nine-center randomized controlled trial (RCT) completed in 2011, compared outcomes including post-operative hospital stay, morbidity, reoperation rate, readmission rate, in-hospital mortality, quality of life, patient satisfaction, and in-hospital costs amongst open or laparoscopic and fast track multimodal management or standard care in the treatment of colon cancer [40]. The primary outcome of total post-operative hospital stay was dependent on the predefined discharge criteria which included adequate pain control with paracetamol and/or nonsteroidal anti-inflammatory drugs (NSAID), ability to tolerate solid foods, lack of nausea, passage of flatus or stool, mobilization, and acceptance of discharge. The laparoscopic/fast track group had a median total post-operative hospital stay of 5 days as compared to 7 days in the open/fast track group, 6 days in the laparoscopic/standard group, and 7 days in the open/standard group ($p < 0.001$) [40]. Those in the laparoscopic/fast track group were meeting the defined discharge criteria earlier than the other categories implying that these fast-track and MIS interventions allowed for adequate pain control earlier in the post-operative course as compared to open and non-multimodal standard of care protocols.

2.2.2 Opioid-sparing pain control and anesthetic management

Pain control begins during the intra-operative period and continues into the post-operative period. Intra-operative pain control involves appropriate anesthetic management, the use of local anesthetics around incisions, and the use of additional pain-relieving adjunctive interventions. ERAS protocol suggests the use of multimodal opioid-sparing pain control regimens.

2.2.3 Avoidance of prophylactic nasogastric (NG) tubes and drains

In the pre-ERAS era, the use of drains and NG tubes were common despite lack of research support for these practices. In fact, the Cochrane review by Verma et al. [41] demonstrated that patients without NG tubes had an earlier return of bowel function and decreased complications. ERAS protocols suggest the avoidance of prophylactic NG tubes or drains given no clear benefit from their use in multiple studies and multiple types of surgery [41–45] as well as potential harms including pain and discomfort from the tube or drain, delayed nutrition, and decreased ambulation.

2.3 Post-operative interventions for pain in ERAS

Following surgery, ERAS guidelines focus on preventing complications and helping with the speed of recovery. The components of ERAS in the post-operative period include post-operative pain control, pain and nausea management, early oral nutrition, early ambulation, early catheter removal, prevention of post-operative ileus, and appropriate discharge criteria. In the post-operative period, it is an expectation that the patient will have some degree of pain because pain is an unavoidable sequelae of surgery. The goal of pain control in ERAS is not complete elimination of pain. Instead, the objective is dynamic pain relief, where pain is controlled to the point of allowing normal function in terms of both physiology and mobility.

2.3.1 Nausea and prevention of post-operative ileus

Post-operative nausea, vomiting, and ileus can be significant causes of patient pain and discomfort. Best practice recommendations for post-operative nausea and vomiting include the use of serotonin antagonists along with avoidance of opioid analgesics given their likelihood to cause GI side effects including nausea, constipation, and ileus. Other antiemetic medications commonly used include dopamine receptor antagonists, benzamides, and antihistamine medications. Other interventions targeted to minimize the risk of post-operative ileus include the use of central neural blocks. The rationale behind these neural blocks is two-fold as a method of pain control and acting as a sympathetic nerve block allowing for increased gastrointestinal motility and reduced rate of post-operative ileus [7].

2.3.2 Early oral nutrition

Historically, surgeons employed prolonged fasting periods after surgery with a gradual return to normal eating habits. Research has shown early nutrition to be associated with reduced rates of infections and decreased duration of hospital stay [46, 47], and demonstrated improvements in immune functioning [48, 49]. During the inflammatory reaction to trauma and surgical stress, hyperglycemia is common due to increased hepatic glucose production and decreased peripheral uptake [3]. This is compounded by relative insulin resistance. When cells do not have glucose readily available for metabolic needs, the body will enter into pathways that promote gluconeogenesis and leads to catabolism of skeletal and visceral protein. Because pain pathways and the immunologic stress response are linked, interventions that addresses insulin resistance would also mitigate pain responses and vice versa.

2.3.3 Early ambulation

Some interventions in ERAS that are designed to improve the rate of recovery may result in increased pain for the patient. ERAS protocols encourage prompt mobilization as early as the day of the operative procedure. Activity targets are dependent on pre-operative functioning and tolerance of physical activity requires adequate pain control. Although evidence of the positive benefits of early mobilization are limited, post-operative bed rest is associated with increased risk of thromboembolism and pulmonary complications. The surgical stress response causes both micro and macroscopic endothelial injury and post-operative immobilization increases venous stasis placing patients at significantly increased risk of thromboembolism regardless of the presence or lack of coagulopathy [7, 50, 51]. Bed rest and maintaining a supine position encourages positional-hypoxemia which may be improved with sitting positioning (>30° from horizontal) that allows for improved oxygenation, functional residual capacity, and decreased work of breathing [52]. Additionally, immobilization contributes to general catabolism and muscle wasting. An understanding of the pathophysiologic processes supports the continued use of this intervention despite its potential to cause patient discomfort.

3. Multimodal pain management

A central tenet of ERAS protocols is the use of multimodal pain management techniques. These techniques can be broken down into multiple subcategories including non-pharmacologic therapy, non-opioid pharmacotherapy, opioid pharmacotherapy, and regional anesthesia techniques. Multimodal pain management takes into consideration the multiple potential points of intervention for pain, targeting both ascending input to the brain and descending pain regulation pathways [53]. Using interventions at multiple points along the pain pathways helps to maximize pain control while minimizing unwanted effects or reliance on one specific strategy. The multimodal approach allows for plans tailored to the needs of the patient that can adapt and change with circumstances, pain control, patient preference, and symptoms.

3.1 Non-pharmacologic pain management

Non-pharmacologic pain management interventions can be used as adjunct therapies to traditional pain management techniques. These interventions can involve cognitive or physical strategies to reduce pain and discomfort. Common cognitive strategies include therapy (cognitive behavioral therapy, psychotherapy, music and art therapy), mindfulness and relaxation techniques, hypnosis, meditation, and virtual reality. Physical strategies include positioning, topical heat or cold application, acupuncture, massage, transcutaneous electrical nerve stimulation, and therapeutic ultrasound [53]. Many of these modalities are low cost interventions that confer minimal risk with potential benefit though quality of evidence of improved efficacy is variable.

3.2 Non-opioid pharmacotherapy

Various non-opioid medications exist and are commonly employed agents in standard pain control regimens. These include, but are not limited to anti-inflammatory

DOI: http://dx.doi.org/10.5772/intechopen.111899

drugs, local and regional anesthetics, gabapentinoids, symptom-driven adjuvant therapy, serotonin-norepinephrine reuptake inhibitors (SNRI), N-methyl-D-aspartate (NMDA) antagonists, and $\alpha 2$-agonists.

3.2.1 Acetaminophen and NSAIDs

Acetaminophen and nonsteroidal anti-inflammatory drugs (NSAIDs) are the mainstay of mild to moderate pain control in outpatient and inpatient settings. They can also be effectively employed in multimodal pain management approaches for more severe pain in the peri-operative period. Acetaminophen functions both as an analgesic and an antipyretic though its exact mechanism of action is unknown. NSAIDs inhibit cyclooxygenase and work as an analgesic, antipyretic, and anti-inflammatory. General best practice recommendations include the use of these medications unless contraindicated. They can be used on an as needed basis or scheduled around the clock. These medications are preferably administered orally, but intravenous (IV) options are available in the setting of poor GI absorption or inability to tolerate oral intake.

3.2.2 Symptom-driven adjuvant therapies

Symptom-driven adjuvant therapies should be employed to target the specific symptoms that a patient is experiencing in the peri-operative period that are causing distress. This may include medications for symptoms including, but not limited to incisional pain, musculoskeletal pain, nausea and vomiting, and anxiety. Medications to consider in this category include lidocaine patches, skeletal muscle relaxants, and anti-nausea and antiemetic therapy.

3.2.3 Neuropathic pain

Most post-surgical pain fits into the category of nociceptive pain, where the pain results from damage to tissue and structures outside of the nervous system. Although to a smaller proportion, some degree of post-surgical pain may be of neuropathic origin. Initial management may include failed attempts with medications such as acetaminophen or NSAIDs, but neuropathic pain may be more responsive to a variety of alternative medications such as the antiepileptic and SNRI medication classes. Medications such as gabapentinoids and $\alpha 2$-agonists target reducing descending pain input through action on the presynaptic neuron.

3.3 Opioid-pharmacotherapy

Opioid medications are synthetic analogues of opiates and act on both ascending and descending pain pathways via action on opioid receptors, primarily μ- and κ-receptors. Opioid medications are incredibly effective methods of pain control, but come with significant risks including respiratory and central nervous system depression, and abuse potential. Other less severe effects include opioid-associated ileus, nausea and vomiting, and urinary retention. These side effects are non-desirable in a post-operative patient with recent abdominal surgery where the goal is to preserve normal physiologic functioning. Therefore, there is significant reason to avoid these medications when possible.

3.4 Local and regional anesthesia techniques

The use of local and regional anesthesia is a common practice that functions well in the multimodal pain management approach and can limit the need for other medications including opioids. Incisional lidocaine and the use of single injection nerve blocks are useful adjuncts that can be employed for short-term pain relief. Other methods include placement of a catheter in a particular region or nerve distribution and analgesic medication is continuously administered. This is generally used when analgesia will be required for greater than 12 hours. Some of the more common regional anesthesia blocks used in abdominal surgeries and trauma include epidural, paravertebral, and transverse abdominis plane (TAP). All of these options provide some relief of abdominal wall pain. The physiologic basis of the use of local and regional anesthetics is centered on the evidence that neural blockade attenuates the hormonal and inflammatory response [54] to surgery.

4. Pain management in trauma patients

Trauma is one of the leading causes of mortality in younger populations [55], but it can affect patients of all ages alike. Unsurprisingly, the most common complaint from trauma patients is pain. The management of this acute pain has been shown to be critical in improving patient outcomes after trauma; poor pain management is associated with longer hospital stays, delays in return to work, decreased quality of life, and increased risk of developing debilitating conditions like post-traumatic stress disorder (PTSD) and chronic pain [55–57]. Traditionally, opiates were one of the main pharmacologic agents used to treat pain caused by traumatic injuries. In recent years, trauma surgeons and emergency medicine physicians have shifted towards a multimodal approach to pain management by including non-opiate pharmacologic agents and regional anesthetics as part of the arsenal of treatments to alleviate acute pain. This shift in paradigm arises in the context of a worsening opioid epidemic in which trauma patients have higher rates of pre-injury opioid use, estimated to be as high as four times that of the average population [58]. The higher prevalence of pre-injury opioid use makes managing acute pain in trauma patients more challenging with patients developing some degree of tolerance to narcotics and putting them at increased risk of withdrawal. Consequently, the higher dose of narcotics required to manage their pain puts them at increased risk of developing dangerous adverse effects including oversedation, urinary retention, nausea, ileus, constipation, and respiratory depression. Considering trauma patients are often critically ill with multiple traumatic injuries, these effects can be deleterious.

4.1 Pharmacologic options

Patients who suffer significant traumatic injuries can present with a wide range of physiologic derangements in response to the acute stress from trauma, which can be far greater than that caused by elective surgery [58–60]. Special attention must be given to a patient's mental, hemodynamic and respiratory status when choosing an appropriate medication for pain relief in order to minimize further physiologic derangements [61]. Additionally, pharmacologic options for pain relief are further limited by route of administration. Oral medications are typically not first-line in the resuscitative period for several reasons including decreased absorption, inability to tolerate enteral intake due to mental status changes or injury to the digestive tract. Intravenously administered drugs are preferred given their rapid onset and more predictable effects. As patients recover from their acute injuries and their physiologic status approximates normalcy, additional pharmacologic and nonpharmacologic options become available.

4.1.1 Opioid analgesics

Although one of the main goals of multimodal analgesia is to optimize pain management while reducing the use of narcotic pain medications, opioids are still the cornerstone of pain management in trauma and critically ill patients given their familiarity, efficacy and known pharmacokinetics. Fentanyl is typically the opioid of choice in the acute resuscitative period, given its minimal effects on hemodynamics, rapid onset and short half-life. However, its short-acting effects means frequent dosing is required for adequate pain relief. Once in the intensive care unit (ICU), continuous infusions of systemic opioids are typically employed for pain management. However, inadequate titration of these medications can cause systemic drug accumulation and result in decreased cognition, ileus, and respiratory depression. A viable option for awake patients is IV narcotics such as hydromorphone or morphine delivered through a patient-controlled analgesic pump. Clinicians should also be aware of the paradoxical syndrome of Opioid-induced hyperesthesia (OIH). Although poorly understood, this syndrome has been observed in patients with chronic opioid use and is characterized by worsening pain with increasing doses of opioids. Furthermore, use of opioid analgesics induces tolerance and exposes patients to possible addiction. Use of other pharmacologic agents for pain relief overall can decrease these adverse effects while improving pain management.

4.1.2 Acetaminophen and nonsteroidal anti-inflammatory drugs (NSAIDs)

Although acetaminophen and NSAIDs may not provide adequate analgesia for severe pain alone, the use of these agents as part of multimodal therapies can be beneficial in pain management. Acetaminophen has been shown to reduce the use of opioids and sedatives in critically ill patients in doses up to 4,000 mg per day. Its availability in oral, rectal and IV formulations make it a viable option as part of a multimodal pain management in most patients.

The efficacy of NSAIDs like ketorolac, celecoxib and ibuprofen in critically ill patients has not been well studied. Their use is often overlooked due to their dose-dependent side effects including gastritis, renal impairment and platelet dysfunction. Specifically in patients with rib fractures, the use of ketorolac has been shown to reduce the risk of pneumonia and ICU length of stays significantly, and use of IV ibuprofen reduces the use of opioids and overall hospital length of stay [62, 63]. Traditionally, some clinicians have been reluctant to prescribe NSAIDs in patients with fractures due to concerns regarding their effects on bone healing. A recent review of the evidence demonstrated that the data supporting the avoidance of NSAIDs in patients with fractures is conflicting and insufficient to formulate clinical recommendations [64–66]. Given their known benefits in relieving pain from musculoskeletal injuriesinjuries, some guidelines actually recommend the routine use of NSAIDs as part of multimodal pain management in patients with non-operative and operative fractures [67].

4.1.3 Anticonvulsants

Gabapentin and pregabalin are two commonly used anticonvulsants in some multimodal pain regimens. The mechanism of their analgesic effects is not entirely understood, but these medications have been effective in treatment of neuropathic pain [68]. Their effects on analgesia related to traumatic injuries is thought to be secondary to their suppression of nociceptive neuronal firing [58]. Their side effect profile which includes dizziness, somnolence, ataxia, convulsions, and visual disturbances, as well as their lack of IV formulations may limit their use in trauma patients. Some studies have shown benefits to using anticonvulsants in patients with phantom limb pain, post-thoracotomy pain, and burns [58, 69, 70]. Furthermore, use of these medications may help prevent transition of acute pain into chronic pain due to their dampening effect on neuronal pathways responsible for the hyperesthesia secondary to nociceptive stimuli [68].

4.1.4 Ketamine

The use of ketamine in the management of acute pain has been studied extensively in recent years. An NMDA receptor antagonist, ketamine has become one of the preferred agents for analgesia in trauma patients for multiple reasons. Its limited effects on hemodynamics, short half-life, quick onset of action, and limited CNS depression have identified it as a favored option in the acute resuscitative period after traumatic injuries [71, 72]. Unlike opioids, ketamine has no effect on the respiratory system and is especially useful in trauma patients who are at high risk of complications from respiratory depression due to multi-system injuries. Studies have shown it to be an effective agent in the treatment of acute pain and reduces the use of opioids in the pre-hospital and emergency room settings [73]. Use of analgesic-dose IV ketamine has been seen to reduce the need for narcotics in the postoperative period as well [74]. Furthermore, its use in traumatic brain injuries has become a preferred agent because of its neuroprotective effects [75].

4.1.5 Other adjuncts

The use of dexmedetomidine has shown promise in the perioperative period for trauma patients, with some studies showing decreased opioid use associated with administration of dexmedetomidine in patients undergoing intra-abdominal surgeries. The addition of dexmedetomidine as part of multimodal pain management is limited by its effects on hemodynamics including bradycardia and hypotension [76]. For this reason, dexmedetomidine is considered a better option for analgesia and sedation during the post-resuscitative phase [77]. Other adjuncts to pain management have been used in some perioperative settings, including IV lidocaine, though studies on its use in trauma populations has been limited [78].

4.2 Non-pharmacologic options

Use of regional analgesia, including peripheral nerve blocks (PNBs), fascial plane blocks and neuraxial blocks, has shown significant promise in the improvement of pain in patients with multiple injuries [79]. When appropriate, implementation of regional analgesia has been shown to decrease requirements for opioid and non-opioid analgesic in trauma patients requiring laparotomies

[80]. Neuraxial blocks have demonstrated a reduction in the postoperative risk of venous thromboembolism and cardiopulmonary complications [81]. The effects of regional analgesia have been best described in cases of thoracic trauma and orthopedic injuries. Specifically, paravertebral blocks in patients with rib fractures have shown significant improvements in pulmonary function, pain control and decreased length of stay. Similar effects have been seen in elderly patients after hip fracture, and in addition, these patients experienced less delirium [82]. Because of these benefits of regional analgesia, early implementation of these modalities should be considered with consultation of an acute pain management service to provide satisfactory pain control in trauma patients.

5. Pain management in cancer patients

One of the most common symptoms for patients with cancer is pain, which can be secondary to the cancer itself or related to the treatment [83]. In the era of the opioid epidemic, there has been a drive to move away from opiate-centered pain management because cancer survivors have a higher risk of opioid misuse due to exposure to opioids during their treatment [84]. The American College of Physicians (ACP), National Comprehensive Cancer Networks (NCCN), the National Cancer Institute (NCI), and the American Society of Clinical Oncology (ASCO) have developed guidelines for the management of cancer-related pain with the overarching concept of using a combination of pharmacologic and nonpharmacologic modalities for pain management. By employing a multimodal approach to pain management clinicians can enhance pain relief and limit side effects from the treatment of pain. This becomes especially important in patients who are already suffering significant side effects from undergoing cancer treatment.

5.1 The WHO analgesic ladder

In an effort to improve cancer-related pain management, the World Health Organization (WHO) developed an "analgesic ladder," a guideline for clinicians to use in their efforts to treat their patients' pain [85]. Originally established in 1986, the analgesic ladder has been modified over the years to include other non-cancer related painful conditions, acute and chronic. The guideline consists of a step-wise approach to pain management starting with non-opioid medications, including NSAIDs and acetaminophen along with other adjuvants, followed by the introduction of weak and then potent opioids. A progressive plan based on pain levels adjusts dosing to balance pain relief with the associated negative side effects these medications may cause. Importantly, this stepwise management is based on the continuous assessment of a patient's level of pain in order to effectively develop individualized, patient-centered treatment plans that can be modified as a patient progresses through the course of the disease.

The first step includes basic non-opioid medications like acetylsalicylic acid (ASA), paracetamol, ibuprofen, indomethacin, and other alternatives. The second step includes "weak" opioids for mild to moderate pain, which include codeine, dihydrocodeine, and tramadol. The third step introduces "potent" opioids, or opioids used for moderate to severe pain. These include morphine, methadone, oxycodone, and buprenorphine. Adjuvant medications are added throughout these steps to manage unwanted side effects, enhance pain relief or for the treatment of concomitant problems like anxiety, insomnia and depression. These medications include antiemetics to treat nausea, laxatives to treat constipation, corticosteroids for the treatment of nerve compression or bone metastases, and psychotropic medications to treat anxiety, depression or other associated conditions. A distinction is also made for neuropathic pain, for which use of tricyclic antidepressants (TCAs) and antiepileptic drugs are recommended [86].

5.2 Nonpharmacologic alternatives to pain management

Initially the analgesic ladder consisted of three steps, each introducing only pharmacologic options for pain management. In recent years, however, the WHO has added a fourth step to include invasive and minimally invasive procedures as a way of managing pain that persists despite optimal pharmacologic therapy. These include epidural and intrathecal analgesia, neurosurgical procedures, neuromodulation strategies, peripheral nerve stimulation, nerve blocks, ablative procedures, and palliative radiotherapy. These techniques have been shown to be effective in the treatment of some cancer-related pain [86–90]. Additionally, integrative medicine therapies like hypnosis, acupuncture and music therapy have also been shown to play a role in the reduction of pain [91].

6. Conclusions

Surgery and traumatic injuries are on a spectrum of energy transfer to the body leading to tissue disruption. As a result of the tissue disruption, multiple responses occur which elaborate a cascade of reactions that cause and augment the pain response. In the management of pain in the peri-operative period, multimodal pain management has evolved as the preferred strategy to control pain and to mitigate the surgical stress response. The ERAS protocols and guidelines for pain control in the injured patient and cancer patient might be summarized in the word "PAIN" itself, now used as a mnemonic. In order, pain control starts with "P" for prevention through use of local anesthesia prior to incision and/or dissection that reduces the endocrine and inflammatory response. Next, patients should be offered "A" for anti-inflammatory agents, followed by "I" for intervention consisting of neural blocks such as epidural or spinal interventions as well as blocking the distribution of named nerve. Finally, "N" for narcotics should be considered for moderate and severe pain and after the previous methods have been attempted so that we move away from opioids as a singular choice. This approach may help to address some of the issues with the opioid crisis.

Conflict of interest

The authors declare no conflict of interest.

Author details

Gustavo Rodriguez[1], Emma Whiting[2] and Juliet Lee[1*]

1 Department of Surgery, George Washington University School of Medicine and Health Sciences, DC, USA

2 George Washington University School of Medicine and Health Sciences, DC, USA

*Address all correspondence to: jclee@mfa.gwu.edu

References

[1] Desborough JP, Hall GM. Endocrine response to surgery. In: Kaufman L, editor. Anaesthesia Review. Vol. 10. Edinburgh: Churchill Livingtone; 1993. pp. 131-148

[2] Desborough JP. The stress response to trauma and surgery. British Journal of Anaesthesia. 2000;**85**(1):109-117

[3] Carli F. Physiologic considerations of enhanced recovery after surgery (ERAS) programs: Implications of the stress response. Canadian Journal of Anaesthesia. 2015;**62**(2):110-119. DOI: 10.1007/s12630-014-0264-0 Epub 2014 Dec 12

[4] Kehlet H. Surgical stress: The role of pain and analgesia. British Journal of Anaesthesia. 1989;**63**:189-195

[5] Wolf G, Livshits D, Beilin B, Yirmiya R, Shavit Y. Interleukin-1 signaling is required for induction and maintenances of postoperative incisional pain: Genetic and pharmacologic studies in mice. Brain, Behavior, and Immunity. 2008;**22**:1072-1077

[6] Griesen J, Juhl CB, Grofte T, Vilstrup H, Jensen TS, Schmitz O. Acute pain induces insulin resistance in humans. Anesthesiology. 2001;**95**(3):578-584

[7] Kehlet H. Multimodal approach to control postoperative pathophysiology and rehabilitation. British Journal of Anaesthesia. 1997;**78**(5):606-617

[8] ERAS® Society. History [Internet]. 2023. Available from: https://erassociety.org/about/history/ [Accessed: April 30, 2023]

[9] Ljungqvist O. ERAS--enhanced recovery after surgery: Moving evidence-based perioperative care to practice. JPEN. Journal of Parenteral and Enteral Nutrition. 2014;**38**(5):559-566

[10] Noba L, Rodgers S, Doi L, Chandler C, Hariharan D, Yip V. Costs and clinical benefits of enhanced recovery after surgery (ERAS) in pancreaticoduodenectomy: An updated systematic review and meta-analysis. Journal of Cancer Research and Clinical Oncology. Advance Online Publication. 2023;**11**:1-22. DOI: 10.1007/s00432-022-04508-x

[11] Noba L, Rodgers S, Chandle C, Balfour A, Hariharan D, Yip VS. Enhanced recovery after surgery (ERAS) reduces hospital costs and improve clinical outcomes in liver surgery: A systematic review and meta-analysis. Journal of Gastrointestinal Surgery. 2020;**24**(4):918-932

[12] Egbert LD, Battit GE, Welch CE, Bartlett MK. Reduction of postoperative pain by encouragement and instruction of patients - a study of doctor-patient rapport. NEJM. 1964;**270**:825-827

[13] Hathaway D. Effect of preoperative instruction on postoperative outcomes: A meta-analysis. Nursing Research. 1986;**35**(5):269-275

[14] Mogan J, Wells N, Robertson E. Effects of preoperative teaching on postoperative pain: A replication and expansion. International Journal of Nursing Studies. 1985;**22**(3):267-280

[15] Stenberg E, dos Reis Falcao LF, O'Kane M, Liem R, Pournaras DJ, Salminen P, et al. Guidelines for perioperative Care in Bariatric Surgery: Enhanced recovery after surgery (ERAS) society. Recommendations:

A 2021 update. World Journal of Surgery. 2022;**46**:729-751

[16] Gustafsson UO, Scott MJ, Hubner M, Nygren J, Demartines N, Francis N, et al. Guidelines for perioperative Care in Elective Colorectal Surgery: Enhanced recovery after surgery (ERAS®) society recommendations: 2018. World Journal of Surgery. 2019;**43**:659-695

[17] Mortensen K, Nilsson M, Slim K, Schäfer M, Mariette C, Braga M, et al. Consensus guidelines for enhanced recovery after gastrectomy. The British Journal of Surgery. 2014;**101**:1209-1229

[18] Ding J, Liao GQ, Liu HL, Liu S, Tang J. Meta-analysis of laparoscopy-assisted distal gastrectomy with D2 lymph node dissection for gastric cancer. Journal of Surgical Oncology. 2012;**105**(3):297-303

[19] Memon MA, Khan S, Yunus RM, Barr R, Memon B. Meta-analysis of laparoscopic and open distal gastrectomy for gastric carcinoma. Surgical Endoscopy. 2008;**22**(8):1781-1789

[20] Ohtani H, Tamamori Y, Noguchi K, Azuma T, Fujimoto S, Oba H, et al. A meta-analysis of randomized controlled trials that compared laparoscopy-assisted and open distal gastrectomy for early gastric cancer. Journal of Gastrointestinal Surgery. 2010;**14**(6):958-964

[21] Viñuela EF, Gonen M, Brennan MF, Coit DG, Strong VE. Laparoscopic versus open distal gastrectomy for gastric cancer: A meta-analysis of randomized controlled trials and high-quality nonrandomized studies. Annals of Surgery. 2012;**255**(3):446-456

[22] Yakoub D, Athanasiou T, Tekkis P, Hanna GB. Laparoscopic assisted distal gastrectomy for early gastric cancer: Is it an alternative to the open approach? Surgical Oncology. 2009;**18**(4):322-333

[23] Zeng YK, Yang ZL, Peng JS, Lin HS, Cai L. Laparoscopy-assisted versus open distal gastrectomy for early gastric cancer: Evidence from randomized and nonrandomized clinical trials. Annals of Surgery. 2012;**256**(1):39-52

[24] Bracale U, Rovani M, Bracale M, Pignata G, Corcione F, Pecchia L. Totally laparoscopic gastrectomy for gastric cancer: Meta-analysis of short-term outcomes. Minimally Invasive Therapy & Allied Technologies. MITAT. 2012;**21**(3):150-160

[25] Martínez-Ramos D, Miralles-Tena JM, Cuesta MA, Escrig-Sos J, Van der Peet D, Hoashi JS, et al. Laparoscopy versus open surgery for advanced and resectable gastric cancer: A meta-analysis. Revista espanola de enfermedades digestivas. 2011;**103**(3):133-141

[26] Huang YL, Lin HG, Yang JW, Jiang FQ, Zhang T, Yang HM, et al. Laparoscopy-assisted versus open gastrectomy with D2 lymph node dissection for advanced gastric cancer: A meta-analysis. International Journal of Clinical and Experimental Medicine. 2014;**7**(6):1490-1499

[27] Luján JA, Frutos MD, Hernández Q, Liron R, Cuenca JR, Valero G, et al. Laparoscopic versus open gastric bypass in the treatment of morbid obesity: A randomized prospective study. Annals of Surgery. 2004;**239**(4):433-437

[28] Nguyen NT, Goldman C, Rosenquist CJ, Arango A, Cole CJ, Lee SJ, et al. Laparoscopic versus open gastric bypass: A randomized study of outcomes, quality of life, and costs. Annals of Surgery. 2001;**234**(3):279-291

[29] Westling A, Gustavsson S. Laparoscopic vs open roux-en-Y gastric bypass: A prospective, randomized trial. Obesity Surgery. 2001;**11**(3):284-292

[30] Buchwald H, Estok R, Fahrbach K, Banel D, Sledge I. Trends in mortality in bariatric surgery: A systematic review and meta-analysis. Surgery. 2007;**142**(4):621-635

[31] Bonjer HJ, Deijen CL, Abis GA, Cuesta MA, van der Pas MH, de Lange-de Klerk ES, Lacy AM, Bemelman WA, Andersson J, Angenete E, Rosenberg J, Fuerst A, Haglind E, COLOR II Study Group. A randomized trial of laparoscopic versus open surgery for rectal cancer. NEJM 2015; 372(14): 1324-1332

[32] Green BL, Marshall HC, Collinson F, Quirke P, Guillou P, Jayne DG, et al. Long-term follow-up of the Medical Research Council CLASICC trial of conventional versus laparoscopically assisted resection in colorectal cancer. The British Journal of Surgery. 2013;**100**(1):75-82

[33] Guillou PJ, Quirke P, Thorpe H, Walker J, Jayne DG, Smith AM, et al. Short-term endpoints of conventional versus laparoscopic-assisted surgery in patients with colorectal cancer (MRC CLASICC trial): Multicentre, randomised controlled trial. Lancet. 2005;**365**(9472):1718-1726

[34] Jeong SY, Park JW, Nam BH, Kim S, Kang SB, Lim SB, et al. Open versus laparoscopic surgery for mid-rectal or low-rectal cancer after neoadjuvant chemoradiotherapy (COREAN trial): Survival outcomes of an open-label, non-inferiority, randomised controlled trial. The Lancet. Oncology. 2014;**15**(7):767-774

[35] Kang SB, Park JW, Jeong SY, Nam BH, Choi HS, Kim DW, et al. Open versus laparoscopic surgery for mid or low rectal cancer after neoadjuvant chemoradiotherapy (COREAN trial): Short-term outcomes of an open-label randomised controlled trial. The Lancet. Oncology. 2010;**11**(7):637-645

[36] Lacy AM, Delgado S, Castells A, Prins HA, Arroyo V, Ibarzabal A, et al. The long-term results of a randomized clinical trial of laparoscopy-assisted versus open surgery for colon cancer. Annals of surgery. 2008;**248**(1):1-7

[37] Weeks JC, Nelson H, Gelber S, Sargent D, Schroeder G. Clinical outcomes of surgical therapy (COST) study group. Short-term quality-of-life outcomes following laparoscopic-assisted colectomy vs open colectomy for colon cancer: A randomized trial. Journal of the American Medical Association. 2002;**287**(3):321-328

[38] Phan K, Kahlaee HR, Kim SH, Toh JW. Laparoscopic vs. robotic rectal cancer surgery and the effect on conversion rates: A meta-analysis of randomized controlled trials and propensity-score-matched studies. Techniques in Coloproctology. 2019;**23**:221-230

[39] Huang YJ, Kang YN, Huang YM, Wu AT, Wang W, Wei PL. Effects of laparoscopic vs robotic-assisted mesorectal excision for rectal cancer: An update systematic review and meta-analysis of randomized controlled trials. Asian Journal of Surgery. 2019;**42**(6):657-666

[40] Vlug MS, Jan W, Hollmann M, Ubbink DT, Cense H, Engel AF, et al. Laparoscopy in combination with fast track multimodal management is the best perioperative strategy in patients undergoing colonic surgery: A randomized clinical trial (LAFA-study). Annals of Surgery. 2011;**254**(6):868-875

[41] Verma R, Nelson RL. Prophylactic nasogastric decompression after abdominal surgery. Cochrane database of systematic reviews. 2007;**3**:CD004929

[42] Rao W, Zhang X, Zhang J, Yan R, Hu Z, Wang Q. The role of nasogastric tube in decompression after elective colon and rectum surgery: A meta-analysis. International journal of colorectal disease. 2011;**26**:423-429

[43] Tanguy M, Seguin P, Mallédant Y. Bench-to-bedside review: Routine postoperative use of the nasogastric tube – Utility or futility? Critical Care. 2007;**11**(1):1-7

[44] Ichida H, Imamura H, Yoshimoto J, Sugo H, Ishizaki Y, Kawasaki S. Randomized controlled trial for evaluation of the routine use of nasogastric tube decompression after elective liver surgery. Journal of Gastrointestinal Surgery. 2016;**20**:1324-1330

[45] Peter SDS, Valusek PA, Little DC, Snyder CL, Holcomb GW III, Ostlie DJ. Does routine nasogastric tube placement after an operation for perforated appendicitis make a difference? Journal of Surgical Research. 2007;**143**(1):66-69

[46] Moore FA, Feliciano DV, Andrassy RJ, McArdle AH, Booth FV, Morgenstein-Wagner TB, et al. Early enteral feeding, compared with parenteral, reduces postoperative septic complications. The results of a meta-analysis. Annals of surgery. 1992;**216**(2):172-183

[47] Carr CS, Ling KD, Boulos P, Singer M. Randomised trial of safety and efficacy of immediate postoperative enteral feeding in patients undergoing gastrointestinal resection. BMJ. 1996;**312**(7035):869-871

[48] Alexander JW. Immunoenhancement via Enteral Nutrition. Archives of Surgery. 1993;**128**(11):1242-1245

[49] Daly JM, Weintraub FN, Shou J, Rosato EF, Lucia M. Enteral nutrition during multimodality therapy in upper gastrointestinal cancer patients. Annals of surgery. 1995;**221**(4):327-338

[50] Convertino VA. Cardiovascular consequences of bed rest: Effect on maximal oxygen uptake. Medicine and Science in Sports and Exercise. 1997;**29**(2):191-196

[51] Kehlet H, Wilmore DW. Multimodal strategies to improve surgical outcome. American Journal of Surgery. 2002;**183**(6):630-641

[52] Mezidi M, Guérin C. Effects of patient positioning on respiratory mechanics in mechanically ventilated ICU patients. Annals of Translational Medicine. 2018;**6**(19):384-392

[53] Best Practice Guidelines for Acute Pain Management in Trauma Patients. American College of Surgeons Trauma Quality Programs. 2020. Available from: https://www.facs.org/media/exob3dwk/acute_pain_guidelines.pdf [Accessed: April 30, 2023]

[54] Uchida I, Asoh T, Shirasaka C, Tsuji H. Effect of epidural analgesia on postoperative insulin resistance as evaluated by insulin clamp technique. The British Journal of Surgery. 1988;**75**:557-562

[55] World Health Organization. 2021. Injuries and Violence. https://www.who.int/news-room/fact-sheets/detail/injuries-and-violence

[56] Visser E, Gosens T, Den Oudsten BL, De Vries J. The course, prediction, and treatment of acute

and posttraumatic stress in trauma patients: A systematic review. Journal of Trauma and Acute Care Surgery. 2017 Jun;**82**(6):1158-1183

[57] Puntillo KA, Naidu R. Chronic pain disorders after critical illness and ICU-acquired opioid dependence: Two clinical conundra. Current Opinion in Critical Care. 2016;**22**(5):506-512

[58] Cohen SP, Christo PJ, Moroz L. Pain management in trauma patients. American Journal of Physical Medicine & Rehabilitation. 2004;**83**(2):142-161

[59] Pandya U, O'Mara MS, Wilson W, Opalek J, Lieber M. Impact of preexisting opioid use on injury mechanism, type, and outcome. The Journal of Surgical Research. 2015 Sep;**198**(1):7-12

[60] Seekamp A, Jochum M, Ziegler M, van Griensven M, Martin M, Regel G. Cytokines and adhesion molecules in elective and accidental trauma- related ischemia/reperfusion. The Journal of Trauma. 1998;**44**(5):874-882

[61] Johnson KB, Egan TD, Kern SE, McJames SW, Cluff ML, Pace NL. Influence of hemorrhagic shock followed by crystalloid resuscitation on propofol: A pharmacokinetic and pharmacodynamic analysis. Anesthesiology. 2004;**101**(3):647-659

[62] Yang Y, Young JB, Schermer CR, Utter GH. Use of ketorolac is associated with decreased pneumonia following rib fractures. American Journal of Surgery. 2014;**207**(4):566-572

[63] Bayouth L, Safcsak K, Cheatham ML, Smith CP, Birrer KL, Promes JT. Early intravenous ibuprofen decreases narcotic requirement and length of stay after traumatic rib fracture. The American Surgeon. 2013;**79**(11):1207-1212

[64] Borgeat A, Ofner C, Saporito A, Farshad M, Aguirre J. The effect of nonsteroidal anti- inflammatory drugs on bone healing in humans: A qualitative, systematic review. Journal of Clinical Anesthesia. 2018;**49**:92-100

[65] Dodwell ER, Latorre JG, Parisini E, Zwettler E, Chandra D, Mulpuri K, et al. NSAID exposure and risk of nonunion: A meta-analysis of case-control and cohort studies. Calcified Tissue International. 2010;**87**:193-202

[66] Kurmis AP, Kurmis TP, O'Brien JX, Dalen T. The effect of nonsteroidal anti-inflammatory drug administration on acute phase fracture-healing: A review. The Journal of Bone and Joint Surgery. American Volume. 2012;**94**:815-823

[67] Hsu JR, Mir H, Wally MK, Seymour RB. Orthopaedic trauma association musculoskeletal pain task force. Clinical practice guidelines for pain Management in Acute Musculoskeletal Injury. Journal of Orthopaedic Trauma. 2019;**33**(5):e158-e182

[68] Tremont-Lukats IW, Megeff C, Backonja MM. Anticonvulsants for neuropathic pain syndromes: Mechanisms of action and place in therapy. Drugs. 2000;**60**:1029-1052

[69] Bone M, Critchley P, Buggy DJ. Gabapentin in postamputation phantom limb pain: A randomized, double-blind, placebo-controlled, cross-over study. Regional Anesthesia and Pain Medicine. 2002;**27**(5):481-486

[70] Sihoe AD, Lee TW, Wan IY, Thung KH, Yim AP. The use of gabapentin for post-operative and post-traumatic pain in thoracic surgery patients. European Journal of Cardio-Thoracic Surgery. 2006;**29**(5):795-799

[71] Karlow N, Schlaepfer CH, Stoll CR, Doering M, Carpenter CR, Colditz GA,

et al. A systematic review and meta-analysis of ketamine as an alternative to opioids for acute pain in the emergency department. Academic Emergency Medicine. 2018;**25**(10):1086-1097

[72] Bowers KJ, McAllister KB, Ray M, Heitz C. Ketamine as an adjunct to opioids for acute pain management in the emergency department: A randomized controlled trial. Academic Emergency Medicine. 2017;**6**:676-685

[73] Motov S, Rosenbaum S, Vilke GM, Nakajima Y. Is there a role for intravenous subdissociative-dose ketamine administered as an adjunct to opioids or as a single agent for acute pain management in the emergency department? The Journal of Emergency Medicine. 2016;**51**(6):752-757

[74] Jouguelet-Lacoste J, La Colla L, Schilling D, Chelly JE. The use of intravenous infusion or single dose of low-dose ketamine for postoperative analgesia: A review of the current literature. Pain Medicine. 2015;**16**(2):383-403

[75] Chang LC, Raty SR, Ortiz J, Bailard NS, Mathew SJ. The emerging use of ketamine for anesthesia and sedation in traumatic brain injuries. CNS Neuroscience & Therapeutics. 2013;**19**(6):390-395

[76] Jessen Lundorf L, Korvenius Nedergaard H, Møller AM. Perioperative dexmedetomidine for acute pain after abdominal surgery in adults. Cochrane Database of Systematic Reviews. 2016;**18**(2):CD010358

[77] Karamchandani K, Klick JC, Linskey Dougherty M, Bonavia A, Allen SR, Carr ZJ. Pain management in trauma patients affected by the opioid epidemic: A narrative review. Journal of Trauma and Acute Care Surgery. 2019;**87**(2):430-439

[78] Weibel S, Jelting Y, Pace NL, Helf A, Eberhart LH, Hahnenkamp K, et al. Continuous intravenous perioperative lidocaine infusion for postoperative pain and recovery in adults. Cochrane Database of Systematic Reviews. 2018;**6**:CD009642

[79] Richman JM, Liu SS, Courpas G, Wong R, Rowlingson AJ, McGready J, et al. Does continuous peripheral nerve block provide superior pain control to opioids? A meta-analysis. Anesthesia & Analgesia. 2006;**102**(1):248-257

[80] Chelly JE, Ghisi D, Fanelli A. Continuous peripheral nerve blocks in acute pain management. British Journal of Anaesthesia. 2010;**105**(Suppl 1):i86-i96

[81] Nishimori M, Low JH, Zheng H, Ballantyne JC. Epidural pain relief versus systemic opioid-based pain relief for abdominal aortic surgery. Cochrane Database of Systematic Reviews. 2012;7:CD005059

[82] Mouzopoulos G, Vasiliadis G, Lasanianos N, Nikolaras G, Morakis E, Kaminaris M. Fascia iliaca block prophylaxis for hip fracture patients at risk for delirium: A randomized placebo-controlled study. Journal of Orthopaedics and Traumatology. 2009;**10**:127-133

[83] Sheinfeld Gorin S, Krebs P, Badr H, Janke EA, Jim HS, Spring B, et al. Meta-analysis of psychosocial interventions to reduce pain in patients with cancer. Journal of Clinical Oncology. 2012;**30**:539-547

[84] SalzT,LaveryJA,Lipitz-SnydermanAN, Boudreau DM, Moryl N, Gillespie EF, et al. Trends in opioid use among older survivors of colorectal, lung, and breast cancers. Journal of Clinical Oncology. 2019;**37**:1001-1011

[85] World Health Organization. Cancer Pain Relief: With a Guide to Opioid Availability. 2nd ed. Geneva, Switzerland: World Health Organization; 1996

[86] Di Napoli R, Esposito G, Cascella M. Intrathecal catheter. In: StatPearls. Treasure Island (FL): StatPearls Publishing; 2022

[87] Cascella M, Muzio MR, Viscardi D, Cuomo A. Features and role of minimally invasive palliative procedures for pain Management in Malignant Pelvic Diseases: A review. The American Journal of Hospice & Palliative Care. 2017;**34**(6):524-531

[88] Kanpolat Y. Percutaneous destructive pain procedures on the upper spinal cord and brain stem in cancer pain: CT-guided techniques, indications and results. Advances and Technical Standards in Neurosurgery. 2007;**32**:147-173

[89] Cahana A, Mavrocordatos P, Geurts JW, Groen GJ. Do minimally invasive procedures have a place in the treatment of chronic low back pain? Expert Review of Neurotherapeutics. 2004;**4**(3):479-490

[90] Zhang H. Cancer pain management-new therapies. Current Oncology Reports. 2022;**24**(2):223-226

[91] Deng G. Integrative medicine therapies for pain Management in Cancer Patients. Cancer Journal. 2019;**25**(5):343-348

Chapter 5

Effectiveness of Ultrasound-Guided Serial Injection Triple Nerve Block before and after Cementless Bipolar Hemiarthroplasty in Femoral Neck Fracture

Dong Ha Lee and Jung Wook Huh

Abstract

Bipolar hemiarthroplasty (BHA) is a common treatment for femoral neck fractures, but post-surgery pain can delay recovery. This study retrospectively analyzed 87 BHA patients from 2016–2020, categorizing them into two groups: Group I (n = 42) received serial injection nerve blocks (SINB) before and after surgery, while Group II (n = 41) did not. Pain was measured using a visual analog scale at multiple time points post-surgery. The groups were also compared for hospital stay length and perioperative complications. Results indicated that Group I patients, who received SINB, had significantly lower pain scores at most time intervals post-surgery and exhibited fewer instances of postoperative nausea, vomiting, and delirium. Using ultrasound-guided SINB not only provided superior pain relief but also minimized the need for narcotics and their side effects, like nausea and delirium.

Keywords: femur neck fracture, bipolar hemiarthroplasty, ultrasonography, peripheral, nerve block

1. Introduction

Bipolar hemiarthroplasty (BHA) is a common surgical intervention used to manage the acute pain associated with femoral neck fractures. While effective, BHA is linked to significant postoperative pain that, if not well-managed, can hinder recovery, lengthen hospitalization, and increase the risk of negative outcomes such as myocardial ischemia, pulmonary dysfunction, and thromboembolism. Therefore, optimal pain management after BHA should prioritize providing potent pain relief while minimizing opioid consumption and supporting recovery. Similarly, total knee arthroplasty (TKA) can also result in significant postoperative pain, and various pain management strategies are available, such as systemic or intrathecal opioids, local infiltration analgesia, and peripheral nerve blocks (PNBs). However, the ideal pain management approach should offer robust analgesia without any unwanted consequences to minimize adverse effects [1–3].

The hip joint receives innervation from multiple nerves. Specifically, the obturator nerve and articular branches of the femoral nerve innervate the anteromedial section of the hip joint, while the lateral femoral cutaneous nerve (LFCN) innervates the anterolateral section [4]. It has been observed that patients undergoing a direct lateral approach for femur neck fracture at our institution often report postoperative pain in both the anteromedial and anterolateral regions of the hip joint [5], which can be attributed to the involvement of these nerves.

Inserting a catheter that can cover all three nerves is a challenging procedure, mainly due to the complexity of the process and the location of the nerves. The femoral nerve seems to be the most feasible option, but the success of the blocks using this technique is unpredictable [4]. Using ultrasound guidance can make the procedure easier, but the results may still be unreliable. The procedure is technically difficult, even for experienced practitioners, as the space lies beyond penetrating a needle through two fascial layers [6].

Capdevila et al. recommend using continuous psoas compartment block for total hip arthroplasty, utilizing modified Winnie's landmark [7] to determine the distance between the lumbar plexus and L4 transverse process accurately [8]. They have found that the fascia iliaca compartment block is more effective than the 3-in-1 block. However, it is worth noting that both techniques provide sensory blockade in only 35% of cases [9]. Therefore, we opted to perform a single injection of each of the three nerves before the BHA procedure, rather than dwelling a catheter on one nerve that innervates the hip joint.

Ensuring that the effects of peripheral nerve blocks are sustained is crucial to reducing opioid use among inpatients, as even small doses (20 to 50 MME/day) may increase the risk of clinical complications and long-term opioid dependence [10–12]. However, the duration of a single injection nerve block is limited to a maximum of 12 hours [13]. To extend the effects beyond 12 hours, we developed a method of serial injection.

An experienced orthopedic surgeon performed an ultrasound-guided block of the lateral femoral cutaneous nerve, obturator nerve, and femoral nerve. The procedure took less than 10 minutes for each nerve block, and it did not significantly add to the perioperative time. Furthermore, there were no local complications, such as infection or hematoma, at the injection site.

In addition to the potential temporary weakness in the quadriceps muscle, a known side effect of femoral nerve blocks [11–13], we made a concerted effort to preserve ankle dorsiflexion and plantarflexion to mitigate the risk of deep vein thrombosis (DVT) during our study.

The purpose of this investigation is to evaluate the clinical benefits of ultrasound-guided serial injection nerve blocks (SINB) targeting the femoral, obturator, and lateral femoral cutaneous nerves in patients undergoing BHA. As these peripheral nerves innervate the proximal femur and hip joint, the study aims to assess the effectiveness of SINB in achieving optimal pain relief while minimizing opioid consumption during the first 48 hours postoperatively. Furthermore, we aim to investigate the extent to which SINB decreases the incidence of postoperative nausea and vomiting (PONV) and delirium, thereby promoting enhanced rehabilitation.

2. Materials and methods

2.1 Trial design and study settings

A direct lateral approach under spinal anesthesia was utilized by a single orthopedic surgeon to perform all BHA procedures in our study. Our study population consisted of 83 patients who underwent BHA between September 2016 and September 2020, all of whom were operated on by the same surgeon. These patients were divided into two groups - those who received SINB and those who did not. The SINB procedure was performed for all patients after January 2018, spanning a period of 2 years and 7 months.

During the BHA procedure, all patients received a standard dose of 0.2 ml/kg of bupivacaine (Heavy MarcaineTM, AstraZeneca, England) intrathecally under spinal anesthesia.

2.2 Participants

In our study, we conducted a retrospective review of the medical records of 87 patients who had undergone BHA for fragility femoral neck fracture at Busan Medical Center between September 2016 and September 2020. The study was approved by the Public Institutional Bioethics Committee designated by the MOHW, and the Institutional Review Board granted approval under the number P01–202011–21-027.

To ensure the validity of our results, patients were excluded from the study if they met certain criteria, including pre-existing immobility prior to the injury, malunion or nonunion resulting from delayed initial treatment, diagnosis of severe dementia or other psychiatric conditions, or signs of delirium within 24 hours of surgery (Delirium Rating Scale >10). In total, four patients were excluded from the study, as shown in **Figure 1**.

2.3 Interventions

Group 1 comprised of the intervention group receiving the saphenous, femoral, and lateral femoral cutaneous nerve blocks (SINB), while Group II was designated as the control group and did not receive any blocks. All SINBs were performed by a single experienced orthopedic surgeon immediately prior to surgery and repeated thrice postoperatively at 12-hour intervals. A 5-cm long, 5–12 MHz linear probe (LOGIQ e, GE, Boston, USA) and 22G spinal needle were used for the nerve blocks under ultrasound guidance. The femoral, obturator, and lateral femoral cutaneous nerves were each blocked with 7.5, 4, and 4 ml respectively of 0.75% ropivacaine mixed with 7.5, 4, and 4 ml of 1% lidocaine at a 1:1 ratio, which is similar to the method used in a previous study. A sensory test including a pin prick test was performed to confirm the efficacy of the blocks. Premedication included 200 mg of Celebrex (celecoxib; Pfizer, NY, USA) and no additional local anesthetics or analgesics were given during surgery.

Postoperative pain management included patient-controlled intravenous analgesia, consisting of a mixture of 2 mg butorphanol tartrate (Myungmoon Pharm., Seoul, Korea), 50 mg tramadol hydrochloride (Yuhan Corp., Seoul, Korea), and 30 mg ketorolac tromethamine (Hanmi Pharm., Seoul, Korea) mixed in 100 mL of saline, with a background infusion rate of 0.05 ml/hr., bolus of 0.2 ml, and lockout of 8 minutes. This regimen was calculated as 19 MME (morphine milligram equivalent), and the number of doses administered was recorded by checking the volume

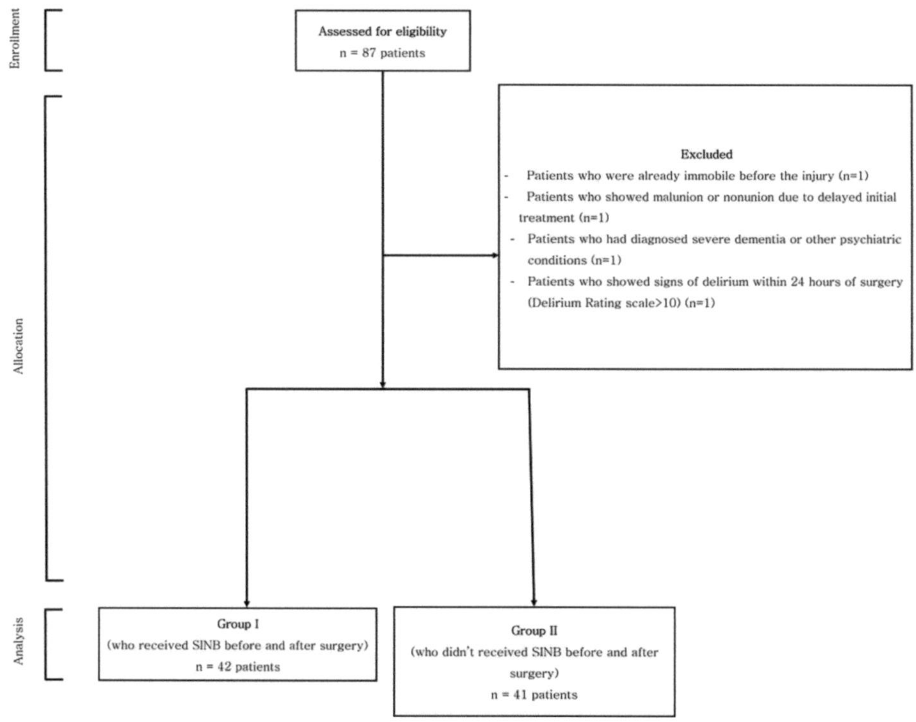

Figure 1.
Flow chart of patient's registration.

remaining on the 3rd postoperative day. Rescue analgesics (50 mg of Tramadol or 90 mg of Diclofenac) were administered to patients as required for postoperative pain control, and anti-emetic injection was only given to those who exhibited symptoms of nausea and vomiting.

Patients were instructed on straight leg raising exercises, knee flexion/extension, and ankle dorsiflexion/plantarflexion exercises prior to surgery and encouraged to continue these exercises postoperatively to facilitate rehabilitation. Additionally, patients were educated on postural changes and were provided with medical compression stockings throughout their hospital stay to help prevent postoperative complications.

2.4 Outcome assessments

The post-operative pain intensity was assessed using the visual analogue scale (VAS) at 6, 12, 24, 48, and 72 hours after the surgery. The medical staff provided a detailed explanation of the meaning of VAS before the initial measurement. The number of doses administered through patient-controlled analgesia (PCA) was recorded for the first 72 hours, along with the amount of rescue analgesics. Additionally, the number of cases of nausea and vomiting was recorded from the electronic medical record. Koval classification grade (ambulatory ability I-VII), T-cane walking (days until the patient was able to walk with the aid of a T-cane after the operation), local complications due to SINB, general postoperative complications (pressure sore, pneumonia, deep vein thrombosis, postoperative nausea and vomiting, delirium), and duration of hospitalization were also compared.

2.5 Statistical methods

The statistical analysis was carried out using the SPSS version 22.0 software (IBM Corporation, Armonk, NY). Patient characteristics were evaluated using frequency analysis and cross analysis. The t-test was used to determine any differences in clinical outcomes and patient demographics between the two groups. Power analysis was conducted, which revealed an effect size of 0.5, statistical significance level of 0.05, and statistical power of 0.90 for both groups.

3. Results

The two groups did not differ significantly in terms of age (Group I: 57–88, Group II: 59–86), gender, sex, BMI (kg/m^2), Charlson Comorbidity Index (CCI), VAS measured in the ward on the day of admission, koval classification grade, blood loss, or urine output. However, the operative time was longer in Group II by an average of 8.58 minutes (**Table 1**). Group I had significantly lower subjective pain scores compared to Group II at 6, 12, 24, and 48 hours after BHA ($p < 0.05$). However, there were no significant differences in post-operative VAS scores at 72 hours (**Table 2**).

	I‡(n = 42)	**II§(n = 41)**	**p-value**
Mean Age (years)	76.24	77.49	0.236
Gender			
Male	17	14	0.846
Female	25	25	
Mean BMI* (kg/m^2)	22.08	22.05	0.484
Mean CCI†	12.45	13.36	0.26
Mean VAS measured in ward on the day of admission	6.76 (1.84)	6.87 (1.75)	0.36
Koval classification (Grade)			
I	27	29	0.262
II	6	3	
III	2	0	
IV	3	6	
V	1	0	
VI	1	2	
VII	2	1	
Mean Operation time (min)	131.57	140.15	0.005*
Mean Blood loss (ml)	343	279	0.065
Mean Urine output (ml)	360.02	279.67	0.051

**BMI: Body mass index.*
†CCI: Charlson Comorbidity Index.
‡I: 3 Nerves block by continuous injection group.
§II: Control group (No injection).
**Significant difference between Group I and Group II.*

Table 1.
Patient demographics.

In terms of pain management, Group I used a smaller volume of PCA solution (65.72 mL) in the first 72 hours after surgery compared to Group II (83.90 mL). The number of injections administered by PCA was also significantly lower in Group I, with an average of 0.65 injections for Group I patients and 0.88 injections for Group II patients (**Table 3**).

	I‡(n = 42)	**II§(n = 41)**	**p-value**
6 hours	1.71 (0.21)	7.38 (2.30)	0.000*
12 hours	3.81 (0.30)	6.49 (1.57)	0.000*
24 hours	1.93 (0.17)	6.41 (1.20)	0.000*
48 hours	3.45 (1.28)	5.82 (1.62)	0.000*
72 hours	4.52 (0.45)	4.62 (0.51)	0.28

**VAS: Visual analog scale at.*
†Hours Post-op: Hours of the post-operative.
‡I: 3 Nerves block by serial injection group.
§II: Control group (No injection).
**Significant difference between Group I and Group II.*

Table 2.
VAS for post-operative (mean, standard deviation).*

	I†(n = 42)	**II‡(n = 41)**	**p-value**
PCA* consumption (ml)	65.72 (8.78)	83.90 (18.39)	0.000*
Additional analgesic injection(number of injection)	0.65	0.88	0.029*

**PCA: patient controlled analgesia.*
†I: 3 Nerves block by serial injection group.
‡II: Control group (No injection).
**Significant difference between Group I and Group II.*

Table 3.
PCA consumption for post-operative 72 hours (mean, standard deviation).*

	I*(n = 42)	**II†(n = 41)**	**p-value**
General Complications			0.571
Pressure sore	1	2	
Pneumonia	2	3	0.875
DVT‡	0	0	-
Postoperative nausea and vomiting	0	6	0.013*
Delirium	3	10	0.032*
Local Complications	0	—	—
Length of stay (day) (mean)	39.26	44.54	0.073
T-cane walking (day) (mean)	11.52	11.97	0.40

**I: 3 Nerves block by serial injection group.*
†II Control group (No injection).
‡DVT: Deep vein thrombosis.
#HHS: Harris Hip Score.
**Significant difference between Group I and Group II.*

Table 4.
Complications & Length of stay & ambulation function.

The incidence of pressure sores, pneumonia, and deep vein thrombosis did not differ significantly between the groups. However, the incidence of postoperative nausea and vomiting (PONV) (0.00%) and delirium (0.07%) in Group I was lower than that in Group II (0.15 and 0.24%, respectively). There were no reports of any local complications due to SINB or any reports of block failure. The length of hospital stay and T-cane walking start day after the operation did not differ significantly between the groups (**Table 4**).

4. Discussion

The limitation of single injection nerve block is that it can manage only post-operative pain after BHA up to 12 hours. Serial injection nerve blocks effectively extended the duration of analgesic effects necessary for postoperative pain management. In this study, SINB can achieve adequate pain control not only for 12 hours after surgery but also up to 48 hours after surgery. Besides pain control, general complications such as the incidence of PONV and delirium were remarkably reduced due to SINB effect. These results are quite different from other studies which demonstrated no significant difference in delirium rate in CFNC (Continuous Femoral Nerve Catheter) treatment [12]. Considering the etiology of delirium is complex and multifactorial, it is remarkable that controlling pain adequately can be a powerful management of delirium.

Performing triple nerve blocks every 12 hours for 2 days can be a labor-intensive process. To address this issue, we implemented a manual approach for serial triple nerve blocks. Prior to the BHA surgery, triple nerve blocks were performed with ultrasound guidance just before spinal anesthesia in the operating room. Following the surgery, we conducted rounds approximately 12 hours later (following the first triple nerve blocks) and performed the triple nerve block at the patient's bedside with the assistance of the ward nurse. On postoperative day 1, we conducted wound dressing and repeated the triple nerve blocks at the bedside. Finally, the last set of triple nerve blocks were performed during the afternoon rounds, following the same protocol as before.

Several advantages of favoring longer-acting regional block techniques were reported besides our study. Based on work by Farrar et al. with the utilization of continuous femoral nerve catheter, 60% pain score was reduced preoperatively, as well as 50 and 54% lower pain scores on postoperative day 1 and 2, respectively [14].

Our study confirms the results of previous studies that serial femoral nerve blocks not only decrease average patient-reported pain scores, morphine consumption in the pre- and postoperative period, but also lower the rate of opioid-related side effects [12]. This is consistent with findings that controlling pain and reducing opioid requirement is associated with reductions in PONV and delirium and adds to the body of evidence that regional techniques can decrease post-operative complications.

Moreover, also found by the chart notes, patients were able to perform postoperative breathing and rehabilitation exercises [12, 13]. However, unlike previous studies we could not find that more patients were discharged with or without home health services [12].

The present study aimed to assess the efficacy of single-injection nerve block (SINB) for managing pain during BHA surgery. Although the study showed that SINB provided effective pain relief, it had certain limitations that require further exploration.

One such limitation was the retrospective nature of the study, indicating the need for a randomized, double-blind trial to validate the results. Additionally, the potential influence of antiemetic medication on postoperative pain and narcotic-related side effects was not considered.

The cost of multiple injections required for SINB was another limiting factor, particularly in patients with low income. Additionally, the procedure duration and the risk of local complications such as infection and hematoma were potential concerns.

The study found that temporary weakness in the quadriceps muscles [11–13] caused by femoral nerve block did not hinder patients undergoing BHA surgery, as they were advised to stay in bed for 72 hours and partial weight-bearing was recommended [15–18] for several weeks after the surgery. Ankle dorsiflexion and plantarflexion exercises were also utilized to prevent deep vein thrombosis.

Although there was no statistically significant difference in hospitalization duration between the two groups, a trend towards shorter hospitalization was observed in the SINB group. Future studies could investigate pain control using continuous femoral nerve catheter dwelling or explore the impact of T-cane walking initialization day on early mobilization between the two groups.

5. Conclusion

Administration of sequential lower limb nerve blocks with the guidance of ultrasound not only yields superior pain relief during the early post-operative phase following BHA, but also has the potential to maintain pain relief, resulting in reduced consumption of narcotics and mitigating associated adverse effects, such as post-operative nausea and vomiting (PONV) and delirium.

Funding

No Funding has been received.

Competing interests

All the other authors declare no conflict of interest.

Consent for publication

Not applicable.

Declarations

Ethics approval and consent to participate

1. Ethics approval was obtained from the Institutional Review Board "Public Institutional Review Board Designated by Ministry of Health and Welfare" (Approval # P01–202201–01-026). The study was carried in accordance with relevant guidelines and regulations, such as Declaration of Helsinki.

2. Not applicable.

   The need for Informed Consent was waived by the Public Institutional Review Board Designated by Ministry of Health and Welfare. All methods were performed in accordance with the relevant guidelines and regulations.

Availability of data and materials

Data availability

The datasets generated during and/or analyzed during the current study are not publicly available due to the IRB ("Public Institutional Review Board Designated by Ministry of Health and Welfare") guideline, it is stipulated that the patient's personal data should be discarded within 6 months after data collection.

Author details

Dong Ha Lee* and Jung Wook Huh
Department of Orthopaedic Surgery, Busan Medical Center, Busan, South Korea

*Address all correspondence to: dlee6808@gmail.com

References

[1] Terkawi AS, Mavridis D, Sessler DI, et al. Pain management modalities after total knee arthroplasty: A network meta-analysis of 170 randomized controlled trials. Anesthesiology. 2017;**126**(5):923-937

[2] Al-Zahrani T, Doais KS, Aljassir F, Alshaygy I, Albishi W, Terkawi AS. Randomized clinical trial of continuous femoral nerve block combined with sciatic nerve block versus epidural analgesia for unilateral total knee arthroplasty. The Journal of Arthroplasty. 2015;**30**(1):149-154

[3] Bendtsen TF, Moriggl B, Chan V, Børglum J. The optimal analgesic block for total knee arthroplasty. Regional Anesthesia & Pain Medicine. 2016;**41**(6):711-719

[4] Birnbaum K, Prescher A, Hessler S, Heller K-D. The sensory innervation of the hip joint-an anatomical study. Surgical and Radiologic Anatomy. 1997;**19**(6):371-375

[5] Spina M, Luppi V, Chiappi J, Bagnis F, Balsano M. Direct anterior approach versus direct lateral approach in total hip arthroplasty and bipolar hemiarthroplasty for femoral neck fractures: A retrospective comparative study. Aging Clinical and Experimental Research. 2020;**33**:1-10

[6] Winnie A, Ramamurthy S, Durrani Z. The inguinal paravascular technic of lumbar plexus anesthesia: The "3-in-1 block". Anesthesia & Analgesia. 1973;**52**(6):989-996

[7] Dupré L. Three-in-one block or femoral nerve block. What should be done and how? Annales Françaises d'Anesthèsie et de Rèanimation. 1996;**15**:1099-1101

[8] Capdevila X, Macaire P, Dadure C, et al. Continuous psoas compartment block for postoperative analgesia after total hip arthroplasty: New landmarks, technical guidelines, and clinical evaluation. Anesthesia & Analgesia. 2002;**94**(6):1606-1613

[9] Capdevila X, Biboulet P, Bouregba M, Barthelet Y, Rubenovitch J, d'Athis F. Comparison of the three-in-one and fascia iliaca compartment blocks in adults: Clinical and radiographic analysis. Anesthesia & Analgesia. 1998;**86**(5):1039-1044

[10] Garlich JM, Pujari A, Debbi EM, et al. Time to block: Early regional anesthesia improves pain control in geriatric hip fractures. JBJS. 2020;**102**(10):866-872

[11] Nie H, Yang Y-X, Wang Y, Liu Y, Zhao B, Luan B. Effects of continuous fascia iliaca compartment blocks for postoperative analgesia in patients with hip fracture. Pain Research and Management. 2015;**20**(4):210-212

[12] Arsoy D, Gardner MJ, Amanatullah DF, et al. Continuous femoral nerve catheters decrease opioid-related side effects and increase home disposition rates among geriatric hip fracture patients. Journal of Orthopaedic Trauma. 2017;**31**(6):e186-e189

[13] Huh J-W, Park M-J, Lee W-M, Lee D-H. Effectiveness of ultrasound-guided single-injection triple nerve block before Cementless bipolar hip Hemiarthroplasty in femoral neck fractures. Hip & Pelvis. 2020;**32**(3):142

[14] Farrar JT. What is clinically meaningful: Outcome measures in pain clinical trials. The Clinical Journal of Pain. 2000;**16**(2 Suppl):S106-S112

[15] Aldinger PR, Thomsen M, Mau H, Ewerbeck V, Breusch SJ. Cementless Spotorno tapered titanium stems: Excellent 10-15-year survival in 141 young patients. Acta Orthopaedica Scandinavica. 2003;**74**(3):253-258

[16] Jacobsen S, Jensen FK, Poulsen K, Stürup J, Retpen J. Good performance of a titanium femoral component in cementless hip arthroplasty in younger patients 97 arthroplasties followed for 5-11 years. Acta Orthopaedica Scandinavica. 2003;**74**(4):380-388

[17] Kim Y-H, Kim J-S, Cho S-H. Primary total hip arthroplasty with a cementless porous-coated anatomic total hip prosthesis: 10-to 12-year results of prospective and consecutive series. The Journal of Arthroplasty. 1999;**14**(5):538-548

[18] Mont MA, Yoon T-R, Krackow KA, Hungerford DS. Clinical experience with a proximally porous-coated second-generation cementless total hip prosthesis: Minimum 5-year follow-up. The Journal of Arthroplasty. 1999;**14**(8):930-939

Chapter 6

Intravenous Lidocaine in Non-Opioid Multimodal Perioperative Pain Management: Current Controversy and Future Perspectives

Dimitar Tonev

Abstract

In the perioperative setting, intravenous lidocaine moderately reduces postoperative pain, opioid consumption and inflammatory response. Under laboratory conditions, lidocaine has been shown to inhibit cancer cell behaviour and exerts beneficial effects on components of the inflammatory and immune responses that are known to affect cancer biology. New evidence suggests that it might minimize the impact of surgery on NK cells and could augment NK cell cytotoxicity and improve survival in patients after pancreatic oncosurgery. Given the narrow therapeutic index, potential toxicity and inconclusive evidence about its Enhanced Recovery After Surgery benefits, however, currently intravenous lidocaine is not routinely use for perioperative pain control. It should be administered after considering with the patient of its clear benefits over risks, in a dose of 1-2 mg/kg/h, not more than 24 hours and under a high dependency unit monitoring. Patients groups where the risk-benefit balance is tilted towards benefit include patients who are already on high doses of opioids, intolerant of opioids, and those who are at high risk of chronic postoperative pain. The upcoming role for intravenous lidocaine in oncosurgery might shift its place from a second line non-opioid adjuvant to a first line option in the context of improving oncological outcomes.

Keywords: lidocaine, perioperative pain management, ERAS, oncosurgery, outcomes

1. Introduction

Lidocaine (Xylocaine®) was first synthesized in 1942, approved for use in human medicine and launched in 1948 in Sweden [1], patented in USA in 1948, and launched in 1949 after Food and Drug Administration approval [2]. Since 1958, intravenous (i.v.) lidocaine infusions have been used for postoperative analgesia as well [3]. The i.v. lidocaine is administered as an adjuvant in multimodal perioperative pain management for its analgesic, anti-inflammatory, and anti-hyperalgesic properties [4] in many clinical settings. They include the operating theater, recovery room, high dependency unit (HDU), intensive care unit (ICU), and surgical ward [5]. Currently, the Enhanced Recovery After Surgery (ERAS) society guidelines recommend lidocaine as a continuous intravenous infusion in some ERAS protocols (colorectal surgery, hysterectomy, and pancreaticoduodenectomy) when epidural regional analgesia is not feasible or opioids may be contraindicated [6]. Under laboratory conditions, lidocaine has been shown to inhibit cancer cell behavior and exerts beneficial effects on components of the inflammatory and immune responses which are known to affect cancer biology [7]. The promising immune-modulatory and antinociceptive properties of i.v. lidocaine expand its role beyond the immediate perioperative period targeting the prevention of chronic postsurgical pain (CPSP) and the improvement of oncological outcomes as well.

In this chapter, the mechanism of action of i.v. lidocaine, its pharmacokinetics, pharmacological and clinical considerations of perioperative i.v. lidocaine infusions in terms of their current controversy and future perspectives in the field of acute and chronic non-opioid multimodal pain management and beyond will be presented.

2. Mechanism of action

2.1 Sodium channels

The primary mechanism of action of i.v. lidocaine is through blockade of voltage-gated sodium channels (VGSCs) leading to reversible block of action potential propagation. After a rapid state of depolarization activated VGSCs pass to a nonconductive state of inactivation, when VGSCs are closed and not capable of opening during a certain period, followed by resting state when VGSCs are still closed but capable of opening. Repetitive pulses from afferent fibers with a high-frequency abnormal firings produce an additional VGSC block, the so-called use-dependent block/frequency-dependent block, when the availability of VGSC to reopen decline [8, 9]. These different states of VGSC (open, resting, and inactivated) have different binding affinity for local anesthetics, and the affinity of the inactivated state is the highest [10]. Thus, i.v. lidocaine preferentially binds to the inactivated state, thereby enhancing use-dependent block and suppressing the high-frequency abnormal firings in injured dorsal root ganglion (DRG) or peripheral nerves [11]. The higher the frequency, the more intense the block is. The i.v. lidocaine blocks the sodium currents during the resting state of VGSC, the so-called tonic block, as well [12].

Ectopic firing could be suppressed by a systemic i.v. dose of lidocaine far below that required to inhibit nerve impulse propagation along an uninjured nerve [13]. To date, nine isoforms of VGSCs (Nav1.1-Nav1.9) have been identified. The Nav1.8 channel is approximately five times more sensitive to lidocaine than other VGSC isoforms [14]. In addition, in isolated Nav1.8, the half-maximal inhibitory concentration (IC_{50}) for low-frequency block is 319 μM, whereas its IC_{50} for high-frequency block is 50 μM. This may explain why i.v. lidocaine blocks ectopic activity in injured nerves, while normal nociception remains unchanged at the same IC_{50} values [15]. Thus, in vivo, systemic lidocaine suppressed the noxious stimulus evoked discharges in dorsal horn-wide dynamic range neurons, while spontaneous action potentials and activity induced by non-noxious stimuli remained unchanged [16]. The experimental evidence to date supports the hypothesis that i.v. lidocaine suppresses the ectopic firing in injured peripheral nerves, DRG, and dorsal-horn cells. These findings, however, could only partially explain the possible mechanisms of i.v. lidocaine inhibitory effect on spontaneous chronic pain in clinical settings. The clinical effects of i.v. lidocaine in chronic pain patients outlast its plasma concentrations [17] which points to a supra-spinal mechanism as well (such as a specific site of action in the thalamic region of the brain [18]), involving targets other than VGSC.

2.2 Calcium channels

The voltage-gated calcium channels (VGCCs) are involved in numerous physiological processes, including neurotransmitter release [19]. Their modulation is a potential target in chronic pain control [20]. Experimental data reveal that lidocaine inhibits VGCC in a dose- and voltage-dependent manner [21]. However, much higher doses (approximately 100-fold higher) of lidocaine are needed in order to inhibit VGCC compared to VGSC [22]. Thus, its degree of VGCC blockade is limited [23].

2.3 Potassium channels

The potassium channels are important regulators of membrane resting potential, firing action potentials, and repolarization in neurotransmission [24]. Certain types of potassium channels are involved in pain modulation and inflammation, such as voltage-gated potassium channels (VGPCs), voltage-independent potassium channels, tandem pore domain potassium channels (2P K^+ channels), and ATP-sensitive potassium channels. Although the affinity of i.v. lidocaine for VGPCs is sixfold lower compared to VGSC, the inhibition of outward potassium currents causes partial membrane depolarization and leads to an increased amount of sodium channels which in turns are more sensitive to lidocaine. Thus, inhibition of outward potassium currents promotes sodium channel inactivation. Lidocaine inhibited tandem pore potassium channels at IC_{50} of 1 mM and voltage-independent potassium channels at IC_{50} of 219 μM [9]. Lidocaine modulates mitochondrial adenosine triphosphate (ATP)-sensitive potassium channels and thus reduces cytokine-induced cell injury. In an experimental model of incubated vascular smooth muscle and endothelial cells, the cell survival improved with increasing dosages of lidocaine [25].

2.4 Nonselective cation channels

The nonselective cation channels are members of the transient receptor potential (TRP) family of ion channels and play a distinct role in nociception and neurogenic inflammation [26–30]. The transient receptor potential vanilloid 1 (TRPV1) and ankyrin 1 (TRPA1) channels as typical members of TRP family are expressed on some sensory and dorsal root ganglia [31], are interrelated functionally each other [32], and are involved into the development and sustainability of chronic pain [33]. Lidocaine at concentrations 10–30 mM (> 100 higher than plasma concentrations of i.v. lidocaine) have a greater inhibitory effect on TRP channels in rodents than in humans and may have a desensitizing effect on TRP channels as well [34]. The desensitized TRP channels could explain i.v. lidocaine prolonged antinociceptive effects in human sural nerve injury, which ameliorate the neuropathic pain well beyond the end of the exposure to lidocaine [35].

2.5 G protein-coupled receptors

The G protein-coupled receptors (GPCRs) consist of a large family of membrane proteins, which are of great importance for intra- and intercellular communication pathways [36]. After injury, their expression on sensory neurons for signaling pain changes considerably [37]. The Gq protein α-subunit ($G_{\alpha q}$) plays a significant role in pain modulation and inflammation [38, 39] and is a potential target for lidocaine antinociceptive and anti-inflammatory modulatory effects. Lidocaine binds with the $G_{\alpha q}$ in certain GPCRs, such as m1 and m3 muscarinic receptors, lysophosphatic acid (LPA), platelet-activating factor (PAF), and thromboxane A2 (TXA2) receptors [9 = E J Pain 2016 – самата статия] and inhibits their receptor signaling in a reversible and time-dependent manner [40]. Prolonged exposure to lidocaine increased the inhibitory potency on m1 and m3 receptors in a biphasic time-dependent manner, with initial inhibition followed by enhanced signaling [41]. However, the observed $G_{\alpha q}$ inhibition in experimental settings was at lidocaine concentrations much lower than those observed clinically [23]. Lidocaine inhibits LPA and PAF-mediated priming of human polymorphonuclear neutrophils (hPMN) and thus hPMN-mediated tissue injury on the site of inflammation in clinically relevant concentrations [42, 43], whereas TXA2 inhibitory concentrations are relatively high (IC_{50} of 1.1 mM) [44].

2.6 N-methyl-D-aspartate receptors

The N-methyl-D-aspartate (NMDA) receptors are heavily involved in excitatory neurotransmission and modulation of nociceptive signaling in the dorsal horn, contributing to the development of hyperalgesia and allodynia and spinal central sensitization [45–47]. Lidocaine inhibits the activation of NMDA receptors in a dose-dependent manner via an intracellular biding site. Therefore, higher lidocaine doses are needed for NMDA receptors blockade (IC_{50} of 0.8–1.2 mM) [9].

2.7 Glycinergic system

Glycine has a dual role in central nervous system neurotransmission. Depending on its extracellular levels, it can be both an obligate inhibitor and an excitatory co-agonist of NMDA receptors. The glycine levels are regulated by glycine transporter 1 (GlyT1) and glycine transporter 2 (GlyT2). GlyT1 removes glycine from the synaptic cleft, whereas GlyT2 reuptakes glycine into nerve terminals by reloading it into synaptic vesicles [48]. During the high-frequency abnormal neuronal activity, glycine released from inhibitory inter-neurons escapes from the synaptic cleft, reaches nearby NMDA receptors, and stimulates them as an excitatory NMDA receptor co-agonist [49]. Lidocaine modulates the glycinergic system in a dose-dependent manner. Low-dose lidocaine (10 μM) enhances, whereas high-dose lidocaine (1 mM) inhibits glycinergic signaling [50]. In addition, lidocaine metabolites monoethylglycinexylidide (MEGX) and N-ethylglicine (NEG), but not lidocaine itself, inhibit the GlyT1 in vitro in clinically relevant concentrations (55 μM) [51]. The i.v. lidocaine metabolites are glycine transporter's substrates that compete with endogenous and synaptically released glycine for reuptake and by blocking the reuptake lead to increased extracellular and synaptic glycine levels. Thus by facilitating the inhibitory neurotransmission, the systemic lidocaine and its metabolites may produce antihyperalgesia [52].

2.8 Analgesic and antihyperalgesic properties

The analgesic and antihyperalgesic effect of i.v. lidocaine infusion is obtained through inhibition of the VGSCs, VGCCs, various potassium channels, NMDA receptors, glycinergic system, and G protein pathways [9], the mechanism of action of which has already been discussed in detail above.

2.9 Anti-inflammatory properties

The neurogenic inflammation is involved into the development and maintenance of chronic pain by means of activation of numerous non-neuronal cells such as monocytes, leukocytes, macrophages, lymphocytes, and peripheral or central glial cells which play a key role in the release of multiple inflammatory mediators (such as pro-inflammatory IL-1β, IL-6, IL-8, and TNF-α or anti-inflammatory IL-1Ra and IL-10, etc.) [23]. Lidocaine can inhibit leukocytes activation, adhesion, and migration, as well as human peripheral polymorphonuclear neutrophils priming (contact of B or T cells with and an antigen) and phagocytosis [42, 43, 53]. Furthermore, it can reduce the release of inflammatory mediators, such as IL-1β, IL-6, IL-8, TNF-α, the expression of intercellular molecule-1 (ICAM-1), the release of prostanoids, thromboxanes, leukotrienes, and histamine release by human leukocytes, mastocytes, and basophils [53, 54]. Animal studies reveal that the anti-inflammatory effects of lidocaine are mediated by VGSC, GCPRs, and ATP-sensitive potassium channels [47 = IntechOpen pediatric i.v. lidocaine - самата статия]. However, just a few human studies demonstrate the anti-inflammatory properties of lidocaine in reducing the surgery-induced release of pro-inflammatory cytokines IL-1, IL-6, IL-8, and TNF-α [55–58], or the TNF-α production in lipopolysaccharide-activated human leukocytes [59].

2.10 Anticancer properties

Laboratory research suggests that perioperative i.v. lidocaine inhibits cancer cell behavior and exerts beneficial effects on components of the inflammatory and immune responses which are known to affect cancer biology [7]. It could be done by using multiple biological pathways, not just by blocking the VGSCs [60]. Several potential mechanisms of its antineoplastic properties are suggested (**Figure 1**). Lidocaine could attack directly the cancer cells via many pathways, such as the inhibition of nuclear factor-KB (NF-KB), epidermal growth factor receptor (EGRF), or Src (oncoprotein tyrosine kinase)-dependent signaling pathway. In addition, i.v. lidocaine could modulate the immune cells by enhancing NK cells cytotoxicity or by preserving Th1 predominance (from shifting Th1/Th2 balance toward a decrease of Th2-dominance, which Th2-dominance protect tumor cells from immune attack). Moreover, it could interfere with tumor angiogenesis by inhibiting the hypoxia-inducible factor (HIF) and the vascular endothelial growth factor (VEGF) signaling pathways. And last but not least, i.v. lidocaine possesses anti-inflammatory properties which may modulate the pro-cancer effects of surgery-induced stress response by inhibiting the expression of pro-inflammatory cytokines (IL-1, IL-6, IL-8, IL-10, TNF-α, and IFN-gamma) [7, 61]. In addition, the lidocaine TRPV6 receptor inhibition [62], the lidocaine dose- and time-dependent demethylation of DNA in different cancer cells [63], and the lidocaine VGSCs inhibition in cancer cells [64] are all involved in reducing tumor cell invasion and migration. In vitro studies are helpful in establishing a multitude of potential underlying mechanisms of i.v. lidocaine

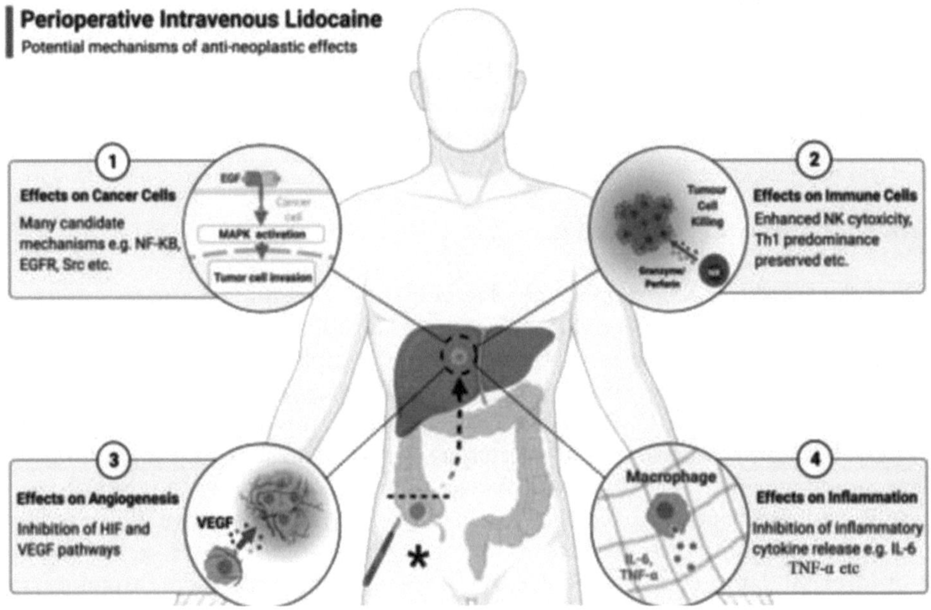

Figure 1.
Potential mechanisms of i.v. lidocaine antineoplastic effects (adapted from [7]).

anticancer effects, but their findings are not directly transferrable to in vivo settings. Preclinical studies usually use human-toxic lidocaine concentrations making their results inapplicable to the real clinical settings. In addition, the in vitro model could not replicate the tumor cells microenvironment with its complex interactions among cells, stroma, and cytokines [7]. Despite the accumulated evidence, different types of tumor cells are unique in their behavior, which further limits reaching a consensus on the exact anticancer mechanism of action of i.v. lidocaine [54].

3. Pharmacokinetics

I.v. lidocaine displays a rapid onset of action (45–90 seconds after i.v. injection), but a very short duration (10–20 min after 50 or 100 mg i.v. boluses) [2, 65]. When administered intravenously, lidocaine initially follows distribution in the highly vascularized organs of the body, such as the liver, heart, lung, and brain with a large volume of distribution of 0.6–4.5 L/kg. Lidocaine metabolism occurs rapidly by the cytochrome P450 system in the liver (90% hepatic biotransformation). It undergoes oxidative N-deakylation to the metabolites monoethylglycinexylidine (MEGX), glycinexylidide (GX), and N-ethylglycine (NEG), all of which possess a glycine moiety. MEGX and GX are active metabolites, whereas NEG is inactive. All lidocaine metabolites are excreted by the kidneys. About 10% of i.v. lidocaine is excreted unchanged by the kidneys as well [47]. Approximately 70% of i.v. lidocaine is bound to plasma proteins. Certain clinical conditions can modify the pharmacokinetics of lidocaine with impact on the lidocaine half-life, such as chronic hepatic diseases like liver cirrhosis where patients require lower doses due to decrease plasma clearance or cardiovascular disorders like congestive heart failure where the volume of distribution and clearance are reduced and patients may require smaller doses as well [8]. The elimination of lidocaine usually follows a linear pharmacokinetic model with a half-life of approximately 1.5–2 hours after bolus or after infusion within 12-hour time frame. After 12-hour infusion, lidocaine exerts time-dependent rather than linear pharmacokinetic model of elimination and may have a half-life up to 4 hours [65].

4. Safety of i.v. lidocaine administration

The therapeutic plasma concentrations of i.v. lidocaine range from 1.5 to 5 μg/ml [2]. In normal adults without co-morbidities, a bolus dose of 100 mg i.v. lidocaine followed by an infusion at 1 mg/kg/h produces a plasma levels slightly above 1 μg/ml [66]. In mainstream clinical practice, the implemented i.v. lidocaine doses for pain management are in the range of 1–2 mg/kg/h. This rate of infusion reaches plasma levels less than 3–5 μg/ml. Even after a bolus administration of 2 mg/kg and a continuous infusion of 2–5 mg/kg/h, the i.v. lidocaine reaches plasma levels of 1–4 μg/ml. After exceeding the upper safety plasma level of 5 μg/ml, the awake patients may exhibit signs and symptoms of local anesthetic systemic toxicity (**Table 1**). Due to the short half-life of lidocaine, however, these symptoms of local anesthetic systemic toxicity are easily reversible by reducing the rate or stopping the infusion. In the presence of severe hepatic dysfunction and renal impairment (impaired lidocaine metabolism and clearance), severe hypoalbuminemia (impaired lidocaine protein binding), severe acidosis (increased lidocaine dissociation from plasma proteins), severe cardiac disease, heart block, or seizures, there are contraindications to i.v. lidocaine administration [2, 47].

Given the narrow therapeutic index of i.v. lidocaine leading to a high risk of reaching toxic plasma levels, the recently published international consensus in the field outlined some controversies regarding its intravenous use . The exact dose of i.v. lidocaine continues to be debated. The dose should be calculated based on the patient's ideal body weight. Systemic lidocaine should be avoided in patients weighing less than 40 kg. The maximum dose for any patients should not exceed 120 mg/h. The initial loading (bolus) dose should be a maximum of 1.5 mg/kg initially over 10 min,

System	Signs and symptoms
Central nervous system	Anxiety Dizziness or light-headed Confusion Euphoria Tinnitus Blurring of vision or diplopia Nausea and vomiting Twitching and tremors Seizures and coma
Cardiovascular	Bradycardia Hypotension Cardiovascular depression Cardiac arrest
Respiratory	Tachypnea Respiratory depression Respiratory arrest

Table 1.
Signs and symptoms of i.v. lidocaine systemic toxicity.

followed by a continuous infusion of 1.5 mg/kg/h under ECG, blood pressure, and pulse oximetry monitoring [68]. The most commonly reported i.v lidocaine doses in clinical settings still range from 1 to 2 mg/kg/h (which probably are too low as could be seen from preclinical research above). According to a Cochrane review subgroup meta-analysis, an early analgesic effect was only apparent with higher dose (≥ 2 mg/kg/h) infusion regimens [69]. The optimal i.v. dosage and postoperative duration continue to be unclear [70], pending the results of the ALLEGRO trial [71]. I.v. lidocaine should be postponed if other local anesthetic blocks are applied at the same time. It should not be used within 4 hours after implementing local anesthetic interventions (and vice versa). I.v. lidocaine should be administered after considering with the patient of its clear benefits over risks, not more than 24 hours and under a high dependency unit monitoring . However, according to the other authors, i.v. lidocaine could be used outside the high dependency unit setting as well. In the Ottawa hospital guidelines, a distinction was made between low-risk patients (American Society of Anesthesiology (ASA) class I and II) and high-risk patients (ASA III or above) in order to decide which ward for i.v. lidocaine infusion patients required [72]. In suitable patients, the postoperative lidocaine infusion could also be applied in surgical wards, as long as there is a well-established acute pain service and a clear protocol to follow [72].

5. Clinical effectiveness in the management of acute postsurgical pain

Until recently data suggest that i.v. lidocaine in the perioperative period results in less postoperative pain and opioid consumption, earlier return of gastro-intestinal tract function, and reduced hospital length of stay following abdominal procedures [69]. It could be a substitute to epidural for laparoscopic colorectal surgery within the ERAS pathways [73, 74]. Similar benefits have been observed after laparoscopic abdominal surgery when compared with systemic opioids, but not when compared to thoracic epidural analgesia, and especially in the absence of an ERAS program [69, 75, 76]. The latest revised Cochrane review concludes that the ERAS pathways benefits of perioperative i.v. lidocaine on reduction of pain, ileus, and PONV were uncertain due to limited quality of evidence [70]. Its conclusions are considered uncertain because of the existing heterogeneity of included trials as well. Thus, i.v. lidocaine may not always be beneficial in an individual setting given the variety of surgical interests. For example, the beneficial effects of i.v. lidocaine on postoperative recovery are of great interest to the colorectal surgeons, but probably of less interest to breast or spine surgeons [77]. Current evidence suggests that i.v. lidocaine alone may provide sufficient antinociceptive effect in patients undergoing abdominal surgery in addition to being an important component of perioperative multimodal analgesia [65]. In this context, the Enhanced Recovery After Surgery society guidelines for perioperative care in elective colorectal surgery (2019) make strong recommendations for lidocaine infusions during colorectal cancer surgery [78]. The following meta-analysis in elective colorectal surgery, however, reveals a statistically significant, but clinically irrelevant (the IASP criteria) reduction of pain after i.v. lidocaine infusion [79]. The less perioperative pain, the more difficult it will be to demonstrate the lidocaine's beneficial effects. This is supported by the results of a recent RCT which indicate that i.v. lidocaine has no significant benefits for patients undergoing robot-assisted colorectal surgery, including cumulated morphine consumption at 24 hours or 72 hours after the end of surgery [80]. To date, there appears to be limited evidence supporting that lidocaine reduces opioid consumption intraoperatively and in the immediate postoperative period in breast and spine surgeries [65, 81]. The same applies to renal and orthopedic surgeries. As far as gynecological operations are concerned, there is some evidence that lidocaine may reduce intraoperative consumption in laparoscopic hysterectomy [82], but there is insufficient evidence to support improved postoperative pain control as a part of perioperative multimodal analgesia or alone [65].

6. Clinical effectiveness in the management of chronic postsurgical pain

Perioperative use of i.v. lidocaine can have a beneficial effect as a prophylactic measure to prevent the development of persistent/chronic postsurgical pain (CPSP). For breast cancer patients, the i.v. lidocaine infusion decreases the incidence and severity of CPSP at 3 months [83, 84] and mastectomy patients have 20 times less the relative risk of the occurrence of CPSP than their placebo controls [85]. Similar benefits of perioperative i.v. lidocaine are observed after complex spinal surgery [86] as well as before spinal surgery in patients with neuropathic radicular pain [87, 88]. According to a recent Cochrane review, there is moderate evidence that i.v. lidocaine may reduce the risk of developing persistent postsurgical pain 3 to 6 months after breast cancer surgery (NNT 3) [89]. Another systematic review and meta-analysis on the efficacy and safety of i.v. lidocaine for the prevention of CPSP concludes that perioperative lidocaine infusions may reduce the incidence of CPSP between 3 and 6 months after surgery. The effect size is considerable for both breast and nonbreast surgical procedures, indicating that for every five patients exposed to lidocaine, at least one will be spared the development of CPSP, an absolute risk reduction about 22% (OR 0.29, 95% CI 0.18-0.48) [90]. The authors described their meta-analysis as a hypothesis-generating project to stimulate future research [91]. The next systematic review corroborates that i.v. lidocaine seems to decrease the incidence of CPSP. However, given the limited evidence, more trials are necessary to define its efficacy and safety [92]. This gap for more strong evidence was partly filled by two recent randomized controlled trials. The first RCT reveals that perioperative lidocaine infusion reduces the incidence of CPSP at 3 months after radical gastrointestinal tumor surgery [93], whereas the second one confirms that intraoperative lidocaine infusion reduces the incidence of CPSP in breast cancer surgery at 3 and 6 months and is effective in relieving acute postoperative pain [94].

7. Clinical effectiveness in the prevention of postoperative cancer recurrence

As has been described above, lidocaine has promising anticancer properties. There is strong in vitro evidence of its protective effect on cancer recurrence. However, there are limited relevant clinical findings in the field. To date, only three recent retrospective clinical studies have shown an association between i.v. lidocaine infusion and improved outcomes after cancer surgery. The first covered 2239 patients who underwent resection of pancreatic carcinomas and found that those who received perioperative i.v. lidocaine had significantly better overall survival at 1 and 3 years, although disease-free survival was unaffected [95]. The second covered 144 patients who underwent radical cystectomy for bladder cancer and revealed that those who received intraoperative i.v. lidocaine (after the implementation of the specially designed urological ERAS protocol) had significantly higher overall survival and lower incidence of cancer recurrence after 2-year follow-up compared to patients who did not received lidocaine [96]. The third covered 702 patients who underwent primary debulking surgery for ovarian cancer and showed that those who received intraoperative i.v. lidocaine had significantly prolonged overall survival and disease-free survival at 3 and 5 years after surgery [97]. Finally, focusing on the effect of implementation of ERAS protocol on 3-year survival after colorectal cancer surgery (with a strong recommendation, grade 1(+), for i.v. lidocaine as an integral part of the protocol [74]), the ERAS was associated with better 3-year survival and was identified as an independent protective factor with a 30% reduction in the risk of death (HR 0.70, 95% CI 0.55-090) [98]. It may be speculated that the strong modulation of the surgical stress response associated with the implemented ERAS protocol, rather than the adjuvant lidocaine therein, most likely led to the observed survival benefits.

8. Summary and future perspectives

Lidocaine is increasingly used by anesthesiologists as an intravenous adjunct to general anesthesia due to its anti-inflammatory, antinociceptive, and opioid-sparing characteristics [99]. Intraoperatively, it could be used as alternative of regional analgesia in the case of contraindication or failed epidural analgesia, in laparoscopic surgery or trauma with multiple significant injuries, and especially as a part of ERAS protocols. The application of i.v. lidocaine may also be continued postoperatively, usually up to 24 hours, in the setting of inadequate or failed epidural analgesia, in conversion from laparoscopic to open surgery, and for the prevention or treatment of postoperative ileus [72]. I.v. lidocaine is a useful option in the prevention and/or treatment of acute hyperalgesia, such as in surgery at a site of chronic pain (spine surgery, limb amputations) or in previous experience of poorly controlled pain, such as in patients who are already on high doses of opioids, intolerant of opioids, and those who are at high risk of chronic postoperative pain [67, 72]. Outside of the context of acute perioperative pain management, future research is needed to explore whether the anti-inflammatory and natural killer cell effects of i.v. lidocaine result in improved oncological outcomes [79]. The question of whether i.v. lidocaine has clinically relevant influence on postoperative cancer surgery outcomes can only be answered by well-designed RCTs. Two ongoing trials, VAPOR-C and ALLEGRO, have oncology outcomes included as primary, secondary, or tertiary end points, which when completed, would partially fill the gap [7, 71]. The upcoming role for intravenous lidocaine in oncosurgery might shift its place from a second-line non-opioid adjuvant to a first-line option in the context of improving oncological outcomes [100].

Acknowledgements

The author has no acknowledgments to make.

Conflict of interest

The author declares no conflict of interest.

Author details

Dimitar Tonev
Medical University of Sofia, University Hospital Tsaritsa Yoanna—ISUL, Clinic of Anesthesiology and Intensive Care, Bulgaria

*Address all correspondence to: dgtsofia@abv.bg

References

[1] Löfgren N. Studies on Local Anaesthetics: Xylocaine, a New Synthetic Drug. [Ph.D. thesis] Stockholm University, Stockholm, Sweden. 1948

[2] Weinberg L, Peake B, Tan C, Nikfarjam M. Pharmacokinetics and pharmacodynamics of lignocaine: A review. World Journal of Anesthesiology. 2015;**4**(2):17-29

[3] de Clive-Lowe SG, Desmond J, North J. Intravenous lignocaine anaesthesia. Anaesthesia. 1958;**13**:138-146

[4] Weibel S, Jokinen J, Pace NL, Schnabel A, Hollmann MW, Hahnenkamp K, et al. Efficacy and safety of intravenous lidocaine for postoperative analgesia and recovery after surgery: A systematic review with trial sequential analysis. British Journal of Anaesthesia. 2016;**116**(6):770-783

[5] Dunn LK, Durieux ME. Perioperative use of intravenous lidocaine. Anesthesiology. 2017;**126**(4):729-737

[6] Beverly A, Kaye AD, Ljungqvist O, Urman RD. Essential elements of multimodal analgesia in enhanced recovery after surgery (ERAS) guidelines. Anesthesiology Clinics. 2017;**35**(2):e115-e143

[7] Wall TP, Buggy DJ. Perioperative intravenous lidocaine and metastatic cancer recurrence - a narrative review. Frontiers in Oncology. 2021;**11**:688896

[8] Marcos Michel-Levy J. Pharmacokinetics and pharmacodynamics of local Anesthetics. In: Whizar-Lugo VM, Hernández-Cortez E, editors. Topics in Local Anesthetics. London, UK London, UK, Rijeka, Croatia: IntechOpen; 2020. DOI: 10.5772/intechopen.91700

[9] van der Wal SE, van den Heuvel SA, Radema SA, van Berkum BF, Vaneker M, Steegers MA, et al. The in vitro mechanisms and in vivo efficacy of intravenous lidocaine on the neuroinflammatory response in acute and chronic pain. European Journal of Pain. 2016;**20**(5):655-674

[10] Hondeghem LM, Katzung BG. Time- and voltage-dependent interactions of antiarrhythmic drugs with cardiac sodium channels. Biochimica et Biophysica Acta. 1977;**472**(3-4):373-398

[11] Courtney KR. Mechanism of frequency-dependent inhibition of sodium currents in frog myelinated nerve by the lidocaine derivative GEA. The Journal of Pharmacology and Experimental Therapeutics. 1975;**195**(2):225-236

[12] Olschewski A, Hempelmann G, Vogel W, Safronov BV. Blockade of Na+ and K+ currents by local anesthetics in the dorsal horn neurons of the spinal cord. Anesthesiology. 1998;**88**(1):172-179

[13] Kirillova I, Teliban A, Gorodetskaya N, Grossmann L, Bartsch F, Rausch VH, et al. Effect of local and intravenous lidocaine on ongoing activity in injured afferent nerve fibers. Pain. 2011;**152**(7):1562-1571

[14] Chevrier P, Vijayaragavan K, Chahine M. Differential modulation of Nav1.7 and Nav1.8 peripheral nerve sodium channels by the local anesthetic lidocaine. British Journal of Pharmacology. 2004;**142**(3):576-584

[15] Leffler A, Reiprich A, Mohapatra DP, Nau C. Use-dependent block by lidocaine but not amitriptyline is more pronounced in tetrodotoxin (TTX)-resistant Nav1.8 than in TTX-sensitive Na+ channels. The Journal of Pharmacology and Experimental Therapeutics. 2007;**320**(1):354-364

[16] Sotgiu ML, Lacerenza M, Marchettini P. Selective inhibition by systemic lidocaine of noxious evoked activity in rat dorsal horn neurons. Neuroreport. 1991;**2**(8):425-428

[17] Hollmann MW, Durieux ME. Prolonged actions of short-acting drugs: Local anesthetics and chronic pain. Regional Anesthesia and Pain Medicine. 2000;**25**(4):337-339

[18] Cahana A, Carota A, Montadon ML, Annoni JM. The long-term effect of repeated intravenous lidocaine on central pain and possible correlation in positron emission tomography measurements. Anesthesia and Analgesia. 2004;**98**(6):1581-1584

[19] Koyanagi Y, Torturo CL, Cook DC, Zhou Z, Hemmings HC Jr. Role of specific presynaptic calcium channel subtypes in isoflurane inhibition of synaptic vesicle exocytosis in rat hippocampal neurones. British Journal of Anaesthesia. 2019;**123**(2):219-227

[20] Patel R, Montagut-Bordas C, Dickenson AH. Calcium channel modulation as a target in chronic pain control. British Journal of Pharmacology. 2018;**175**(12):2173-2184

[21] Oyama Y, Sadoshima J, Tokutomi N, Akaike N. Some properties of inhibitory action of lidocaine on the Ca2+ current of single isolated frog sensory neurons. Brain Research. 1988;**442**(2):223-228

[22] Lingamaneni R, Hemmings HC Jr. Differential interaction of anaesthetics and antiepileptic drugs with neuronal Na+ channels, Ca2+ channels, and GABA(a) receptors. British Journal of Anaesthesia. 2003;**90**(2):199-211

[23] Hermanns H, Hollmann MW, Stevens MF, Lirk P, Brandenburger T, Piegeler T, et al. Molecular mechanisms of action of systemic lidocaine in acute and chronic pain: A narrative review. British Journal of Anaesthesia. 2019;**123**(3):335-349

[24] Takeda M, Tsuboi Y, Kitagawa J, Nakagawa K, Iwata K, Matsumoto S. Potassium channels as a potential therapeutic target for trigeminal neuropathic and inflammatory pain. Molecular Pain. 2011;7:5

[25] de Klaver MJM, Buckingham MG, Rich GF. Lidocaine attenuates cytokine-induced cell injury in endothelial and vascular smooth muscle cells. Anesthesia and Analgesia. 2003;**97**(2):465-470

[26] Montell C. The history of TRP channels, a commentary and reflection. Pflügers Archiv : European Journal of Physiology. 2011;**461**(5):499-506

[27] Nilius B, Owsianik G. The transient receptor potential family of ion channels. Genome Biology. 2011;**12**(3):218

[28] Damann N, Voets T, Nilius B. TRPs in our senses. Current Biology. 2008;**18**(18):R880-R889

[29] Geppetti P, Nassini R, Materazzi S, Benemei S. The concept of neurogenic inflammation. BJU International. 2008;**101**(Suppl 3):2-6

[30] Fernandes ES, Russell FA, Spina D, McDougall JJ, Graepel R, Gentry C, et al. A distinct role for transient receptor potential ankyrin 1, in addition to transient receptor potential vanilloid

1, in tumor necrosis factor α-induced inflammatory hyperalgesia and Freund's complete adjuvant-induced monarthritis. Arthritis and Rheumatism. 2011;**63**(3):819-829

[31] Anand U, Otto WR, Facer P, Zebda N, Selmer I, Gunthorpe MJ, et al. TRPA1 receptor localisation in the human peripheral nervous system and functional studies in cultured human and rat sensory neurons. Neuroscience Letters. 2008;**438**(2):221-227

[32] Fernandes E, Fernandes M, Keeble J. The functions of TRPA1 and TRPV1: Moving away from sensory nerves. British Journal of Pharmacology. 2012;**166**(2):510-521

[33] Dai Y. TRPs and pain. Seminars in Immunopathology. 2016;**38**:277-291

[34] Leffler A, Lattrell A, Kronewald S, Niedermirtl F, Nau C. Activation of TRPA1 by membrane permeable local anesthetics. Molecular Pain. 2011;**7**:62

[35] Docherty RJ, Ginsberg L, Jadoon S, Orrell RW, Bhattacharjee A. TRPA1 insensitivity of human sural nerve axons after exposure to lidocaine. Pain. 2013;**154**(9):1569-1577

[36] Hollmann MW, Wieczorek KS, Berger A, Durieux ME. Local anesthetic inhibition of G protein-coupled receptor signaling by interference with Galpha(q) protein function. Molecular Pharmacology. 2001;**59**(2):294-301

[37] Geppetti P, Veldhuis NA, Lieu T, Bunnett NW. G protein-coupled receptors: Dynamic machines for signaling pain and itch. Neuron. 2015;**88**(4):635-649

[38] Malin SA, Molliver DC. Gi- and Gq-coupled ADP (P2Y) receptors act in opposition to modulate nociceptive signaling and inflammatory pain behavior. Molecular Pain. 2010;**6**:21

[39] Tappe-Theodor A, Constantin CE, Tegeder I, Lechner SG, Langeslag M, Lepcynzsky P, et al. Gα(q/11) signaling tonically modulates nociceptor function and contributes to activity-dependent sensitization. Pain. 2012;**153**(1):184-196

[40] Hollmann MW, Herroeder S, Kurz KS, Hoenemann CW, Struemper D, Hahnenkamp K, et al. Time-dependent inhibition of G protein-coupled receptor signaling by local anesthetics. Anesthesiology. 2004;**100**(4):852-860

[41] Picardi S, Stevens MF, Hahnenkamp K, Durieux ME, Lirk P, Hollmann MW. Time-dependent modulation of muscarinic m1/m3 receptor signalling by local anaesthetics. British Journal of Anaesthesia. 2014;**112**(2):370-379

[42] Fischer LG, Bremer M, Coleman EJ, Conrad B, Krumm B, Gross A, et al. Local anesthetics attenuate lysophosphatidic acid-induced priming in human neutrophils. Anesthesia and Analgesia. 2001;**92**(4):1041-1047

[43] Hollmann MW, Gross A, Jelacin N, Durieux ME. Local anesthetic effects on priming and activation of human neutrophils. Anesthesiology. 2001;**95**(1):113-122

[44] Hönemann CW, Hahnenkamp K, Podranski T, Strumper D, Hollmann MW, Durieux ME. Local anesthetics inhibit thromboxane A2 signaling in Xenopus oocytes and human k562 cells. Anesthesia and Analgesia. 2004;**99**(3):930-937

[45] Nishizawa N, Shirasaki T, Nakao S, Matsuda H, Shingu K. The inhibition of the N-methyl-D-aspartate receptor channel by local anesthetics in mouse

CA1 pyramidal neurons. Anesthesia and Analgesia. 2002;**94**(2):325-330

[46] Vranken JH. Elucidation of pathophysiology and treatment of neuropathic pain. Central Nervous System Agents in Medicinal Chemistry. 2012;**12**(4):304-314

[47] Lauder GR. A review of intravenous lidocaine infusion therapy for paediatric acute and chronic pain management. In: Maldonado C, editor. Pain Relief - from Analgesics to Alternative Therapies. London, UK London, UK, Rijeka, Croatia: IntechOpen; 2017. DOI: 10.5772/66771

[48] Vandenberg RJ, Ryan RM, Carland JE, Imlach WL, Christie MJ. Glycine transport inhibitors for the treatment of pain. Trends in Pharmacological Sciences. 2014;**35**(8):423-430

[49] Ahmadi S, Muth-Selbach U, Lauterbach A, Lipfert P, Neuhuber WL, Zeilhofer HU. Facilitation of spinal NMDA receptor currents by spillover of synaptically released glycine. Science. 2003;**300**(5628):2094-2097

[50] Hara K, Sata T. The effects of the local anesthetics lidocaine and procaine on glycine and gamma-aminobutyric acid receptors expressed in Xenopus oocytes. Anesthesia and Analgesia. 2007;**104**(6):1434-1439

[51] Werdehausen R, Kremer D, Brandenburger T, Schlösser L, Jadasz J, Küry P, et al. Lidocaine metabolites inhibit glycine transporter 1: A novel mechanism for the analgesic action of systemic lidocaine? Anesthesiology. 2012;**116**(1):147-158

[52] Werdehausen R, Mittnacht S, Bee LA, Minett MS, Armbruster A, Bauer I, et al. The lidocaine metabolite N-ethylglycine has antinociceptive effects in experimental inflammatory and neuropathic pain. Pain. 2015;**156**(9):1647-1659

[53] Missair A, Cata JP, Votta-Velis G, Johnson M, Borgeat A, Tiouririne M, et al. Impact of perioperative pain management on cancer recurrence: An ASRA/ESRA special article. Regional Anesthesia and Pain Medicine. 2019;**44**(1):13-28

[54] Lee IW, Schraag S. The use of intravenous lidocaine in perioperative medicine: Anaesthetic, analgesic and immune-modulatory aspects. Journal of Clinical Medicine. 2022;**11**(12):3543

[55] Herroeder S, Pecher S, Schönherr ME, Kaulitz G, Hahnenkamp K, Friess H, et al. Systemic lidocaine shortens length of hospital stay after colorectal surgery: A double-blinded, randomized, placebo-controlled trial. Annals of Surgery. 2007;**246**(2):192-200

[56] Yardeni IZ, Beilin B, Mayburd E, Levinson Y, Bessler H. The effect of perioperative intravenous lidocaine on postoperative pain and immune function. Anesthesia and Analgesia. 2009;**109**(5):1464-1469

[57] Yon JH, Choi GJ, Kang H, Park JM, Yang HS. Intraoperative systemic lidocaine for pre-emptive analgesics in subtotal gastrectomy: A prospective, randomized, double-blind, placebo-controlled study. Canadian Journal of Surgery. 2014;**57**(3):175-182

[58] Xu S, Hu S, Ju X, Li Y, Li Q, Wang S. Effects of intravenous lidocaine, dexmedetomidine, and their combination on IL-1, IL-6 and TNF-α in patients undergoing laparoscopic hysterectomy: A prospective, randomized controlled trial. BMC Anesthesiology. 2021;**21**(1):3

[59] Weinschenk S, Weiss C, Benrath J, von Baehr V, Strowitzki T, Feißt M. Anti-inflammatory characteristics of local Anesthetics: Inhibition of TNF-α secretion of lipopolysaccharide-stimulated leucocytes in human blood samples. International Journal of Molecular Sciences. 2022;**23**(6):3283

[60] Chamaraux-Tran TN, Piegeler T. The amide local Anesthetic lidocaine in cancer surgery-potential Antimetastatic effects and preservation of immune cell function? A narrative review. Frontiers in Medicine (Lausanne). 2017;**4**:235

[61] Cassuto J, Sinclair R, Bonderovic M. Anti-inflammatory properties of local anesthetics and their present and potential clinical implications. Acta Anaesthesiologica Scandinavica. 2006;**50**(3):265-282

[62] Piegeler T, Votta-Velis EG, Liu G, Place AT, Schwartz DE, Beck-Schimmer B, et al. Antimetastatic potential of amide-linked local anesthetics: Inhibition of lung adenocarcinoma cell migration and inflammatory Src signaling independent of sodium channel blockade. Anesthesiology. 2012;**117**(3):548-559

[63] House CD, Vaske CJ, Schwartz AM, Obias V, Frank B, Luu T, et al. Voltage-gated Na+ channel SCN5A is a key regulator of a gene transcriptional network that controls colon cancer invasion. Cancer Research. 2010;**70**(17):6957-6967

[64] Brackenbury WJ. Voltage-gated sodium channels and metastatic disease. Channels (Austin, Tex.). 2012;**6**(5):352-361

[65] Lockwood N, Misra L. Efficacy of perioperative intravenous lidocaine for multimodal analgesia. Open Journal of Anesthesiology. 2020;**10**:299-312

[66] Rowland M, Thomson PD, Guichard A, Melmon KL. Disposition kinetics of lidocaine in normal subjects. Annals of the New York Academy of Sciences. 1971;**179**:383-398

[67] Foo I, Macfarlane AJR, Srivastava D, Bhaskar A, Barker H, Knaggs R, et al. The use of intravenous lidocaine for postoperative pain and recovery: International consensus statement on efficacy and safety. Anaesthesia. 2021;**76**(2):238-250

[68] Weinberg L, Rachbuch C, Ting S, et al. A randomised controlled trial of peri-operative lidocaine infusions for open radical prostatectomy. Anaesthesia. 2016;**71**(4):405-410

[69] Kranke P, Jokinen J, Pace NL, Schnabel A, Hollmann MW, Hahnenkamp K, et al. Continuous intravenous perioperative lidocaine infusion for postoperative pain and recovery. Cochrane Database of Systematic Reviews. 2015;7:CD009642. [Accessed 29 May 2023]

[70] Weibel S, Jelting Y, Pace NL, Helf A, Eberhart LH, Hahnenkamp K, et al. Continuous intravenous perioperative lidocaine infusion for postoperative pain and recovery in adults. Cochrane Database of Systematic Reviews. 2018;**6**(6):CD009642

[71] Paterson HM, Cotton S, Norrie J, Nimmo S, Foo I, Balfour A, et al. The ALLEGRO trial: A placebo controlled randomised trial of intravenous lidocaine in accelerating gastrointestinal recovery after colorectal surgery. Trials. 2022;**23**(1):84

[72] Eipe N, Gupta S, Penning J. Intravenous lidocaine for acute pain: An evidence-based clinical update. BJA Education. 2016;**16**(9):292-298

[73] Wongyingsinn M, Baldini G, Charlebois P, Liberman S, Stein B,

Carli F. Intravenous lidocaine versus thoracic epidural analgesia: A randomized controlled trial in patients undergoing laparoscopic colorectal surgery using an enhanced recovery program. Regional Anesthesia and Pain Medicine. 2011;**36**(3):241-248

[74] Alfonsi P, Slim K, Chauvin M, Mariani P, Faucheron JL, Fletcher D. Working Group of Société française d'anesthésie et réanimation (SFAR); Société française de chirurgie digestive (SFCD). French guidelines for enhanced recovery after elective colorectal surgery. Journal of Visceral Surgery. 2014;**151**(1):65-79

[75] Sun Y, Li T, Wang N, Yun Y, Gan TJ. Perioperative systemic lidocaine for postoperative analgesia and recovery after abdominal surgery: A meta-analysis of randomized controlled trials. Diseases of the Colon and Rectum. 2012S;**55**(11):1183-1194

[76] Feldheiser A, Aziz O, Baldini G, Cox BP, Fearon KC, Feldman LS, et al. Enhanced recovery after surgery (ERAS) for gastrointestinal surgery, part 2: Consensus statement for anaesthesia practice. Acta Anaesthesiologica Scandinavica. 2016;**60**(3):289-334

[77] Paterson HM. Continuous intravenous lidocaine infusion for postoperative pain and recovery in adults. Techniques in Coloproctology. 2019;**23**:69-71

[78] Gustafsson UO, Scott MJ, Hubner M, Nygren J, Demartines N, Francis N, et al. Guidelines for perioperative Care in Elective Colorectal Surgery: Enhanced recovery after surgery (ERAS®) society recommendations: 2018. World Journal of Surgery. 2019;**43**(3):659-695

[79] Rollins KE, Javanmard-Emamghissi H, Scott MJ, Lobo DN. The impact of peri-operative intravenous lidocaine on postoperative outcome after elective colorectal surgery: A meta-analysis of randomised controlled trials. European Journal of Anaesthesiology. 2020;**37**(8):659-670

[80] Herzog J, Schou M, Jensen KM, Lauridsen JT, Jensen AG. A randomised controlled trial of lidocaine infusion on post-operative opioid consumption in patients undergoing robotic colorectal surgery. Danish Medical Journal. 2020;**67**(1):A06190342

[81] Haratian A, Musa A, Field R, Farhan S, Bennett C, Cooke C, et al. Intravenous lidocaine in spine surgery: A meta-analysis of randomized controlled trials. North American Spine Society Journal. 2021;7:100079

[82] Grady MV, Mascha E, Sessler DI, Kurz A. The effect of perioperative intravenous lidocaine and ketamine on recovery after abdominal hysterectomy. Anesthesia and Analgesia. 2012;**115**(5):1078-1084

[83] Grigoras A, Lee P, Sattar F, Shorten G. Perioperative intravenous lidocaine decreases the incidence of persistent pain after breast surgery. The Clinical Journal of Pain. 2012;**28**(7):567-572

[84] Chang YC, Liu CL, Liu TP, Yang PS, Chen MJ, Cheng SP. Effect of perioperative intravenous lidocaine infusion on acute and chronic pain after breast surgery: A meta-analysis of randomized controlled trials. Pain Practice. 2017;**17**(3):336-343

[85] Terkawi AS, Sharma S, Durieux ME, et al. Perioperative lidocaine infusion reduces the incidence of post-mastectomy chronic pain: A double-blind, placebo-controlled randomized trial. Pain Physician. 2015;**18**(2):E139-E146

[86] Farag E, Ghobrial M, Sessler DI, Dalton JE, Liu J, Lee JH, et al. Effect of perioperative intravenous lidocaine administration on pain, opioid consumption, and quality of life after complex spine surgery. Anesthesiology. 2013;**119**(4):932-940

[87] Tremont-Lukats IW, Hutson PR, Backonja MM. A randomized, double-masked, placebo-controlled pilot trial of extended IV lidocaine infusion for relief of ongoing neuropathic pain. The Clinical Journal of Pain. 2006;**22**(3):266-271

[88] Tonev D, Radeva S. Radiculopathy: Causes, diagnosis and treatment. In: Berhardt LV, editor. Advances in Medicine and Biology. Vol. 158. New York: Nova Science Publishers, Inc.; 2020. pp. 43-116

[89] Weinstein EJ, Levene JL, Cohen MS, Andreae DA, Chao JY, Johnson M, et al. Local anaesthetics and regional anaesthesia versus conventional analgesia for preventing persistent postoperative pain in adults and children. Cochrane Database of Systematic Reviews. 2018;**6**(6):CD007105

[90] Bailey M, Corcoran T, Schug S, Toner A. Perioperative lidocaine infusions for the prevention of chronic postsurgical pain: A systematic review and meta-analysis of efficacy and safety. Pain. 2018;**159**(9):1696-1704

[91] Bailey M. Reply. Pain. 2019;**160**(3):754-755

[92] Ramos LMF. The role of intravenous lidocaine in preventing chronic post-operative pain. Research and Practice in Anesthesiology – Open Journal. 2021;**5**(1):1-4

[93] Dai Y, Jiang R, Su W, Wang M, Liu Y, Zuo Y. Impact of perioperative intravenous lidocaine infusion on postoperative pain and rapid recovery of patients undergoing gastrointestinal tumor surgery: A randomized, double-blind trial. Journal of Gastrointestinal Oncology. 2020;**11**(6):1274-1282

[94] Xia M, Wei Q, Zhang Q, Jiang H. Effect of intravenous lidocaine on chronic postoperative pain in patients undergoing breast cancer surgery: A prospective, double-blind, randomized, placebo-controlled clinical trial. Annals of Translational Medicine. 2022;**10**(14):803

[95] Zhang H, Yang L, Zhu X, Zhu M, Sun Z, Cata JP, et al. Association between intraoperative intravenous lidocaine infusion and survival in patients undergoing pancreatectomy for pancreatic cancer: A retrospective study. British Journal of Anaesthesia. 2020;**125**(2):141-148

[96] Cazenave L, Faucher M, Tourret M, Marques M, Tezier M, Mokart D. Intravenous lidocaine and cancer outcomes after radical cystectomy. European Journal of Anaesthesiology. 2022;**39**(4):396-399

[97] Zhang H, Gu J, Qu M, Sun Z, Huang Q, Cata JP, et al. Effects of intravenous infusion of lidocaine on short-term outcomes and survival in patients undergoing surgery for ovarian cancer: A retrospective propensity score matching study. Frontiers in Oncology. 2022;**11**:689832

[98] Tidadini F, Bonne A, Trilling B, Quesada JL, Sage PY, Foote A, et al. Effect of implementation of enhanced recovery after surgery (ERAS) protocol and risk factors on 3-year survival after colorectal surgery for cancer-a retrospective cohort of 1001 patients. International Journal of Colorectal Disease. 2022;**37**(5):1151-1159

[99] Bailey MA, Toner AJ, Corcoran TB. A survey of perioperative intravenous lidocaine use by anaesthetists in Australia and New Zealand. Anaesthesia and Intensive Care. 2020;**48**(1):53-58

[100] Koepke EJ, Manning EL, Miller TE, Ganesh A, Williams DGA, Manning MW. The rising tide of opioid use and abuse: The role of the anesthesiologist. Perioperative Medicine (London, England). 2018;7:16

Chapter 7

Perspective Chapter: Interdisciplinary Pain Rehabilitation Programs – Evidence and Clinical Real-World Results

Björn Gerdle, Marcelo Rivano Fischer and Åsa Ringqvist

Abstract

Chronic pain conditions are influenced by and interact with physical, psychological, social, and contextual factors. These conditions are associated with psychological distress, poor health, sick leave, and high socio-economic costs. Therefore, modern clinical practice applies a biopsychosocial (BPS) framework. Interdisciplinary pain rehabilitation programs (IPRPs) for chronic pain distinguish themselves as well-coordinated complex interventions. This chapter describes the contents of such programs. We will briefly review the evidence for IPRPs and discuss problems when evaluating these complex interventions. Furthermore, we will report practice-based results from a large Swedish pain registry—the Swedish Quality Registry for Pain Rehabilitation (SQRP). The SQRP collects data from a relevant special clinical department in Sweden—i.e., real-life outcomes will be depicted. Characteristics of patients that benefit the most from IPRPs will be described and discussed. The indications for IPRPs will also be presented. Finally, we will discuss how to improve rehabilitation for chronic pain patients.

Keywords: complex, chronic pain, interdisciplinary, multimodal, outcome, rehabilitation

1. Introduction

Today, there is no controversy about considering acute and chronic pain based on a foundation of neurobiology influenced by and interacting with biological, psychological, and social/contextual factors [1–3]. Hence, modern clinical practice applies a biopsychosocial (BPS) framework in assessments and treatments [4, 5]. This approach is the result of developments that have occurred over the past 70 years.

Units dedicated to treat pain were developed in the USA based on physicians' experiences with chronic pain in soldiers during and after World War Two. During this period, surgeons and anaesthesiologists attempted to alleviate both chronic and acute pain mainly using blockades and local anaesthesia [6]. Later, this type of unit expanded into Europe and Sweden. The first multidisciplinary pain clinic opened in the 1960s as a development of the pain clinic founded by John Bonica in the 1950s at the University of

IntechOpen

Washington in Seattle (USA) [7]. Bonica realised that patients with complex pain problems were not helped by single specialties, and during the 1950s he brought neurosurgeons, psychiatrists, and anaesthesiologists to his clinic. In 1959, Wilbert Fordyce, a psychologist hired by the Department of Physical Medicine and Rehabilitation at the same hospital, became interested in applying behavioural strategies in the assessments and treatments of chronic pain. Their collaboration led to the incorporation of psychologists in pain clinics and later other health care providers trained in different but related areas [6]. Bonica also led an international initiative that resulted in the formation of an association of researchers and clinicians dedicated to the understanding and treatment of pain (International Association for the Study of Pain, IASP).

In 1982, Fordyce's psychological program and Bonica's pain clinic merged under the direction of John Loeser [6]. Under this new arrangement, patients were evaluated and treated by teams, and the BPS model started to be used in pain programs. These early programs had to deal with medication problems and addiction, so inpatient treatment became the standard. During the 1970s, the number of multidisciplinary pain clinics following the example of Seattle's clinic grew in the USA and later in Australia, New Zealand, and Europe. During the 1980s, psychologists began to add cognitive treatment strategies to the programs, which opened up treatment to a broader mix of patients. By 1990, cognitive-behavioural pain management programs were widespread and became the golden standard of care. During the 1980s and the 1990s, many studies focused on interdisciplinary pain programs (IPRPs), and new theories were launched [6, 8, 9].

The positive development in the USA slowed down at the beginning of 2000, and most units offering IPRPs closed their operations in the following decade, except for units in the Department of Veterans Affairs (VA). The Commission for the Accreditation of Rehabilitation Facilities (CARF) offers a specific set of standards that emphasise the interdisciplinary setting and the BPS model for the treatment of chronic pain. As the CARF standards remained focused on the BPS framework, the number of accredited programs illustrates the development in the USA. In 1998, there were 205 accredited chronic pain programs in the USA. By 2004, the number decreased to 125, 11 of which were VA programs [6]. These programs, excluding the VA IPRPs, decreased to 63 in 2010, 53 in 2015, and 32 in 2020 (Carolan Terrence, CARF, personal communication). However, outside the USA, the development has gone in the opposite direction. By the end of 1990 outside the USA, fewer than five tertiary pain units with CARF accredited pain programs were in operation; however, by 2021, this number had increased to 140 (CARF, personal communication). According to many reports, the decline in the USA was due to opioid use as a medication for chronic pain, but this approach, as the result of the opioid pandemic, is currently being replaced by initiatives to re-start IPRP.

Both evidence and clinical practice guided the development of how to face the problem of chronic pain—from viewing chronic pain as a symptom of underlying causes to viewing chronic pain as a dysfunction (i.e., from a biomedical approach to a biopsychosocial approach). Therefore, treatments have evolved from monodisciplinary to multidisciplinary treatments and from multidisciplinary treatments to interdisciplinary programs.

During the 1970s and 1980s, the novel approaches to chronic pain developed slowly in Sweden. As new methods and treatments were developed, national guidelines for chronic pain treatment were warranted. In 1994, an expert group formed by the Swedish National Board of Health and Welfare summarised the recommendations for treatment of chronic pain based on the International Association for the Study of Pain (IASP) guidelines and available evidence at the time. In 2006 and 2010, two compilations of evidence for chronic pain treatments, commissioned by the Swedish Agency for Health Technology Assessment and Assessment of Social Services (SBU; see below), confirmed the conclusions of the 1994 report about appropriate methods and lack of evidence for methods still being used. In the 2006 and 2010 reports, one method was singled out as an evidence-based approach, the IPRP. These reports contributed to a governmental decision to financially support the development of IPRPs throughout Sweden. During this period, a registry for pain rehabilitation was formed through an initiative of the professions with the aim to analyse outcomes of pain rehabilitation. The registry with the support of the affiliated units and the national organisation of county councils (SKL) developed into a national quality registry that included all tertiary pain rehabilitation units as well as units operating at the primary care level.

2. Indications for IPRP

In clinical practise, patients with complex chronic pain conditions with difficulties coping with their condition in daily life are referred to an IPRP. These patients' ability to cope with their pain can be compromised by co-morbidities and/or their work situation. Often, these patients have tried monodisciplinary interventions and/or pharmacological treatments without marked improvements. The Swedish guidelines regarding indications for IPRP, which have been approved by several authorities and professional organisations, recommend that IPRP be offered to chronic pain patients with complex clinical presentations and when monodisciplinary interventions have not been effective [10].

In 2011, the IASP stated in the Declaration Montreal that 'access to pain management is a fundamental human right' [11]. This humanitarian approach is important; however, availability to IPRP is scarce, as mentioned above, in several parts of the world, and chronic pain is common in the general population—approximately 20% of the European and North American population has a significant chronic pain condition [12, 13]. In addition, as many patients with chronic pain rarely seek health care services, these patients seem to have adapted to their pain condition to lead lives with minor consequences to their function and well-being. This needs to be considered as IPRP is costly interventions in the short run and patients need to be fully invested in the process and very possibly have a sense of urgency to benefit from treatment and be motivated to engage in behavioural and cognitive change. The motivation to behavioural and cognitive change is fundamental as an indication for IPRP. For IPRP to be used with an ethical and humanitarian perspective, it needs to prioritise individuals who suffer from substantial consequences of their chronic pain condition regarding function, social, and/or psychological well-being.

3. Basic contents of IPRP

The idea of treating chronic diseases with a broader approach than the biomedical approach was first launched by Engel in a biopsychosocial (BPS) model for the treatment of diseases, especially chronic diseases [14]. The model emphasises the mutual interactions between biological, psychological, and experiential or social factors that impact people's perceptions of their overall health. This model lies at the core of the multidisciplinary and interdisciplinary approaches to the treatment of chronic pain.

Similarities and differences between these approaches are described in detail elsewhere [7]. Although both rely on the BPS model, they differ regarding whether the goals of the professionals are integrated, whether professionals work collaboratively in teams, and whether their treatments are provided simultaneously or sequentially [9, 15]. The interdisciplinary treatment, which is based on the BPS approach [1], is the standard treatment used in IPRPs. According to IASP, interdisciplinary treatment is a:

> *Multimodal treatment provided by a multidisciplinary team collaborating in assessment and treatment using a shared biopsychosocial model and goals.*
>
> *For example: the prescription of an anti-depressant by a physician alongside exercise treatment from a physiotherapist, and cognitive behavioural treatment by a psychologist, all working closely together with regular team meetings (face to face or online), agreement on diagnosis, therapeutic aims and plans for treatment and review*[1].

The programs usually include experts working in an integrated manner with physical, social, psychological, and medical aspects to diminish the consequences of chronic pain in these or other areas [7, 16]. The principal components of IPRP are as follows:

1. a team assessment of the chronic pain problem and its consequences;

2. the establishment of a treatment plan, including interventions by different professions with goals to be achieved during the program;

3. communication between team members and between the team, the patient, and significant others;

4. deliveries of the different synchronised interventions of IPRP;

5. evaluation of the interventions;

6. documentation; and

7. a discharge process, including interaction with other stakeholders.

Other researchers have also identified the same content [17]. Although the areas covered by the interdisciplinary programs are well described elsewhere, there are very few descriptions of the interventions used in clinical practice in IPRPs, usually describing the interventions used in specific centres, such as Mayo Clinic or Chicago University Hospital [16]. In Sweden, it is possible to gather information on the interventions used in clinical practice from most of the IPRPs affiliated with the Swedish National Registry. Of the 39 affiliated units, 31 were included [18]. The usual contents of IPRP described by Swedish units are as follows:

1. dialogue and education (e.g., education, training in wellness and healthy living habits, meetings with families, video feedback, and couples therapy) and

---

[1] From Terminology|International Association for the Study of Pain (iasp-pain.org).

self-training (e.g., home lessons, activity diary, physical self-training, reflection time, and self-analysis);

2. activity training (activity training, graded activity training, and exposure training);

3. meetings (conferences with patients, rehabilitation team, vocational guidance, rehabilitation coordinator, goal-setting meetings, and meetings to check goal achievement);

4. cognitive behavioural therapy, other psychological treatments (e.g., supervised group therapy, pain or a stress coping course, psychological and social aspects, post-traumatic stress disorder (PTSD) treatment, and psychodynamic methods) and Acceptance and Commitment Therapy (ACT) (e.g., goal compass, training in ACT principles, and mindfulness);

5. relaxation techniques; and

6. physical exercise.

Only 14 of 31 programs reported using interventions in the workplace. All programs reported having follow-ups (1-year follow-up by mail or at the unit for completing the registry's questionnaires). Usually, extra follow-up meetings were scheduled two to three months after discharge from rehabilitation (21 of 31 units).

The optimal composition of IPRP with respect to length, contacts with therapists, and intensity are insufficiently known according to a systematic review (SR) [19] and a meta-analysis (MA) [20]. The former concluded that because dose variables were not investigated separately in the RCTs, the reviewers could not disentangle the interrelationships between dose, content, and effects of IPRP on disability, work, and quality of life. Similarly, a longitudinal study of IPRP dosage (i.e., duration) could not establish an optimal dosage [21].

4. The general and specific goals of IPRP

Generally, IPRP goals include improving important outcomes (4,5). There are several simultaneous general goals to be considered—decreased pain intensity and increased mental health; increased participation in work/studies and social life; and increased health and quality of life. These general goals are combined with the specific goals of the individual with chronic pain. Thus, goals should ideally be set at the level of the individual, the rehabilitation teams, and the socio-economic constraints. The latter is essential since IRRPs historically have been financial failures. For IRRP to prosper and receive funding, the considerable socio-economic costs of chronic pain need to be considered. Goals, such as return to work/studies and decrease in medication use, health care use, and surgery, will in the long run also benefit the individual move towards an active, independent lifestyle.

As chronic pain is a complex experience with possible adverse effects on function and social and psychological well-being, goal setting should include several aspects and involve a BPS perspective. The general goals for IPRPs are mentioned above. In addition to these goals, there is an increasing emphasis on cognitive areas that could mediate positive changes, such as catastrophizing, acceptance of the pain condition, avoidance of activity due to unrealistic concerns about harm, and expectations of pain treatment [22].

Researchers have debated whether pain intensity aspects should be amongst the main outcomes of pain treatments included in IPRP [23–26]. Many patients consider reducing pain to be the most important aspect of treatments with respect to regaining a normal lifestyle; however, changing this view is considered an intrinsic component of IPRP. Many chronic pain patients eligible for IPRP have experienced how short-sighted attempts to control only pain intensity can lead to vicious cycles of increased physical and psychological disability and reduced quality of life. Thus, many IPRPs have largely adopted the idea of introducing acceptance as a cornerstone of the psychological component of IPRP (i.e., the willingness to experience pain as it is) and encouraging patients to set up activity-related rehabilitation goals and to risk initial pain flare-ups. This means that patients are advised against establishing pain reduction as the only or the most important goal. Paradoxically, in the long run, pain reduction is one of the more robust results of IPRP [27]. Nevertheless, in traditional CBT, a cornerstone and mainstream in IRPs, an array of strategies is presented, strategies that target the consequences of pain with non-pharmaceutical techniques for pain control.

The process of goal setting is vital and fundamental both for the individual and the team as goal setting has been shown to promote greater behavioural change across a wide range of behaviours [28]. At the individual level, a thorough assessment that is communicated to the patient and a collaborative goal-setting process will increase engagement and adherence to treatment. In addition, the rehabilitation team will benefit from formulating common goals for treatment, reviewing results, and improving plans to stay engaged and to be flexible. The latter should constitute an important goal for the team as role models for patients. Often, the goal is to attain goals that are SMART—i.e., Specified, Measurable, Attractive, Realistic, and Time-limited [29, 30]. However, possibly the most important quality for goals is to be personalised and agreed upon by the patient. The team should strive for a collaborative approach but must always bear in mind that the patient is in a more vulnerable position and might easily give in to goals that might, for example, not feel relevant or feel too demanding. Motivational Interviewing (MI) can be used to discover a patient's motivation for a specific goal when a patient finds it difficult to specify goals. Patients are often more focused on avoiding unpleasant experiences and frequently the main wish of the patient is to be free of pain. As such, the goal-setting can constitute an acceptance of intervention as it models how to focus on the attainable and let go of the difficult to achieve a goal—i.e., pain relief.

Nevertheless, the SMART model for goal setting has lately been challenged by Acceptance and Commitment Therapy (ACT), the third wave CBT. ACT, which has increasingly been introduced in IRRP, emphasises identifying important values and not primarily setting specified, time-limited goals. However, the SMART model can be used as a step towards identifying important values.

5. Consensus approaches to identify relevant domains and variables in IPRPs

The variety of interventions used at most IPRPs in a single country [18] is in itself a challenge when it comes to measuring the outcomes of IPRPs delivered in clinical settings. Nevertheless, the areas addressed correspond to the areas proposed by the BPS model. In addition to the variety of interventions within IPRPs, many tools have been used both by researchers and clinicians to assess patients and to measure IPRP outcomes. Two well-known initiatives to bring consensus into the areas of evaluating clinical trials, including IPRP are the Initiative on Methods, Measurement, and Pain Assessment in Clinical Trials (IMMPACT) [4, 31] and the validation and application of a patient-relevant core set of outcome domains to assess multimodal PAIN therapy (VAPAIN) initiatives (**Table 1**) [32].

IMMPACT identifies relevant outcome domains for clinical studies and proposes reliable measurement tools for the study of treatments of chronic pain, including all possible modalities and approaches. IMMPACT has resulted in several studies evaluating clinical treatments. VAPAIN specifically targets IPRPs. These initiatives have some overlapping domains that are included in clinical trials (**Table 1**). VAPAINs focused on IPRPs led to the addition of two domains considered critical when the treatment is interdisciplinary—productivity and patient satisfaction with social roles and activities. VAPAIN renamed certain domains and extended their scope (e.g., the more inclusive 'emotional well-being' rather than 'emotional function').

A different approach taken by a Canadian research group focuses on the variables of interest for health care providers and the variables of interest for patients, according to lists of parameters from the Patient-Reported Outcomes Measurement Information System (PROMIS), the International Classification of Functioning, Disability and Health (ICF), and current guidelines [33]. Here, the initiative was to identify the set of variables that are important to both providers and patients. They triangulated the ICF and the PROMIS frameworks with the perspectives (both the patients' and clinicians' perspectives) and found a common list of ten variables—pain interference, pain intensity, physical function, sleep disturbance, anxiety, depression, ability to participate in social roles and activities, fatigue, sleep-related impairments, and self-efficacy. The authors conclude that these variables mirror the BPS model covering the physical, psychological, and social consequences of chronic pain on an individual's life both from the perspective of people with chronic pain and the perspective of health care providers.

IMMPACT's domains	VAPAIN's domains
Pain	Pain intensity and frequency
Emotional function	Emotional well-being
Physical function	Physical activity
	Productivity
	Satisfaction with social roles and activities
Self-evaluation on overall improvement and satisfaction with the intervention	Patient's perception of achieved treatments goals
Symptom and side-effects of intervention	
Participant disposition (including participation and discontinuation of participation)	Reasons for discontinuation of treatment

Table 1.
Domains of IMMPACT and VAPAIN.

6. How to evaluate the complex IPRP intervention

There is a need to develop clinically applicable, standardised, and accepted ways to evaluate IPRP. IPRP is a complex intervention with several general goals (see above) and is delivered by an interdisciplinary team of professionals in close collaboration with the patient and considering the patient's specific goals. This is entirely different from a pharmacological intervention, which aims to alter a biochemical process to decrease pain intensity (**Figure 1**). In fact, an IPRP tries to influence several levels, including the behaviours of the patient with chronic pain. Hence, in clinical practice, there are several outcomes and to make things, even more, complicated the important goals for the individual patients may differ. Due to these circumstances, the concept of one or two primary outcomes and a few secondary outcomes applied in pharmacological randomised controlled trials (RCTs) do not reflect the complexity of IPRP. In a systematic review (SR) by SBU, the included RCTs on average had nine outcome variables and the variables were seldom divided into primary and secondary outcomes [23].

The evaluation of complex interventions, such as IPRP is not clear-cut [34]. Clinically applicable, standardised, and accepted ways to evaluate the multiple outcomes of IPRP in individual patients clinically and in trials, SRs/meta-analysis (MAs) and observational studies are lacking. If the changes in outcomes are intercorrelated (they often are, see below), it may be problematic to evaluate the outcome measures separately as sometimes is done [35]. In contrast, SBU defined a positive outcome of an RCT when the *majority of outcomes* were significantly better for the control intervention [23, 36]. Another approach was chosen by a group of reviewers [37]. They predetermined *primary* and *secondary outcomes* and what was necessary to classify an intervention as positive before reviewing the RCTs. Recently, we suggested how simultaneous goals can be handled using scores from Principal Component Analysis (PCA) in RCTs and observational studies [27]. For fibromyalgia, OMERACT[2] and

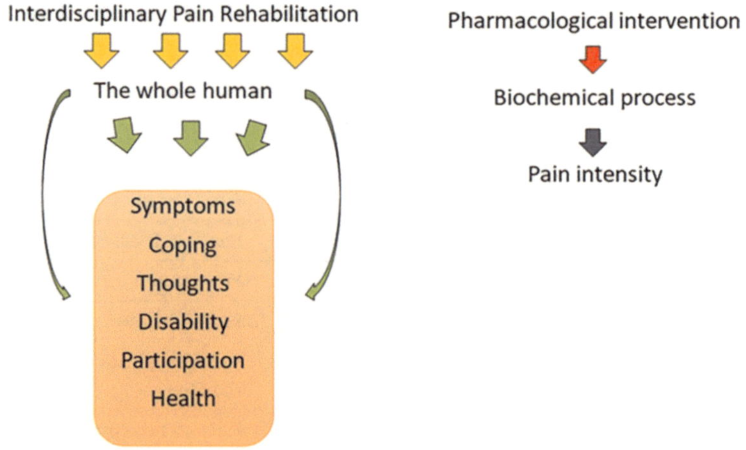

Figure 1.
The complexity of IPRP versus a pharmacological intervention.

---

[2] An international, informally-organized network initiated in 1992 aimed at improving outcome measurement in rheumatology.

others have suggested preliminary responder criteria based on several variables [38–40]. A similar approach that defines a total improvement variable based on the dichotomizing six variables was used by Grimby-Ekman et al. [41].

Because evaluations of several outcomes often raise an issue of multiple comparisons, Bonferroni corrections may be recommended [42, 43]. This is a conservative approach when the number of tests increases and can reduce the chances to detect real treatment effects [42, 44, 45]. Moreover, such corrections are intended for corrections of *independent* comparisons [44]; however, this situation is not present when evaluating the outcomes of IPRPs. Hierarchical or 'gatekeeping' procedures that do not require adjustment for multiplicity have been presented [43], but a natural hierarchy of outcomes must be present. Outcomes may be combined into a single composite outcome [46], but this may be problematic with respect to missing values for different variables and when the components of the composite endpoint are measured on different scales such as non-commensurate outcomes [46]. Multivariate methods that can handle non-commensurate outcomes in one analysis have been presented [46]. In studies from the Swedish Quality Registry for Pain Rehabilitation (SQRP, reported below), advanced multivariate methods such as PCA and Orthogonal Partial Least Square regression have been applied and can handle non-commensurate outcomes in one analysis.

7. Evidence according to systematic reviews

The available SRs and MAs indicate that IPRP is an evidence-based intervention. **Table 2** lists and briefly describes the results of available SRs and MAs based on only RCTs according to Dragioti et al.'s [47] search strategy.

SRs and MAs using several simultaneous outcomes report positive outcomes for IPRP for chronic pain conditions [23, 35–37, 48, 49, 52, 53, 55]. Studies using overall assessments of outcomes and therefore considering that IPRP is a complex intervention agree that IPRP has positive outcomes with moderate to strong evidence [23, 36, 37]. There is no consensus regarding the duration of the effects after IPRP (follow-up time) [23, 35–37, 48, 52–55]. When outcome variables are evaluated independently, the outcomes associated with positive effects differ across studies [50, 53, 56–58]. Articles reporting results for fibromyalgia separately reported positive outcomes for IPRP. However, both evidence levels and follow-up periods (short, medium, or long term) differed [23, 36, 37, 52, 58]. The conclusions regarding the effects of IPRP on vocational variables, such as return to work (RTW) and sick leave were heterogenous according to these reviews [23, 35, 36, 48–51].

The authors of these reviews identify several problems and limitations. Most SRs report that there is heterogeneity in study settings, interventions, and control groups. It is difficult to compare the patient groups included in the identified RCTs since there is no internationally accepted way to describe the patient groups. In addition, the number of comorbidities and duration of sick leave can differ, and external factors, such as the social security situation can differ considerably across studies from different countries and years. Some of the variables suggested by IMMPACT and VAPAIN can be useful for the development of a standardised set of variables that can be used to describe chronic pain patient cohorts [4, 31, 32]. Moreover, because there is no internationally accepted definition of IPRP, authors of SRs and MAs must create their own operational definitions to identify the relevant RCTs. In the quality assessments of RCTs, the issue of blinding might be problematic, and IPRP studies may be

First author, year, and reference	Type	Patients	No. of RCTs*	Main results and comments
Nielson 2001 [48]	SR	CP with separate analysis for CLBP, FM, and other	21	• IPRP is effective in CLBP conditions in intermediate to long-term – moderate evidence. • Contradictory for RTW in CLBP. • IPRP is effective in other pain conditions in the short to intermediate term – moderate evidence.
Guzman 2002 [49]	SR +MA	CLBP	10	• Strong evidence that IPRP improved function compared with inpatient or outpatient non-multidisciplinary treatments. • Contradictory for vocational outcomes (RTW) in CLBP.
SBU 2006 [23]	SR	CP with separate analysis for FM	46	• Strong evidence that IPRP in long term has better overall results in CP than less intensive interventions. • Strong evidence that IPRP is associated with positive effects upon RTW and sick leave in long term. • Moderate evidence that IPRP in long term has better overall results in FM than less intensive interventions.
van Geen 2007 [50]	SR	CLBP	10	• A positive effect of IPRP on work participation and quality of life in the long term. • No long-term effects on pain and functional status.
Scascighini 2008 [37]	SR	CP with separate analyses for CBLP and FM	36	• Compared to non-multidisciplinary control, moderate evidence of higher effectiveness for IPRP. • Compared to no treatment or TAU, strong evidence of higher effectiveness for IPRP in CP; for CBLP and FM, moderate evidence. • No evidence that a special kind, duration, or setting of IPRP was superior to any of the other study regimens.
Norlund 2009 [51]	SR +MA	CLBP	7	• For the Scandinavian studies (n=5), the effects on RTW had clinical relevance.
Häuser 2009 [52]	SR +MA	FM	9	• Strong evidence that IPRP has beneficial short-term effects on the key symptoms of FM. • Strong evidence that the positive effects on key symptoms decline with time.
SBU 2010 [36]	SR	CP with separate analyses for CLBP and FM		Partial update of 2006 SBU** • Moderate evidence that IPRP in the long term has better overall results in chronic back pain (neck, shoulder, and low back together) than less intensive interventions. • Moderate evidence that IPRP in the long term has better overall results in CBLP than less intensive interventions. • Lack of studies for only chronic neck and shoulder pain. • Moderate evidence that IPRP in the long term has better overall results in generalised pain (FM) than less intensive interventions.

First author, year, and reference	Type	Patients	No. of RCTs*	Main results and comments
				• Low evidence that IPRP improves RTW/sick leave compared to less intensive interventions.
van Middelkoop 2011 [53]	SR +MA	CLBP	83	• IPRP was found to reduce pain intensity and disability at short-term follow-up compared to no treatment/WLC. • There was moderate evidence for not finding an effect on disability and long-term outcomes.
Kamper 2014 [35]	SR +MA	CBLP	41	• IPRP is more effective than TAU (moderate evidence) and physical treatments (low-quality evidence) in decreasing pain and disability in long term. • For work outcomes, IPRP was more effective than physical treatment but not more effective than TAU.
Gianola 2018 [54]	SR +MA	CBLP	22	Partial reanalyses of Kamper et al.'s review [35] using minimal important differences units (MIDs). Using this approach, they concluded that IPRP led to improvements in an appreciable number of patients in the short- and medium-term after IPRP. In the long term, IPRP probably had little or no benefit for most patients.
Casey 2020 [55]	SR +MA	CP	27	• For pain intensity and disability, IPRP the effects (low-quality evidence) were better than active physical interventions at the short-term and long-term but not the medium-term follow-up.
Martinez-Calderon 2020 [56]	SR +MA	CP	60	Investigates the outcome pain self-efficacy. • IPRP improved pain self-efficacy with small effects at the short-term, medium-term, and long-term follow-up (low-quality evidence).
Martinez-Calderon 2020 [57]	SR	CLBP	61	Investigates outcomes of fear. • IPRP reduced kinesiophobia (moderate evidence). • IPRP altered fear-avoidance beliefs (very low evidence).
Martinez-Calderon 2021 [58]	SR	FM	12	Investigates the outcome of pain-related fear. • IPRP reduced kinesiophobia (very low evidence).

**Not all RCTs may be used for the analyses of IPRP outcomes.*
***Note that GRADE was used in the 2010 SBU report but not in the 2006 SBU report.*
SR = Systematic Review with narrative synthesis of data; MA = Meta-Analysis; RCT = Randomised Controlled Trial; IPRP = Interdisciplinary Pain Rehabilitation; CLBP = chronic low back pain; FM = fibromyalgia; CP = non-specific chronic pain conditions; TAU = treatment as usual; and WLC = waiting list controls.

Table 2.
Brief conclusions from Systematic Reviews (SR) and Meta-Analyses (MA) of IPRP identified using Dragioti et al.'s search strategy [47].

classified with lower quality since it is impossible to blind IPRP for patients. Different results in the reviews might also depend on the specific criteria for inclusion and the fact that parts of reviews are based on judgements of researchers.

8. Why registry studies?

The results from RCTs, SRs, and MAs must be confirmed in real-life consecutive flow of patients in clinical settings. Direct clinical application of the results from RCTs is not suitable in all situations as these studies might be associated with bias and the patients investigated in RCTs might not represent real-world patients (i.e., insufficient external validity) [59]. Hence, the results from RCTs and SRs must be confirmed in real-life settings, for example, using registry data. This methodology is labelled *practice-based evidence (PBE)* and has been applied in rehabilitation research [60]. An increasing interest in such clinical registries is noted and the International Association for the Study of Pain (IASP) has a special interest group (Pain Registries SIG), which is designed to further increase the interest for evaluating real-world data.

Most real-world observational evaluations of IPRP are based on within-group analyses over time. However, such observational studies are often associated with bias. Creating an objection-free control group in clinical practice in association with registries of IPRP is ethically, economically, and practically impossible. To date, attempts using other types of registries for creating a control group have not been successful [61]. Fortunately, methods have been developed that emulate randomisations based on observational data, which allows comparisons between interventions [62]. Target trial emulations are increasingly applied (e.g., in clinical pharmacology, oncology, cardiovascular diseases, critical care, and rheumatology) and can under appropriate circumstances give valid effect estimations compared to RCTs [63, 64]. When target trial emulations can be adequately performed, they generally yield stronger evidence than other types of observational research designs [63]. However, these are not simple methods or without limitations and biases [65–67]. Although criticised, a first attempt has been made that focuses on sick leave associated with IPRP using data from the SQRP (see below) [68]. If further research and refinements of registries covering IPRP conclude that this methodology is applicable, it would be a great advantage. It would further increase the importance of registries for improving the clinical results of IPRP and other complex interventions for patients with serious chronic pain conditions.

9. The Swedish Quality Registry for Pain Rehabilitation (SQRP) and its goals

9.1 Why a registry?

There are usually two approaches to building a registry, and both influence the architecture and content of the registry. Registries are either built to answer research questions or to provide clinical evaluations to providers at each site. SQRP was built primarily around the second approach. The initiative to start SQRP was taken within the professionals' network, the decision made by the leadership of the units delivering IPRP around 1997. Since its inception, in 1998, the registry has addressed the description of what was being offered at the clinical settings, the overall situation of the patients being admitted, and the changes reported in the included instruments at discharge and 1-year follow-up. Therefore, the SQRP has always worked very closely with the clinicians providing treatment as they are a source of knowledge to be used in the assessment of patients and the evaluation of their progress in the programs as well as describe data at the organization's level. The general goals are given in **Table 3**.

• Develop and secure the quality of care
• Compare outcomes at group level between the Swedish units
• Allow for the participating units to follow-up on their delivery of care
• Based on adequate comparisons with other units, facilitate discussions about improvement plans and practices within each unit

Table 3.
General goals of SQRP.

The registry aims to highlight data on structure, processes, and outcomes. Outcomes are retrieved at the individual, group, unit, and national levels (**Table 4**).

Every year SQRP follows how the registry is used at the clinical level and promotes plans for improvements. Examples of improvement work, using measures of the registry (according to answers to the 2019 survey) are presented in **Table 5**.

9.2 Variables and instruments included in the SQRP in 2021

An overview of the variables and instruments included in the registry (2021) is presented in **Table 6**. Hence, SQRP is mainly a patient-reported registry, including mostly patient-related outcome measures (PROM data) as well as patient-related evaluation measures (PREM data). The PREM variables concern satisfaction with reception/encounter, the site information, degree of participation in the rehabilitation plan, teamwork, and family participation in the program.

Structure			
	Type of intervention		
		Only screening/pain analysis	
		IPRP	
		Other interventions	
	Number of registrations		
Process			
	Time		
	Reasons for discharge		
Results			
	Level of the individual (patient profile and reports)		
	Level of the unit (group reports)		
	Level of the country (yearly reports)		
		Discharge	R 1
		One-year follow-up	R 2
		Analysis (optional)	R 3
		Analysis (optional)	R 4
R = Report.			

Table 4.
Clinical evaluations (levels of analysis).

• Increased patient participation in their rehab and more effective treatment schedules during follow-up
• Increased focus on sick-leave process, contact with the workplace, and physical activity in the program
• Shortened waiting lists
• Increased feedback to patients by means of SQRP data which led to increased motivation to actively work towards a healthier lifestyle
• Focused work on fear of movement to increase physical activity
• Remodelling rehabilitation services to meet patient individual needs
• Broader perspective to increase participation of significant others in rehabilitation
• Regular extraction of the group and individual reports with a focus on results to design specific improvement plans

Table 5.
Examples of improvement work using measures of the registry.

The registry also includes self-reported background information. There are some variables that are evaluated by the professionals in the program (**Table 6**).

Some other Swedish quality registries were built to answer research questions and are now working to adapt the output of information to the needs of clinicians at the sites where healthcare is provided. On the other hand, SQRP has been working to improve its operations to allow for research questions to be explored by improving the validity of its information, reducing dropouts, and enhancing routines to avoid missing values and registration errors. In 2011, a national research network (SQRP research group) was formed through initiatives developed by the SQRP's steering group. This group has developed different research programs focused on the registry, leading to grants from different research funds, dissertations, and many publications. In this way, SQRP is becoming a source of knowledge for researchers interested in finding answers to the complex interventions included and the heterogeneous group receiving treatment.

10. Clinical presentations – results from SQRP

SQRP collects a large amount of self-reported mandatory data concerning pain aspects, psychological distress, interference, health aspects, etc. together with background data from patients referred to specialist pain care in Sweden. The information covering the BPS framework complements information included in the clinical assessments. To determine which variables are generally important in patients with chronic pain, one approach investigates variables important for health aspects.

Pain severity, pain interference, and pain intensity were the most important regressors of health (N > 37 000 patients at baseline) followed by two variables that focus on control of pain and coping with pain, and four variables (also significant) reflecting mood aspects according to a cross-sectional SQRP study (**Figure 2**) [69]. Extent and duration of pain, age, gender, and background variables were not significant regressors.

Another approach is to use PCA to identify variables associated with prominent variations—i.e., high scores. Pain aspects, such as intensity and interference, psychological distress, coping, and health aspects, are the most important and therefore carry the most information for the clinical presentation according to SQRP studies [70, 71].

Type	Variables and instruments
Self-report and background information	
	Socio-demographic data
	Work
	Sick leave
	Pain duration Pain extent
	Attitude towards the future
Self-report, Instruments, and variables	
	Numeric Rating Pain Scale (NRPS)
	The Hospital Anxiety and Depression Scale (HAD)
	Multidimensional Pain Inventory (MPI)
	Health-related life quality (RAND-36)
	Perceived health (the EuroQol Group) (EQ-5D)
	Chronic Pain Acceptance Questionnaire (CPAQ 8)
	Insomnia Severity Index (ISI)
	Perceived work ability index (WAI)
	Kinesiophobia (TAMPA)
	Perceived physical activity (3 items)
	Changes in pain experience (retrospective items)
	Changes in ability to handle life situations (retrospective items)
	Patient satisfaction (six items)
Professional-evaluated variables	
	Diagnosis
	Pain mechanisms
	Expected future financial-support form
	Swedish language ability
	Rehabilitation plan

Table 6.
Variables of SQRP.

It is a clinical experience that patients with the same diagnosis show considerable variations in their presentations and consequences. Therefore, in the context of improving outcomes of interventions, there is a great interest to identify relevant subgroups of chronic pain patients. Most studies have been hypothesis-driven with respect to the input variables for subgrouping. Based on some mandatory variables covering the BPS framework, two subgroups/clusters of patients have been identified from SQRP data (N = 37 100) [70]. The subgroup with the most intense pain intensity/severity had the worst situation regarding psychological distress, interference in daily life, and least life control [70]. Furthermore, according to variables not used as input variables, this subgroup had more pain extent (spreading of pain) and more

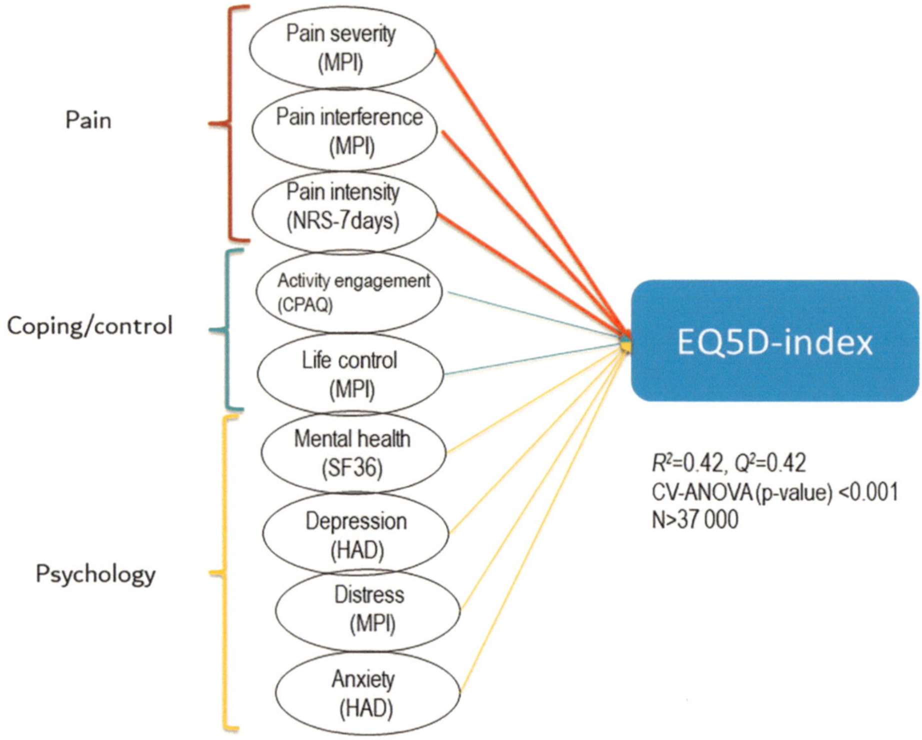

Figure 2.
OPLS regression of health (EQ5D index) using other self reported variables at baseline as regressors. Only significant variables are shown. Data are from [69]. EQ5D-index = The European Quality of Life instrument index; MPI = Multidimensional Pain Inventory; NRS-7days = Average pain intensity the last week rated using a numeric rating scale; CPAQ = Chronic Pain Acceptance Questionnaire; SF36 = The Short Form Health Survey; and HAD = Hospital Anxiety and Depression Scale.

people born outside Europe. Also, smaller SQRP studies report that the patient group is not homogenous and different subgroups have been identified [71, 72].

The Multidimensional Pain Inventory (MPI) classifies patients into subgroups [73, 74]. These subgroups—Adaptive Coper (AC), Dysfunctional (DYS), and Interpersonally Distressed (ID)—were identified in a large cohort from the SQRP (N = 34 513) and the validity of these subgroups of MPI was partially confirmed [75]. However, in contrast to results reported by Turk and Rudy, the subgroups differed in socio-demographic characteristics, pain duration, and pain extent [73]. Hence, factors other than psychosocial may be important for understanding MPI responses.

In an SQRP sample (N > 38 000), the presence of severe anxiety symptoms was detected in 39.5% and the corresponding outcome for depression was 35.2% according to established cut-offs for the Hospital Anxiety and Depression Scale (HAD) [70]. Although psychological distress was common, the strength of the intercorrelations between pain intensity and anxiety and depression scales of HAD were low. The explained variations (r^2) were between 3 and 11%. Two SQRP studies from different times investigated the prevalence of clinical insomnia according to Insomnia Severity Index (ISI) and reported a prevalence between 65 and 66% [76, 77]. Hence, it is important to assess insomnia in patients with complex chronic pain. A network analysis (N = 2 241) reported that psychological variables, such as acceptance and depression mainly were associated with pain interference, whereas the associations with pain intensity and extent together with insomnia were weak [78]. These results taken together may be important for expectations about treatment results (i.e., improvements in psychological distress may not necessarily lead to important improvements in pain intensity).

The pain extent is registered using 36 predetermined anatomical regions in the SQRP, which were summarised and divided into four categories: 1–6 regions with pain (20.6% of patients), 7–12 regions (26.8%), 13–18 regions (22.0%), and 19–36 regions (30.6%) (N = 39 916) [79]. A higher extent of pain spreading was associated with a more severe clinical picture at baseline and longer pain duration with the strongest associations emerging in relation to health and pain aspects (pain intensity, pain interference, and pain duration) [79]; generally, there were at least medium effects sizes (ESs) when comparing the two extreme groups. A cross-sectional multivariate analysis found that pain spreading correlated strongest with general health, vitality, female gender, physical function, pain interference, pain intensity aspects, and pain duration [79].

Patients with chronic pain generally have a higher Body Mass Index (BMI) than healthy controls. Obese patients had a worse pain profile (e.g., pain intensity, pain extent, and pain duration) and more depressive and insomnia symptoms than normal-weight patients according to another SQRP study (N = 3 310) [80].

Most patients referred to the specialist departments in Sweden are women (about 70%). The reasons for this overrepresentation are unclear and are only partially explained by the higher chronic pain prevalence in the population [81, 82]. It is unclear whether sex/gender differences for pain severity exist [83–85]. According to SQRP data, there were generally small differences (generally insignificant ESs) in clinical presentation according to self-reported data between the two genders [86, 87]. Generally, patients born outside Europe had a more severe clinical picture than those born in Europe, for example, with respect to pain intensity and psychological distress (medium ESs) [87]. Patients with only an elementary school education generally reported a worse clinical situation than those with a university education (most variables small to medium ESs).

A cluster analysis using gender, country of birth (Europe vs. outside Europe), and education level (three categories) as input variables identified five subgroups—three subgroups of European women and different education levels, one subgroup of European men, and one subgroup of non-European men and women and different education levels [87]. Prominent differences in clinical presentations, such as pain intensity, psychological distress, interference, life control, and health aspects, were noted between European women with university education and the non-European subgroup (worst situation) (ESs generally medium to large). European women with only elementary school also displayed a worse situation than those with university education.

To summarise, patient groups referred to specialist pain care in Sweden are not homogenous with respect to clinical presentations as distinct subgroups are evident. The clinical presentations show clear associations with pain extent, BMI, and socio-demographic variables.

11. Who participates in IPRP?

Not all patients assessed and registered at baseline in SQRP are selected or choose to participate in IPRP. Unfortunately, the registry does not contain data that can separate these two reasons and other possible reasons, nor does it collect detailed information about assessments, all interventions offered (including IPRP), the interventions' contents and dosages, and patient-related preferences and choices. Assessments of patients, including establishing treatment plans, are clinically necessary and perceived as important by patients. The assessment including a treatment plan with follow-up in primary care per se appears to be associated with positive significant effects on several aspects of the clinical presentation [88]. However, the ESs were insignificant to small.

The Swedish guidelines recommend that IPRP at the specialist level is offered to chronic pain patients with complex clinical presentations, for example, with respect to comorbidities [10]. However, the subgroup with the most severe clinical situation was somewhat underrepresented [70, 89]. Similar results were found for the DYS subgroup of MPI, male gender, and the non-European subgroup [75, 87]. In agreement with this SQRP, data from two university hospital departments showed negative correlations between participation/selection and pain intensity but positive correlations with pain extent [90]. The reasons for these selections are currently unclear and further research is needed.

12. Outcomes of IPRP – based on SQRP studies mainly for the period 2009–2016

IPRP in clinical settings is associated with improvements on the group level with small to medium effect sizes for the majority of the mandatory self-reported outcome variables, for an overall score and retrospective items. Sick-leave data retrieved from the Swedish Social Insurance Agency database show important decreases after IPRP.

12.1 The 22 mandatory outcome variables in SQRP

The outcomes of IPRP were investigated in a study of more than 14 000 patients (**Table 7**) [27]. Significant improvements were generally found except for one or two of the three scales of the second part of MPI (how husband/wife reacts when a patient has pain). Most outcomes showed small ESs and some outcomes were associated with moderate ESs (**Table 2**). For the pre vs. post-IPRP comparisons, three variables had moderate effects sizes—two pain intensity variables and vitality (**Table 7**). At the 12-month follow-up, the same pain intensity variables were associated with moderate effect sizes; this was also the case for pain interference and a health aspect (**Table 6**). The variables of the second part of MPI had insignificant ESs both post IPRP and at the 12-month follow-up.

In 2008, the Swedish government introduced a rehabilitation guarantee to enhance, for example, the implementation of IPRP in primary care. The SQRP created a module to collect data from IPRP in primary care. A relatively small study (N = 397) of the clinical presentation of the patients treated at this care level found that patients presented a considerable complexity [91]. A small study (N = 234) evaluated the outcomes of IPRP in primary care 1 year after discharge for 10 of the 11 variables selected. Eleven outcomes reflecting a BPS approach were evaluated 1 year after IPRP and 10 of these showed significant improvements although ESs were small (0.20–0.49) [92]. A cost-utility analysis indicated that IPRP in primary care was cost-effective [93].

12.2 Overall outcomes of IPRP

The intercorrelations of changes in the 22 mandatory outcome variables (cf. **Table 7**) were investigated using PCAs [27]. Two groups of variables (components), which were not correlated, were identified; the first showed significant intercorrelations between changes in 18 of the outcomes and the second mainly reflected the changes in the second part of MPI together with changes in social support of MPI. Using the score of the first component, a Multivariate Improvement Score (MIS) was defined reflecting changes in the 18 variables [27]. A cluster analysis of MIS was made, and three clusters were identified; retrospectively their baseline situation was analysed. Cluster 1—overall the worst situation pre IPRP—showed the most positive improvements in MIS. Cluster 3—no changes or deterioration in MIS—had the best situation at baseline. Cluster 2 was an intermediary group at baseline and was associated with overall slightly positive MIS improvements [27].

Both post-IPRP and at 12-month follow-up patients retrospectively estimate the degree of positive change in pain and in their ability to handle life situations in general (both rated on five-point Likert scales from markedly increased pain/markedly worsened life situation (score 0) to markedly decreased pain/markedly improved (score 4) [27]. At both time points, most patients reported that their pain situation (57% at both time points), as well as their ability to handle their life situation, had improved (84 and 77%); the two most positive alternatives were added [27].

12.3 Sick leave

All patients undergoing IPRP registered in SQRP between 2007 and 2011 (n=7 297) were linked to the Swedish Social Insurance Agency database and the development of sick leave was analysed [94]. Sick-leave benefits increased during the year before IPRP and decreased after IPRP (analysed up to 2 years after) (**Figure 3**). These reductions in benefits were significant for both men and women. It was concluded that IPRP could positively influence sick-leave benefits for these patients regardless of their sick-leave situation, sex/gender, or policy changes.

A larger study of sick absence for patients included in SQRP (N = 44 241) showed similar results—i.e., sick absence increased from 17% 5 years before to 48% at assessment at the specialist department and thereafter decreased to 38% [95]. Sickness absence history was the strongest predictor of future sickness. Decreases in pain intensity/severity and pain interference but not increases in life control and social support or reduced affective stress during IPRP were associated with decreased risk of being on full-time sick leave 1 year later according to another SQRP study (N = 1 468) from a university department [96]. The same authors reported from a cohort of 2 784 patients that the subgroup DYS of MPI decreased after IPRP [97]. Those belonging to AC or ID had less full-time sick leave 1 year later and therefore the DYS profile was associated with long-term sick leave.

Decreases in sick leave after IPRP were reported in a target trial emulation study using SQRP data (N = 25 613) [68], but the results were not significantly better than for the comparison group. The article was the first target trial emulation attempt using SQRP data (see above). This study has been criticised for its heterogenous comparator group and lack of data concerning other interventions and patient preferences [98]. In addition, this critique emphasised that very complex processes may exist after the assessment when preparing and establishing the rehabilitation/treatment plan. Hence, registries such as SQRP need to collect detailed data concerning assessments, all

Pre vs. post-IPRP							Pre vs. FU					
	Pre		Post IPRP				Pre		FU			
Outcome variables	**Mean**	**SD**	**Mean**	**SD**	***P*-value**	**ES**	**Mean**	**SD**	**Mean**	**SD**	**P-value**	**ES**
NRS-7days	6.86	1.72	5.95	2.09	<0.001	0.45	6.84	1.72	5.78	2.32	<0.001	0.47
HADS-Anxiety	9.00	4.76	7.78	4.55	<0.001	0.32	8.73	4.69	7.38	4.70	<0.001	0.33
HADS-Depression	8.49	4.44	6.70	4.31	<0.001	0.47	8.18	4.37	6.74	4.66	<0.001	0.35
MPI-Pain-severity	4.39	0.93	3.87	1.16	<0.001	**0.52**	4.36	0.91	3.71	1.33	<0.001	**0.56**
MPI-Pain-interference	4.38	1.02	3.94	1.19	<0.001	0.49	4.34	1.02	3.73	1.37	<0.001	**0.54**
MPI-Life Control	2.72	1.10	3.30	1.18	<0.001	0.47	2.77	1.10	3.28	1.27	<0.001	0.40
MPI-Distress	3.46	1.26	2.89	1.38	<0.001	0.42	3.42	1.27	2.92	1.45	<0.001	0.35
MPI-Social support	4.16	1.34	3.95	1.35	<0.001	0.21	4.17	1.33	3.77	1.42	<0.001	0.35
MPI-punish	1.74	1.36	1.72	1.33	0.037	0.02	1.69	1.34	1.69	1.35	0.676	0.01
MPI-protect	2.98	1.40	2.85	1.38	<0.001	0.12	2.96	1.39	2.78	1.40	<0.001	0.16
MPI-distract	2.54	1.19	2.56	1.17	0.043	0.02	2.52	1.17	2.45	1.17	<0.001	0.06
MPI-General activity index	2.44	0.84	2.63	0.82	<0.001	0.26	2.47	0.83	2.64	0.86	<0.001	0.20
EQ-5D-index	0.26	0.31	0.39	0.33	<0.001	0.40	0.27	0.31	0.44	0.34	<0.001	**0.50**
EQ-VAS	41.22	19.09	50.99	21.38	<0.001	0.44	41.90	19.29	52.96	22.87	<0.001	0.46
sf36-pf	52.76	20.58	57.67	21.17	<0.001	0.30	53.07	20.30	59.73	22.57	<0.001	0.36
sf36-rp	12.53	24.40	22.46	33.12	<0.001	0.30	13.07	24.91	27.74	36.32	<0.001	0.39
sf36-bp	24.36	14.49	32.96	17.41	<0.001	**0.52**	24.60	14.11	35.41	20.05	<0.001	**0.56**
sf36-gh	41.70	20.22	46.69	21.88	<0.001	0.29	42.59	20.49	47.35	23.52	<0.001	0.25
sf36-vt	23.95	18.48	35.67	22.76	<0.001	**0.54**	24.96	18.79	34.41	23.85	<0.001	0.41
sf36-sf	47.29	25.19	54.93	25.91	<0.001	0.30	48.95	25.50	57.66	27.05	<0.001	0.32
sf36-re	42.77	42.92	51.15	43.48	<0.001	0.18	44.69	43.17	55.60	43.53	<0.001	0.22
sf36-mh	55.03	21.35	62.55	21.55	<0.001	0.38	56.34	21.15	62.70	22.53	<0.001	0.30

The effect sizes >0.50 are given in bold. The significance (p-values) are reported in the columns to the left of the columns concerning effect sizes. NRS-7days = Pain intensity as measured by a numeric rating scale for the previous 7 days; HADS = Hospital Anxiety and Depression Scale; MPI = Multidimensional Pain Inventory; EQ-5D-index = The index of the European quality of life instrument; EQ-VAS = The European quality of life instrument thermometer-like scale; sf36 = The Short Form (36) Health Survey; subscales; pf = physical functioning; rp = role limitations due to pf physical functioning; bp = bodily pain; gh = general health; vt = vitality; sf = social functioning; re = role limitations due to emotional problems; and mh = mental health.

Table 7.
Mandatory outcome variables at baseline (pre) and immediately after IPRP (post IPRP) (left part; N = 12 999–14 772) and at baseline and at 12-month follow-up (FU) (right part; N = 7 784–8 904). Statistical comparisons are presented with effects sizes (ES, i.e., Cohen's d). Effect sizes in bold were moderate, i.e., Cohen's d ≥ 0.50. These data have been reported in Ringqvist et al. [27].

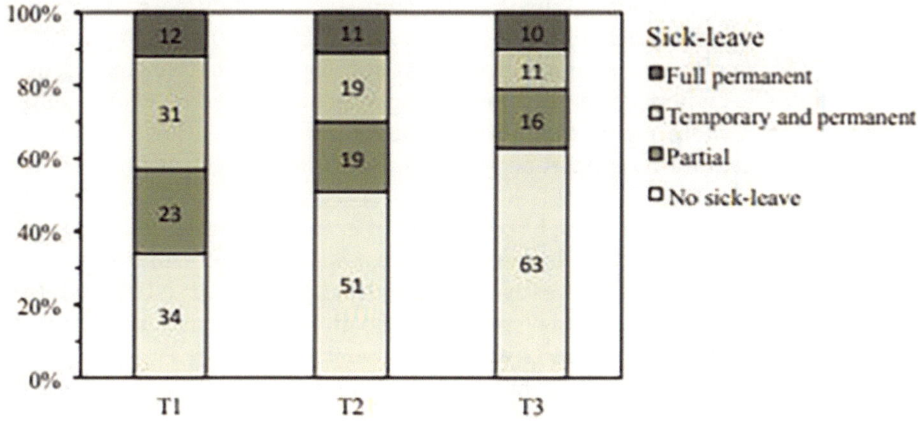

Figure 3.
Level of sick leave at 90–0 days before (T1) IPRP, 320–410 days after (T2) IPRP, and 775–985 days after (T3) IPRP; N = 7 297 (Rivano Fischer et al. [94].

interventions offered (including contents and dosages), as well as patient-related preferences. More details about the clinical departments might also be beneficial [18]. Perhaps one might expect more prominent decreases of sick leave in IPRP than in the comparison group. According to Swedish guidelines, IPRP should be offered to the most complex chronic pain patients, but those participating in IPRP had gross sick leave days the year before IPRP, so that is necessarily not a correct expectation.

12.4 Long-term consequences of unmet needs?

Long-term opioid therapy (LTOT) for chronic pain is unfortunately common in clinical practise despite lack of evidence and serious adverse consequences [99–103]. At a university hospital reporting to SQRP, 30% of the patients referred to a clinical department used opioids daily [104]. These patients had higher pain intensity, more pain interference, lower quality of life, lower activity engagement, and less satisfaction with life than the other patients referred (medium ESs) [104]. Svanberg et al. investigated the opioid prescriptions 2 years after chronic pain patients were assessed for IPRP [105]. Opioid prescriptions were prescribed for 55% of the cohort (N = 1334). The odds of receiving LTOT were similar for those participating and not participating in IPRP. Patient characteristics at baseline/assessment in both these groups could predict LTOT. In those participating in IPRP, dysfunctional pain coping was a predictor; however, in those not participating in IPRP, pain intensity and depressive symptoms were predictors. Taken together, these studies indicate that long-term pharmacological treatment is not optimal for patients who are eligible for IPRP.

13. Who benefits the most from IPRP?

13.1 In relation to clinical presentation and profile

Evidence is contradictory when it comes to clinical presentation pre-treatment. A recent meta-analysis on prognostic factors for IPRP outcome demonstrated that both higher levels of general emotional distress and pain-specific cognitive behavioural factors were related to worse long-term (>6 months) physical functioning post-treatment [106]. However, a similar pattern was not displayed in two large-scale SQRP cohort studies where patients reporting higher levels of perceived disability and suffering displayed slightly greater improvement [27, 70]. Hence, those with the most severe clinical presentations at baseline will display the largest improvements found in SQRP studies [70, 71, 75].

Pain distribution (i.e., spreading of pain) is another factor that needs consideration. Cross-sectional population studies have reported that spreading of pain is significantly associated with pain intensity, depressive disorders, and poor health [107, 108]. In a recent large-scale SQRP cohort study, spreading of pain was associated with poorer outcomes of treatment, but the effects were in the small range [79]. Thus, spreading of pain is important for understanding chronic pain as an indicator of severity, as previously described, and to some extent as a predictor of the poorer outcome of IPRPs.

Psychosocial coping profiles with three subgroups have been derived from the MPI and are commonly used to aid in the assessment of patients with chronic pain. Based on a BPS approach to chronic pain, MPI and its subscales are sensitive to changes in the severity of chronic pain and predict sick leave. The dysfunctional (DYS) subgroup reports high pain severity, marked interference in daily life, high affective distress, low perception of life control, and low levels of activity. The adaptive coper (AC) subgroup is characterised by less severe pain, less interference with activities, less affective distress, and positive perceptions of life control and activity level. The interpersonally distressed (ID) subgroup has been described as perceiving low social support and non-supporting behaviours from significant others [109–111]. Some reports suggest that the DYS and/or ID subgroups have better treatment outcomes than the AC group [109, 112–116], whereas other studies have found no significant differences in outcomes amongst subgroups [110, 111, 117–121]. These results are supported by a large-scale cohort study from the SQRP: DYS and ID subgroups that had the most severe clinical presentation at baseline showed the largest improvement following IPRP [75].

13.2 In relation to socio-demographic variables

The existing literature regarding sex differences in outcomes of IPRP is conflicting—women benefit more [84, 122, 123], no sex differences [124–126], and men benefit more [127, 128]. The outcomes of IPRPs in a primary care study were better in women than in men [92]. A recent large-scale cohort study from SQRP found sex differences in outcomes—women had slightly better results than men [87]. The conflicting results in the literature may be due to different cohorts investigated as well as the choice of outcomes.

An important principle in healthcare is equity (i.e., prioritization of healthcare based on the need of the patient); however, social contexts are seldom considered in studies [129]. Several studies have reported that prevalence of chronic pain, the severity of pain, and disability are inversely related to the socio-economic position and low education, male sex, and/or non-European origin (in European studies), which appear to be associated with lower participation rates and worse IPRP results [129–132].

14. Shortcomings and possible improvements of IPRP

One-fifth of the European adult population lives with at least *moderate* intense chronic pain [12]. Patients with chronic pain describe wide consequences, such as intense and disturbing pain, psychological distress, and insomnia, reduced workability and sick leave, ill health, and low quality of life. Pain conditions caused 21% of all Years Lived with Disability (YLDs), which is a measure of non-fatal health outcomes, globally ahead of 287 other conditions [133]. These striking effects of chronic pain on both the individual and the family and society emphasise the need to improve and develop new treatment methods. Both the systematic reviews and the results from real-world settings indicate the need to improve IPRP.

As described in previous passages, results from IPRP demonstrate low to moderate effect sizes on outcomes with conflicting results concerning effects on RTW. Possible gains for the individual and society might be accomplished with improvements of routines and contents of IPRP. It is thus problematic that IPRP is somewhat heterogenous as this can constitute problems establishing strategies for improvements. As a comparison, *in vitro* fertilization (IVF) has been able to increase success rates from single digits to nearly 50% in largely the same time frames as IPRP have existed, which at least partly can be attributed to registries with clear and transparent descriptions of different protocols and results [134]. It could be advantageous for a registry such as the SQRP to specify protocols to increase transparency when interpreting results, which might possibly inspire evolvement and larger effect sizes on outcomes of IPRP. Currently, IPRP has different approaches and might or might not include, for example, sleep interventions, opioid tapering, workplace interventions, and treatments for psychiatric comorbidities. Moreover, CBT is a large umbrella entailing a multitude of techniques, one of which is exposure. Interventions using exposure have shown beneficial results and it is possible that IPRP, including exposure, might produce better results. Therefore, registries should specify the CBT techniques used [135].

The results obtained by the SQRP show that the subgroup of patients with a relatively better clinical picture before IPRP had worse IPRP results than those with a more severe clinical picture [70]. The patient group with the more difficult clinical picture is most improved by IPRP but not so much that they reach the subgroup with a better clinical picture. Both circumstances indicate a need for the development of IPRP so that IPRP better matches the clinical picture. For example, individual treatments, short interventions, small group activities with different content to be selected for individual patients, individual treatments with the team as a backup, and closer communication with primary care to ensure that recommendations can improve the lives of patients without going through extensive IPRPs, which might be more appropriate for the less severe subgroups [15]. In the long run, this could mean that different IPRPs are available in clinical settings. In addition, the activated, mainly unknown, neurobiological pain mechanisms might not be sufficiently targeted by the various interventions in IPRP.

Early interventions might also improve results. The association between prominent pain extent (i.e., widespread pain) and pain duration supports the concept of early intervention as clinically important and an opportunity to possibly change prognosis with conceivable gains for the individual and society. Early interventions with psychological risk factor screening combined with protocols for active collaboration between caregivers and key stakeholders have been demonstrated to positively impact return to work [136].

Poorer results of IPRP in socially more challenged populations might suggest that equal care is not delivered. For example, IPRP in Sweden may not meet the needs of patients outside Europe. It has been suggested that in particularly non-Western backgrounds might be associated with other attitudes towards self-management interventions, passive symptom-focused management strategies, as well as pharmacological treatments [137], which could influence IPRP outcomes. Selection to participation in IPRP and outcomes might also be disadvantaged by different biases of professionals towards non-European patients and/or insufficient knowledge about immigration and other cultures. Lower socio-economic groups may differ from health professionals in culture, beliefs, and communication style, resulting in disadvantages and possibly feelings of inferiority. Carr and Moffet provocatively suggest that CBT interventions designed by middle-class health professionals are more suitable for middle-class patients [130]. Also, a common goal of IPRP is increased physical functioning; however, exercise and sports activities are less likely to be adopted by people in lower socio-economic groups than by people in higher socio-economic groups [138–140].

This raises important questions concerning fairness and equality. The combination of sex, education, and country of birth needs to be considered in the assessment of chronic pain patients and is important to consider when optimising the content and delivery of IPRP in clinical practice. IPRPs need to be adapted and educational elements fitted to meet different learning styles using techniques to increase retention of new information as described in textbooks, such as 'Explain pain supercharged' [141]. In addition, Carr and Moffet suggest that a useful starting point when considering how to improve treatments is the knowledge that people in socially-deprived areas endure higher levels of stress and lower perceived control [130]. Techniques are suggested to reduce stress and learned helplessness and include involving patients in shared decision-making of treatment, increased social support, incorporating individual coaching where the individual can learn to take more control, and additional validation where IPRPs are supplemented by phone calls between sessions. When attendance is challenged, audio and video material could be provided for patients unable to attend.

15. Conclusions

The patient group with chronic/persistent pain conditions referred to specialist care in Sweden are heterogenous and different subgroups exist. The clinical presentations show clear associations with the extent of pain spreading, BMI, and socio-demographic variables. IPRP is an evidence-based intervention for chronic pain patients who suffer from substantial consequences of their chronic pain condition regarding function, social, and/or psychological well-being. The intervention is complex and is delivered by an interdisciplinary team of professionals in close collaboration with the patient. Observational analyses of IPRP in clinical settings agree with the evidence presented in SRs and MAs. However, results differ amongst subgroups and benefits are not present for all patients. Interestingly, those with the most severe clinical presentation, according to registry data, an assessment benefit most from IPRP. Also, socio-economic factors can influence results and need to be addressed to warrant more equal opportunities for improvement in IPRP.

Units offering IPRPs differ in their strategies, services, and resources, both in intensity and duration, as well as in the degree of individual interventions opposed to group treatment. This diversity should be addressed by researchers and incorporated in studies by looking into the impact of referral flow, traditions, and the heterogeneity of the patients assessed. Methods other than randomised studies, such as emulated trials, repeated measured for patients (patients as controls) should be refined to enhance the potential gaining of analysing real-life information in registries.

There is thus room for enhancement of IPRP possibly by a more structured use of registries. Furthermore, pain registries should expand to cover a variety of clinical efforts designed to meet the individual needs of people with chronic pain and to deliver information about the effectiveness of these measures.

Conflict of interest

The authors declare no conflict of interest.

Author details

Björn Gerdle[1]*, Marcelo Rivano Fischer[2,3] and Åsa Ringqvist[3]

1 Pain and Rehabilitation Centre, and Department of Health, Medicine and Caring Sciences, Linköping University, Linköping, Sweden

2 Faculty of Medicine, Department of Clinical Sciences, Lund University, Lund, Sweden

3 Department of Neurosurgery and Pain Rehabilitation, Skåne University Hospital, Lund, Sweden

*Address all correspondence to: bjorn.gerdle@liu.se

References

[1] Gatchel R, Peng Y, Peters M, Fuchs P, Turk D. The biopsychosocial approach to chronic pain: Scientific advances and future directions. Psychological Bulletin. 2007;**133**:581-624

[2] Linton S, Bergbom S. Understanding the link between depression and pain. Scandinavian Journal of Pain. 2011;**2**: 47-54

[3] Ossipov MH, Dussor GO, Porreca F. Central modulation of pain. The Journal of Clinical Investigation. 2010;**120**(11): 3779-3787

[4] Dworkin RH, Turk DC, Farrar JT, Haythornthwaite JA, Jensen MP, Katz NP, et al. Core outcome measures for chronic pain clinical trials: IMMPACT recommendations. Pain. 2005;**113**(1–2):9-19

[5] WHO. International Classification of Functioning, Disability and Health (ICF). 2001. Available from: https://apps.who.int/iris/handle/10665/42407

[6] Loeser J. Multidisciplinary pain management. In: Merskey H, Loeser J, Dubner R, editors. The Paths of Pain 1975–2005. Seattle: IASP; 2005. p. 511

[7] Turk D, Stanos S, Palermo T, Paice J, Jaminson R, Gordon D, et al. Interdisciplinary Pain Management. Available from: http://www.americanpainsociety.org/uploads/pdfs/2010%20Interdisciplinary%20White%20Paper-FINAL.pdf2010

[8] Kaiser U, Treede RD, Sabatowski R. Multimodal pain therapy in chronic noncancer pain-gold standard or need for further clarification? Pain. 2017; **158**(10):1853-1859

[9] Brecht D, Stephens J, Gatchel R. Interdisciplinary pain management programs in the treatment of pain conditions. In: Noe C, editor. Pain Management for Clinicians. Cham: Springer; 2020

[10] Gerdle B, Stålnacke B-M, Söderlund A, Åsenlöf P. Indikation för multimodal rehabilitering vid långvarig smärta. Stockholm: Nationella Medicinska Indikationer (Svenska Läkaresällskapet, Sveriges Kommuner och Landsting, Socialstyrelsen och SBU); 2011. Document no: 2011:02

[11] Cousins MJ, Lynch ME. The declaration Montreal: Access to pain management is a fundamental human right. Pain. 2011;**152**(12):2673-2674

[12] Breivik H, Collett B, Ventafridda V, Cohen R, Gallacher D. Survey of chronic pain in Europe: Prevalence, impact on daily life, and treatment. European Journal of Pain. 2006;**10**(4):287-333

[13] Dahlhamer J, Lucas J, Zelaya C, Nahin R, Mackey S, DeBar L, et al. Prevalence of chronic pain and high-impact chronic pain among adults – United States, 2016. MMWR. Morbidity and Mortality Weekly Report. 2018; **67**(36):1001-1006

[14] Engel G. The need for a new medical model: A challenge for biomedicine. Science. 1977;**196**:129-136

[15] McGeary D, McGeary C, Nabity P, Villarreal R, Kivisalu T, Gatchel R. Improving stress reduction and wellness in interdisciplinary chronic pain management: Is transdisciplinary care a better option? Journal of Applied Biobehavioral Research. 2016;**21**:205-215

[16] Stanos S. Focused review of interdisciplinary pain rehabilitation programs for chronic pain management.

Current Pain and Headache Reports. 2012;**16**:147-152

[17] Garschagen A, Steegers MA, van Bergen AH, Jochijms JA, Skrabanja TL, Vrijhoef HJ, et al. Is there a need for including spiritual care in interdisciplinary rehabilitation of chronic pain patients? Investigating an Innovative Strategy. Pain Practice. 2015; **15**(7):671-687

[18] Rivano Fischer M, Schults M, Stålnacke B, Ekholm J, Persson E, Löfgren M. Variability in patient characteristics and service provision of interdisciplinary pain rehabilitation: A study using the Swedish national quality registry for pain rehabilitation. Journal of Rehabilitation Medicine. 2020;**52**(11): jrm00128

[19] Waterschoot FPC, Dijkstra PU, Hollak N, de Vries HJ, Geertzen JHB, Reneman MF. Dose or content? Effectiveness of pain rehabilitation programs for patients with chronic low back pain: A systematic review. Pain. 2014;**155**(1):179-189

[20] Dragioti E, Bjork M, Larsson B, Gerdle B. A meta-epidemiological appraisal of the effects of interdisciplinary multimodal pain therapy dosing for chronic low back pain. Journal of Clinical Medicine. 2019;**8**(6):871

[21] Tseli E, LoMartire R, Vixner L, Grooten WJA, Gerdle B, Ang BO. What is the effectiveness of different duration interdisciplinary treatment programs in patients with chronic pain? A large-scale longitudinal register study. Journal of Clinical Medicine. 2020;**9**(9):2788

[22] Vowles KE, McCracken LM, Eccleston C. Processes of change in treatment for chronic pain: The contributions of pain, acceptance, and catastrophizing. European Journal of Pain. 2007;**11**(7):779-787

[23] SBU. Methods for treatment of chronic pain a systematic review of the literature (In Swedish: Metoder för behandling av långvarig smärta: En systematisk litteraturöversikt). Vol. 177. No. 1. Stockholm: SBU – Swedish Council on Health Technology Assessment; 2006. pp. 1-504

[24] Henry SG, Bell RA, Fenton JJ, Kravitz RL. Goals of chronic pain management: Do patients and primary care physicians agree and does it matter? The Clinical Journal of Pain. 2017;**33**(11): 955-961

[25] McCracken LM, Zhao-O'Brien J. General psychological acceptance and chronic pain: There is more to accept than the pain itself. European Journal of Pain. 2010;**14**(2):170-175

[26] Thompson M, McCracken LM. Acceptance and related processes in adjustment to chronic pain. Current Pain and Headache Reports. 2011;**15**(2):144-151

[27] Ringqvist Å, Dragioti E, Björk M, Larsson B, Gerdle B. Moderate and stable pain reductions as a result of Interdisciplinary Pain Rehabilitation—A cohort study from the Swedish quality registry for pain rehabilitation (SQRP). Journal of Clinical Medicine. 2019;**8**:905

[28] Epton T, Currie S, Armitage CJ. Unique effects of setting goals on behavior change: Systematic review and meta-analysis. Journal of Consulting and Clinical Psychology. 2017;**85**(12):1182-1198

[29] Schut HA, Stam HJ. Goals in rehabilitation teamwork. Disability and Rehabilitation. 1994;**16**(4):223-226

[30] Doran G. There's a S.M.A.R.T. way to write management's goals and

objectives. Management Review. 1981; **70**(11):35-36

[31] Turk DC, Dworkin RH, Allen RR, Bellamy N, Brandenburg N, Carr DB, et al. Core outcome domains for chronic pain clinical trials: IMMPACT recommendations. Pain. 2003;**106**(3): 337-345

[32] Kaiser U, Kopkow C, Deckert S, Neustadt K, Jacobi L, Cameron P, et al. Developing a core outcome-domain set to assessing effectiveness of interdisciplinary multimodal pain therapy: The VAPAIN consensus statement on core outcome-domains. Pain. 2018;**159**(4):673-683

[33] Zidarov D, Zidarova-Carrié A, Visca R, Miller J, Brecht K, Viens N, et al. Core patient-reported outcome domains for routine clinical care in chronic pain management: Patients' and healthcare professionals' perspective. Quality of Life Research. 2020;**29**(7):2007-2020

[34] Gerdle B, Molander P, Stenberg G, Stalnacke BM, Enthoven P. Weak outcome predictors of multimodal rehabilitation at one-year follow-up in patients with chronic pain—A practice based evidence study from two SQRP centres. BMC Musculoskeletal Disorders. 2016;**17**(1):490

[35] Kamper SJ, Apeldoorn AT, Chiarotto A, Smeets RJ, Ostelo RW, Guzman J, et al. Multidisciplinary biopsychosocial rehabilitation for chronic low back pain. Cochrane Database of Systematic Reviews. 2014;**9**: Cd000963

[36] SBU. Rehabilitation of chronic pain [In Swedish: Rehabilitering vid långvarig smärta. En systematisk litteraturöversikt]. Vol. 198. Stockholm: SBU – Swedish Council on Health Technology Assessment; 2010. pp. 1-286

[37] Scascighini L, Toma V, Dober-Spielmann S, Sprott H. Multidisciplinary treatment for chronic pain: A systematic review of interventions and outcomes. Rheumatology. 2008;**47**(5):670-678

[38] Papadopoulou D, Fassoulaki A, Tsoulas C, Siafaka I, Vadalouca A. A meta-analysis to determine the effect of pharmacological and non-pharmacological treatments on fibromyalgia symptoms comprising OMERACT-10 response criteria. Clinical Rheumatology. 2016;**35**(3):573-586

[39] Arnold LM, Williams DA, Hudson JI, Martin SA, Clauw DJ, Crofford LJ, et al. Development of responder definitions for fibromyalgia clinical trials. Arthritis and Rheumatism. 2012;**64**(3):885-894

[40] Vervoort VM, Vriezekolk JE, van den Ende CH. Development of responder criteria for multicomponent non-pharmacological treatment in fibromyalgia. Clinical and Experimental Rheumatology. 2017;**35**:86-92

[41] Grimby-Ekman A, Kim M, Stankovic N, Mannheimer C. Multidimensional health changes after a multimodal pain rehabilitation program: A registry-based study. Pain reports. 2021;**6**(2):e938

[42] Feise RJ. Do multiple outcome measures require p-value adjustment? BMC Medical Research Methodology. 2002;**2**:8

[43] Turk DC, Dworkin RH, McDermott MP, Bellamy N, Burke LB, Chandler JM, et al. Analyzing multiple endpoints in clinical trials of pain treatments: IMMPACT recommendations. Initiative on methods, measurement, and pain assessment in clinical trials. Pain. 2008;**139**(3):485-493

[44] Bagiella E. Clinical trials in rehabilitation: Single or multiple

outcomes? Archives of Physical Medicine and Rehabilitation. 2009;**90** (Suppl. 11):S17-S21

[45] Tyler KM, Normand SL, Horton NJ. The use and abuse of multiple outcomes in randomized controlled depression trials. Contemporary Clinical Trials. 2011;**32**(2):299-304

[46] Teixeira-Pinto A, Mauri L. Statistical analysis of noncommensurate multiple outcomes. Circulation. Cardiovascular Quality and Outcomes. 2011;**4**(6): 650-656

[47] Dragioti E, Dong HJ, Larsson B, Gerdle B. Reported outcomes in published systematic reviews of interdisciplinary pain treatment: Protocol for a systematic overview. JMIR Research Protocols. 2020;**9**(5):e17795

[48] Nielson WR, Weir R. Biopsychosocial approaches to the treatment of chronic pain. The Clinical Journal of Pain. 2001;**17** (Suppl. 4):S114-S127

[49] Guzmán J, Esmail R, Karjalainen K, Malmivaara A, Irvin E, Bombardier C. Multidisciplinary bio-psycho-social rehabilitation for chronic low back pain. Cochrane Database of Systematic Reviews. 2002;**1**:Cd000963

[50] van Geen JW, Edelaar MJ, Janssen M, van Eijk JT. The long-term effect of multidisciplinary back training: A systematic review. Spine (Phila Pa 1976). 2007;**32**(2):249-255

[51] Norlund A, Ropponen A, Alexanderson K. Multidisciplinary interventions: Review of studies of return to work after rehabilitation for low back pain. Journal of Rehabilitation Medicine. 2009;**41**(3):115-121

[52] Häuser W, Bernardy K, Arnold B, Offenbächer M, Schiltenwolf M. Efficacy of multicomponent treatment in fibromyalgia syndrome: A meta-analysis of randomized controlled clinical trials. Arthritis and Rheumatism. 2009;**61**(2): 216-224

[53] van Middelkoop M, Rubinstein SM, Kuijpers T, Verhagen AP, Ostelo R, Koes BW, et al. A systematic review on the effectiveness of physical and rehabilitation interventions for chronic non-specific low back pain. European Spine Journal. 2011;**20**(1):19-39

[54] Gianola S, Andreano A, Castellini G, Moja L, Valsecchi MG. Multidisciplinary biopsychosocial rehabilitation for chronic low back pain: The need to present minimal important differences units in meta-analyses. Health and Quality of Life Outcomes. 2018;**16**(1):91

[55] Casey MB, Smart KM, Segurado R, Doody C. Multidisciplinary-based rehabilitation (MBR) compared with active physical interventions for pain and disability in adults with chronic pain: A systematic review and meta-analysis. The Clinical Journal of Pain. 2020;**36**(11):874-886

[56] Martinez-Calderon J, Flores-Cortes M, Morales-Asencio JM, Fernandez-Sanchez M, Luque-Suarez A. Which interventions enhance pain self-efficacy in people with chronic musculoskeletal pain? A systematic review with meta-analysis of randomized controlled trials, including over 12000 participants. The Journal of Orthopaedic and Sports Physical Therapy. 2020; **50**(8):418-430

[57] Martinez-Calderon J, Flores-Cortes M, Morales-Asencio JM, Luque-Suarez A. Conservative interventions reduce fear in individuals with chronic low back pain: A systematic review. Archives of Physical Medicine and Rehabilitation. 2020;**101**(2):329-358

[58] Martinez-Calderon J, Flores-Cortes M, Morales-Asencio JM, Luque-Suarez A. Intervention therapies to reduce pain-related fear in fibromyalgia syndrome: A systematic review of randomized clinical trials. Pain Medicine. 2021;**22**(2): 481-498

[59] Hong JC. Strategies to turn real-world data into real-world knowledge. JAMA Network Open. 2021;**4**(10): e2128045

[60] Whiteneck GG, Gassaway J. SCIRehab uses practice-based evidence methodology to associate patient and treatment characteristics with outcomes. Archives of Physical Medicine and Rehabilitation. 2013;**94**(Suppl. 4):S67-S74

[61] Sennehed CP, Stigmar K, Grahn B, Fischer MR, Forsbrand M, Nyberg A, et al. Evaluation of a multimodal pain rehabilitation programme in primary care based on clinical register data: A feasibility study. Primary Health Care Research & Development. 2020;**21**:e2

[62] Hernan MA, Robins JM. Using big data to emulate a target trial when a randomized trial is not available. American Journal of Epidemiology. 2016;**183**(8):758-764

[63] Admon AJ, Donnelly JP, Casey JD, Janz DR, Russell DW, Joffe AM, et al. Emulating a novel clinical trial using existing observational data. Predicting results of the prevent study. Annals of the American Thoracic Society. 2019; **16**(8):998-1007

[64] Matthews AA, Szummer K, Dahabreh IJ, Lindahl B, Erlinge D, Feychting M, et al. Comparing effect estimates in randomized trials and observational studies from the same population: An application to percutaneous coronary intervention. Journal of the American Heart Association. 2021;**10**(11):e020357

[65] Franklin JM, Patorno E, Desai RJ, Glynn RJ, Martin D, Quinto K, et al. Emulating randomized clinical trials with nonrandomized real-world evidence studies: First results from the RCT duplicate initiative. Circulation. 2021;**143**(10):1002-1013

[66] Groenwold RHH. Trial emulation and real-world evidence. JAMA Network Open. 2021;**4**(3):e213845

[67] Zhao SS, Lyu H, Solomon DH, Yoshida K. Improving rheumatoid arthritis comparative effectiveness research through causal inference principles: Systematic review using a target trial emulation framework. Annals of the Rheumatic Diseases. 2020;**79**(7): 883-890

[68] LoMartire R, Bjork M, Dahlstrom O, Constan L, Frumento P, Vixner L, et al. The value of interdisciplinary treatment for sickness absence in chronic pain: A nationwide register-based cohort study. European Journal of Pain. 2021;**25**(10): 2190-2201

[69] Molander P, Dong HJ, Ang B, Enthoven P, Gerdle B. The role of pain in chronic pain patients' perception of health-related quality of life: A cross-sectional SQRP study of 40,000 patients. Scandinavian Journal of Pain. 2018; **18**(3):417-429

[70] Gerdle B, Akerblom S, Brodda Jansen G, Enthoven P, Ernberg M, Dong HJ, et al. Who benefits from multimodal rehabilitation—An exploration of pain, psychological distress, and life impacts in over 35,000 chronic pain patients identified in the Swedish Quality Registry for Pain Rehabilitation. Journal of Pain Research. 2019;**12**:891-908

[71] Gerdle B, Åkerblom S, Stålnacke B-M, Brodda Jansen G, Enthoven P, Ernberg M, et al. The importance of emotional distress, cognitive behavioural factors and pain for life impact at baseline and for outcomes after rehabilitation – A SQRP study of more than 20000 chronic pain patients. Scandinavian Journal of Pain. 2019;**19**(4):693-711

[72] Backryd E, Persson EB, Larsson AI, Fischer MR, Gerdle B. Chronic pain patients can be classified into four groups: Clustering-based discriminant analysis of psychometric data from 4665 patients referred to a multidisciplinary pain centre (a SQRP study). PLoS One. 2018;**13**(2):e0192623

[73] Turk D, Rudy T. Toward an empirically derived taxonomy pf chronic pain patients: Integration of psychological assessment data. Journal of Consulting and Clinical Psychology. 1988;**56**:233-238

[74] Turk DC. The potential of treatment matching for subgroups of patients with chronic pain: Lumping versus splitting. The Clinical Journal of Pain. 2005;**21**(1):44-55

[75] Gerdle B, Cervin M, Rivano Fischer M, Ringqvist A. Outcomes of interdisciplinary pain rehabilitation across subgroups of the multidimensional pain inventory—A Study from the Swedish quality registry for pain rehabilitation. Pain Practice. 2021;**21**(6):662-679

[76] Alfoldi P, Wiklund T, Gerdle B. Comorbid insomnia in patients with chronic pain: A study based on the Swedish quality registry for pain rehabilitation (SQRP). Disability and Rehabilitation. 2014;**36**(20):1661-1669

[77] Lind J, Andrell P, Grimby-Ekman A. Insomnia symptoms and chronic pain among patients participating in a pain rehabilitation program—A registry study. Journal of Clinical Medicine. 2021;**10**(18):4040

[78] Akerblom S, Cervin M, Perrin S, Rivano Fischer M, Gerdle B, McCracken LM. A network analysis of clinical variables in chronic pain: A study from the Swedish quality registry for pain rehabilitation (SQRP). Pain Medicine. 2021;**22**(7):1591-1602

[79] Gerdle B, Rivano Fischer M, Cervin M, Ringqvist A. Spreading of pain in patients with chronic pain is related to pain duration and clinical presentation and weakly associated with outcomes of interdisciplinary pain rehabilitation: A cohort study from the Swedish quality registry for pain rehabilitation (SQRP). Journal of Pain Research. 2021;**14**:173-187

[80] Dong HJ, Larsson B, Rivano Fischer M, Gerdle B. Facing obesity in pain rehabilitation clinics: Profiles of physical activity in patients with chronic pain and obesity—A study from the Swedish quality registry for pain rehabilitation (SQRP). PLoS One. 2020;**15**(9):e0239818

[81] Bergman S, Herrstrom P, Hogstrom K, Petersson IF, Svensson B, Jacobsson LT. Chronic musculoskeletal pain, prevalence rates, and sociodemographic associations in a Swedish population study. The Journal of Rheumatology. 2001;**28**(6):1369-1377

[82] Gerdle B, Bjork J, Henriksson C, Bengtsson A. Prevalence of current and chronic pain and their influences upon work and healthcare-seeking: A population study. The Journal of Rheumatology. 2004;**31**(7):1399-1406

[83] Bartley EJ, Fillingim RB. Sex differences in pain: A brief review of

clinical and experimental findings. British Journal of Anaesthesia. 2013; **111**(1):52-58

[84] Pieh C, Altmeppen J, Neumeier S, Loew T, Angerer M, Lahmann C. Gender differences in outcomes of a multimodal pain management program. Pain. 2012; **153**(1):197-202

[85] Unruh AM. Gender variations in clinical pain experience. Pain. 1996;**65** (2–3):123-167

[86] Rovner GS, Sunnerhagen KS, Bjorkdahl A, Gerdle B, Borsbo B, Johansson F, et al. Chronic pain and sex-differences; women accept and move, while men feel blue. PLoS One. 2017; **12**(4):e0175737

[87] Gerdle B, Boersma K, Asenlof P, Stalnacke BM, Larsson B, Ringqvist A. Influences of sex, education, and country of birth on clinical presentations and overall outcomes of interdisciplinary pain rehabilitation in chronic pain patients: A cohort study from the Swedish quality registry for pain rehabilitation (SQRP). Journal of Clinical Medicine. 2020;**9**(8):2374

[88] Merrick D, Sundelin G, Stalnacke BM. An observational study of two rehabilitation strategies for patients with chronic pain, focusing on sick leave at one-year follow-up. Journal of Rehabilitation Medicine. 2013;**45**(10):1049-1057

[89] Svanberg M, Stalnacke BM, Enthoven P, Brodda-Jansen G, Gerdle B, Boersma K. Impact of emotional distress and pain-related fear on patients with chronic pain: Subgroup analysis of patients referred to multimodal rehabilitation. Journal of Rehabilitation Medicine. 2017;**49**(4):354-361

[90] Enthoven P, Molander P, Oberg B, Stalnacke BM, Stenberg G, Gerdle B. Do pain characteristics guide selection for multimodal pain rehabilitation? Journal of Rehabilitation Medicine. 2017;**49**(2): 161-169

[91] Stenberg G, Enthoven P, Molander P, Gerdle B, Stalnacke BM. Patients selected to participate in multimodal pain rehabilitation programmes in primary care—A multivariate cross-sectional study focusing on gender and sick leave. Scandinavian Journal of Pain. 2020; **20**(3):511-524

[92] Pietila-Holmner E, Enthoven P, Gerdle B, Molander P, Stalnacke BM. Long-term outcomes of multimodal rehabilitation in primary care for patients with chronic pain. Journal of Rehabilitation Medicine. 2020;**52**(2): jrm00023

[93] Eklund K, Stalnacke BM, Stenberg G, Enthoven P, Gerdle B, Sahlen KG. A cost-utility analysis of multimodal pain rehabilitation in primary healthcare. Scandinavian Journal of Pain. 2021;**21**(1):48-58

[94] Rivano Fischer M, Persson E, Stålnacke B, Schult M, Löfgren M. Return to work after interdisciplinary pain rehabilitation: One- and two-years follow-up based on the Swedish quality registry for pain rehabilitation. Journal of Rehabilitation Medicine. 2019;**51**: 281-289

[95] LoMartire R, Dahlstrom O, Bjork M, Vixner L, Frumento P, Constan L, et al. Predictors of sickness absence in a clinical population with chronic pain. The Journal of Pain. 2021;**22**(10): 1180-1194

[96] Nyberg VE, Novo M, Sjolund BH. Do Multidimensional Pain Inventory scale score changes indicate risk of receiving sick leave benefits 1 year after

a pain rehabilitation programme? Disability and Rehabilitation. 2011;**33** (17–18):1548-1556

[97] Nyberg VE, Novo M, Sjolund BH. Changes in multidimensional pain inventory profile after a pain rehabilitation programme indicate the risk of receiving sick leave benefits one year later. Journal of Rehabilitation Medicine. 2014;**46**(10):1006-1013

[98] Rivano Fischer M, Stalnacke BM. Comment on 'The value of interdisciplinary treatment for sickness absence in chronic pain: A nationwide register-based cohort study'. European Journal of Pain. 2022;**26**(2):543-544

[99] Chaparro LE, Furlan AD, Deshpande A, Mailis-Gagnon A, Atlas S, Turk DC. Opioids compared with placebo or other treatments for chronic low back pain: An update of the Cochrane review. Spine (Phila Pa 1976). 2014;**39**(7):556-563

[100] Krebs EE, Gravely A, Nugent S, Jensen AC, DeRonne B, Goldsmith ES, et al. Effect of opioid vs nonopioid medications on pain-related function in patients with chronic back pain or hip or knee osteoarthritis pain: The SPACE randomized clinical trial. Journal of the American Medical Association. 2018; **319**(9):872-882

[101] Chou R, Turner JA, Devine EB, Hansen RN, Sullivan SD, Blazina I, et al. The effectiveness and risks of long-term opioid therapy for chronic pain: A systematic review for a national institutes of health pathways to prevention workshop. Annals of Internal Medicine. 2015;**162**(4):276-286

[102] Sullivan MD. Depression effects on long-term prescription opioid use, abuse, and addiction. The Clinical Journal of Pain. 2018;**34**(9):878-884

[103] Von Korff M, Kolodny A, Deyo RA, Chou R. Long-term opioid therapy reconsidered. Annals of Internal Medicine. 2011;**155**(5):325-328

[104] Kallman TF, Backryd E. Prevalence of analgesic use in patients with chronic pain referred to a multidisciplinary pain centre and its correlation with patient-reported outcome measures: A cross-sectional, registry-based study. Journal of Rehabilitation Medicine. 2020;**52**(11): jrm00126

[105] Svanberg M, Stalnacke BM, Quinn PD, Boersma K. Opioid prescriptions in chronic pain rehabilitation. A prospective study on the prevalence and association between individual patient characteristics and opioids. Journal of Clinical Medicine. 2021;**10**(10):2130

[106] Tseli E, Boersma K, Stalnacke BM, Enthoven P, Gerdle B, Ang BO, et al. Prognostic factors for physical functioning after multidisciplinary rehabilitation in patients with chronic musculoskeletal pain: A systematic review and meta-analysis. The Clinical Journal of Pain. 2019;**35**(2):148-173

[107] Dragioti E, Larsson B, Bernfort L, Levin LA, Gerdle B. Prevalence of different pain categories based on pain spreading on the bodies of older adults in Sweden: A descriptive-level and multilevel association with demographics, comorbidities, medications, and certain lifestyle factors (PainS65+). Journal of Pain Research. 2016;**9**:1131-1141

[108] Dragioti E, Larsson B, Bernfort L, Levin LA, Gerdle B. A cross-sectional study of factors associated with the number of anatomical pain sites in an actual elderly general population: Results from the PainS65+ cohort. Journal of Pain Research. 2017;**10**:2009-2019

[109] Riipinen M, Niemisto L, Lindgren KA, Hurri H. Psychosocial differences as predictors for recovery from chronic low back pain following manipulation, stabilizing exercises and physician consultation or physician consultation alone. Journal of Rehabilitation Medicine. 2005;**37**(3): 152-158

[110] Gatchel RJ, Noe CE, Pulliam C, Robbins H, Deschner M, Gajraj NM, et al. A preliminary study of multidimensional pain inventory profile differences in predicting treatment outcome in a heterogeneous cohort of patients with chronic pain. The Clinical Journal of Pain. 2002;**18**(3): 139-143

[111] Persson E, Eklund M, Lexell J, Rivano-Fischer M. Psychosocial coping profiles after pain rehabilitation: Associations with occupational performance and patient characteristics. Disability and Rehabilitation. 2017; **39**(3):251-260

[112] Turk D, Okifuji A, Sinclair J, Starz T. Differential responses by psychosocial subgroups of fibromyalgia syndrome patients to an interdisciplinary treatment. Arthritis Care and Research. 1998;**11**(5):397-404

[113] Turk DC, Zaki HS, Rudy TE. Effects of intraoral appliance and biofeedback/ stress management alone and in combination in treating pain and depression in patients with temporomandibular disorders. The Journal of Prosthetic Dentistry. 1993; **70**(2):158-164

[114] Harlacher U, Persson A, Rivano-Fischer M, Sjölund B. Using data from multidimensional pain inventory subscales to assess functioning in pain rehabilitation. International Journal of Rehabilitation Research. 2011;**34**:14-21

[115] Strategier LD, Chwalisz K, Altmaier EM, Russell DW, Lehmann TR. Multidimensional assessment of chronic low back pain: Predicting treatment outcomes. Journal of Clinical Psychology in Medical Settings. 1997;**4**(1):91-110

[116] Soderlund A, Denison E. Classification of patients with whiplash associated disorders (WAD): Reliable and valid subgroups based on the multidimensional pain inventory (MPI-S). European Journal of Pain. 2006; **10**(2):113-119

[117] van der Hulst M, Vollenbroek-Hutten MM, Groothuis-Oudshoorn KG, Hermens HJ. Multidisciplinary rehabilitation treatment of patients with chronic low back pain: A prognostic model for its outcome. The Clinical Journal of Pain. 2008;**24**(5):421-430

[118] Davis PJ, Reeves JL, Graff-Radford SB, Hastie BA, Naliboff BD. Multidimensional subgroups in migraine: Differential treatment outcome to a pain medicine program. Pain Medicine. 2003;**4**(3):215-222

[119] Bergstrom C, Jensen I, Hagberg J, Busch H, Bergstrom G. Effectiveness of different interventions using a psychosocial subgroup assignment in chronic neck and back pain patients: A 10-year follow-up. Disability and Rehabilitation. 2012;**34**(2):110-118

[120] Verra ML, Angst F, Staal JB, Brioschi R, Lehmann S, Aeschlimann A, et al. Differences in pain, function and coping in multidimensional pain inventory subgroups of chronic back pain: A one-group pretest-posttest study. BMC Musculoskeletal Disorders. 2011; **12**:145

[121] Asih S, Mayer TG, Williams M, Choi YH, Gatchel RJ. Does classification of chronic musculoskeletal disorder

patients into psychosocial subgroups predict differential treatment responsiveness and 1-year outcomes after a functional restoration program? The Clinical Journal of Pain. 2015;**31**(12): 1036-1045

[122] Jensen IB, Bergstrom G, Ljungquist T, Bodin L, Nygren AL. A randomized controlled component analysis of a behavioral medicine rehabilitation program for chronic spinal pain: Are the effects dependent on gender? Pain. 2001;**91**(1–2):65-78

[123] Krogstad BS, Jokstad A, Dahl BL, Vassend O. The reporting of pain, somatic complaints, and anxiety in a group of patients with TMD before and 2 years after treatment: Sex differences. Journal of Orofacial Pain. 1996;**10**(3): 263-269

[124] Keogh E, McCracken LM, Eccleston C. Do men and women differ in their response to interdisciplinary chronic pain management? Pain. 2005; **114**(1–2):37-46

[125] Scascighini L, Litschi M, Walti M, Sprott H. Effect of an interdisciplinary outpatient pain management program (IOPP) for chronic pain patients with and without migration background: A prospective, observational clinical study. Pain Medicine. 2011;**12**(5):706-716

[126] Tseli E, Vixner L, LoMartire R, Grooten WJA, Gerdle B, Ang BO. Prognostic factors for improved physical and emotional functioning one year after interdisciplinary rehabilitation in patients with chronic pain: Results from a national quality registry in Sweden. Journal of Rehabilitation Medicine. 2020; **52**(2):jrm00019

[127] Hooten WM, Townsend CO, Decker PA. Gender differences among patients with fibromyalgia undergoing multidisciplinary pain rehabilitation. Pain Medicine. 2007;**8**(8):624-632

[128] Murphy JL, Phillips KM, Rafie S. Sex differences between Veterans participating in interdisciplinary chronic pain rehabilitation. Journal of Rehabilitation Research and Development. 2016;**53**(1):83-94

[129] Ahlgren C, Fjellman-Wiklund A, Hamberg K, Johansson EE, Stalnacke BM. The meanings given to gender in studies on multimodal rehabilitation for patients with chronic musculoskeletal pain—A literature review. Disability and Rehabilitation. 2016;**38**(23):2255-2270

[130] Carr JL, Moffett JA. The impact of social deprivation on chronic back pain outcomes. Chronic Illness. 2005;**1**(2): 121-129

[131] Hammarstrom A, Haukenes I, Fjellman Wiklund A, Lehti A, Wiklund M, Evengard B, et al. Low-educated women with chronic pain were less often selected to multidisciplinary rehabilitation programs. PLoS One. 2014;**9**(5):e97134

[132] Jordan KP, Thomas E, Peat G, Wilkie R, Croft P. Social risks for disabling pain in older people: A prospective study of individual and area characteristics. Pain. 2008;**137**(3): 652-661

[133] Vos T, Flaxman AD, Naghavi M, Lozano R, Michaud C, Ezzati M, et al. Years lived with disability (YLDs) for 1160 sequelae of 289 diseases and injuries 1990–2010: A systematic analysis for the global burden of disease study 2010. Lancet. 2012;**380**(9859): 2163-2196

[134] Eskew A, Jungheim E. A History of developments to improve in vitro

fertilization. Missouri Medicine. 2017; **114**(3):156-159

[135] Batho A, Kneale D, Sutcliffe K, Williams A. Sufficient conditions for effective psychological treatment of chronic pain: A qualitative comparative analysis. Pain. 2021; **162**(10):2472-2485

[136] Nicholas MK, Costa DSJ, Linton SJ, Main CJ, Shaw WS, Pearce G, et al. Implementation of early intervention protocol in Australia for 'High Risk' injured workers is associated with fewer lost work days over 2 years than usual (stepped) care. Journal of Occupational Rehabilitation. 2020;**30**(1):93-104

[137] Stalnacke BM, Haukenes I, Lehti A, Wiklund AF, Wiklund M, Hammarstrom A. Is there a gender bias in recommendations for further rehabilitation in primary care of patients with chronic pain after an interdisciplinary team assessment? Journal of Rehabilitation Medicine. 2015; **47**(4):365-371

[138] Bauman A, Owen N, Rushworth RL. Recent trends and socio-demographic determinants of exercise participation in Australia. Community Health Studies. 1990;**14**(1):19-26

[139] Lantz PM, House JS, Lepkowski JM, Williams DR, Mero RP, Chen J. Socioeconomic factors, health behaviors, and mortality: Results from a nationally representative prospective study of US adults. Journal of the American Medical Association. 1998;**279**(21):1703-1708

[140] Lindstrom M, Hanson BS, Ostergren PO. Socioeconomic differences in leisure-time physical activity: The role of social participation and social capital in shaping health related behaviour. Social Science & Medicine. 2001;**52**(3):441-451

[141] Butler D, Moseley L. Explain Pain Super Charged. Adelaide City West: Neuro Orthopaedic Institute, Australia; 2017

Chapter 8

Pain Management in Palliative Care: What Is Significant?

Boris Hait

"Divinum est sedare dolorem"
Galen of Pergamon (129 – 199 A.D.)

Abstract

In pain management of advanced ill patients, various factors appear to be of significance: multidimensional approach and realisation of pain as a complex perception (Total Pain). Existential fear and an exceptional role of pain as a leading symptom in palliative patients ought to be mentioned—chronification of pain progresses rapidly, oftentimes with less preconditions. In advanced ill patients, even the slightest pain stimulus may result in a sensation of total pain. We discuss mechanisms-centred pain therapy (opioid therapy in particular), depending on the pain character—nociceptive, inflammatory, neuropathic, dysfunctional, mixed pain—as a challenge in palliative care: -contemporary understanding of the significance and role of WHO pain management—genetically determined polymorphism of (opioid) receptors and enzyme systems—problems of plasma protein binding and interactions of analgetic drugs—differences in the elimination of various opioid drugs—active metabolites of opioids, peculiarities of the onset, duration and regulation of action—asymmetric pain distribution, breakthrough pain, end-of-dose failure, opioid-induced hyperalgesia—practical considerations on preferred choice of analgetics in patients with different comorbidities and of advanced age.

Keywords: advanced ill patients, multidimensional approach to pain assessment, total pain, chronification of pain, mechanisms-centred pain therapy, opioid therapy, nociceptive pain, neuropathic pain, mixed pain, WHO scheme on pain management, opioid receptor

1. Introduction

In a British study, doctors and nurses were asked only one simple question: How often do you look your patients directly in the eye during a conversation? Most of the answers were anything but satisfactory. Nevertheless, our experiences clearly testify that adequate and dignified care of an advanced ill person is only possible under the precondition of a proper physician-patient relationship – when we meet our patients at eye level (**Figure 1**).

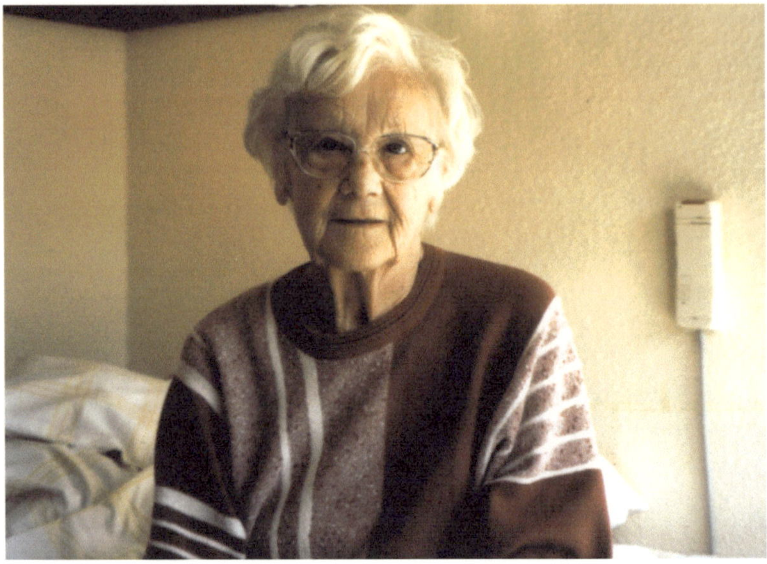

Figure 1.
Meeting at eye level. Courtesy of Centre for Palliative Care, Unna, Germany. 2002.

Especially when treating palliative care patients (PCP), it becomes obvious how important it is to perceive the patient holistically in his or her uniqueness, with all of his or her particularities, concerns and values. Pain in particular, as an extremely complex phenomenon, can only be understood on the condition that we include all dimensions of the person we are facing. Only then can we truly strive for success in pain therapy.

With the expression of our respect and our understanding towards the person who entrusts us with so much he or she holds dear, the construction of our relationship with the patient begins. Without this relationship, the process of treatment cannot take place. This is the fundamental aspect of the palliative attitude.

The specifics of pain management in palliative care patients will be discussed in the chapter at hand.

2. Palliative care and advanced illness patients

The World Health Organisation (WHO) defines [1] palliative care (PC) as follows:

> *"PC is an approach that improves the quality of life of patients and their families facing the problem associated with life-threatening illness, through the prevention and relief of suffering by means of early identification and impeccable assessment and treatment of pain and other problems, physical, psychosocial, and spiritual.*

Palliative Care:

- Provides relief from pain and other distressing symptoms;
- Affirms life and regards dying as a normal process;
- Intends neither to hasten or postpone death;

- Integrates the psychological and spiritual aspects of patient care;
- Offers a support system to help patients live as actively as possible until death;
- Offers a support system to help the family cope during the patient's illness and in their own bereavement;
- Uses a team approach to address the needs of patients and their families, including bereavement counselling, if indicated;
- Will enhance quality of life and may also positively influence the course of illness;
- Is applicable early in the course of illness, in conjunction with other therapies that are intended to prolong life, such as chemotherapy or radiation therapy, and includes those investigations needed to better understand and manage distressing clinical complications".

Taking into account the WHO's definition of palliative care, the basics and main principles of PC can be inferred:

- Treating with a "high-person, low-technology" approach. The patients' needs are given priority, and the patient takes an active role in the mutual decision-making process himself (cf. concept of shared decision-making);
- Interdisciplinary approach (involving different occupational groups, including volunteers);
- Continuity of care (inpatient—day-care—outpatient), ensuring adequate care for patients at home as well;
- Excellent symptom control with the aim of alleviating symptoms;
- PC offers are not limited to the last days and weeks of life. For the benefit of the patient, many principles of palliative care can be applied in the early stages of disease, alongside an effective causal treatment directed at the underlying disease;
- Commitment to the care for loved ones ("the Significant Others"). Supporting the bereaved even after the patient's death.

Thus, the scope of palliative care extends to various settings, clinical pictures and can be applied in different stages of an incurable disease. In this context, the definition of a palliative care patient is important.

We define a patient as a palliative care patient if at least the following conditions are met:

- The patient has an incurable disease;
- He suffers from a high symptom burden, which may include somatic, psychosocial and various other problems;
- The patient has consented to palliative care (**Figure 2**).

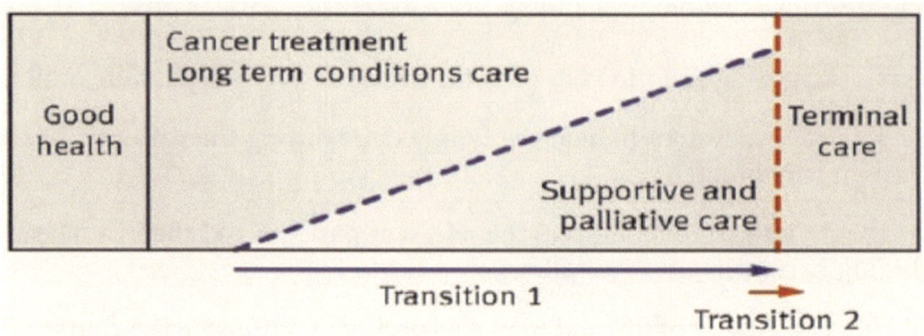

Figure 2.
When do we offer palliative care services? [2].

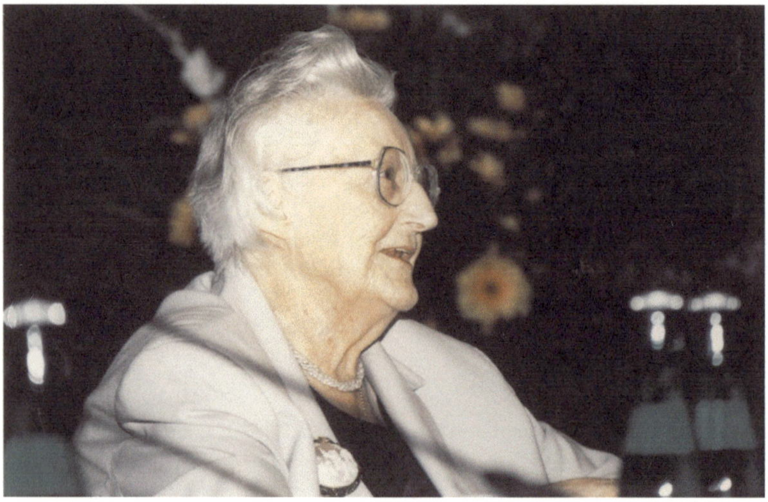

Figure 3.
Dame Cicely Saunders. Courtesy of Centre for Palliative Care, Unna, Germany. 2001.

There are various criteria serving as indicators for the initiation of palliative care. However, Boyd et al. refer to the so-called "surprise question," a question that helps us to identify the right moment to admit the patient to the palliative care setting. The question is: Would I, as a caregiver, be surprised for the patient to die within 6 to 12 months? If this is not the case, then the time has come to provide my patient with palliative care. Nevertheless, the practitioner can only answer such a question with certainty if he (1) has known the patient long enough and (2) is adequately familiar with patient's situation, that is, by being intensively involved in caring for the patient. Caregiver and patient have to be close to each other.

The foundations of PC were laid down by the grande dame of palliative care and the hospice movement, Dame Cicely Saunders (**Figure 3**).

3. The concept of "total pain"

"The death of a loved one is an extreme experience of death and radically demands grief. At the same time, however, this experience is also a challenge to self-realisation in the face of change. Grief in particular can trigger a piece of self-realisation" [3].

Grief entails a kaleidoscope of feelings, a chaos of emotions (see **Figure 4**) [5].

However, grief affects not only the relatives but primarily the patients who are confronted with a fatal diagnosis. The process of dealing with grief usually begins at the time when the patient learns about his or her diagnosis. In this context, we are talking about anticipatory grief.

This means that the advanced ill is constantly in a state of existential threat and stress. Consequences and expected reactions of this state include:

- Severe psychological stress (approx. 70% of those affected are afraid of pain);
- Previous living habits, circumstances and goals can be questioned extensively;
- Solutions are necessary but not included in a person's previous coping repertoire;
- Confronting death and dying is often associated with existential fear;
- **Existential fear cannot be reduced or eliminated, but dealing with it must rather be learned;**
- The gradual processing of the diagnosis begins;
- The illness is accompanied by new perceptions that can contribute to further uncertainty.

The person affected comes to terms with his or her life identity and takes stock.

It is beyond question that all these factors strongly influence the processing of pain and ultimately decide the picture of pain that develops within the patient. Thus, in addition to the physical, psychological and emotional factors, the patient's social environment and spiritual aspects also play a major role. This is especially true for chronic pain.

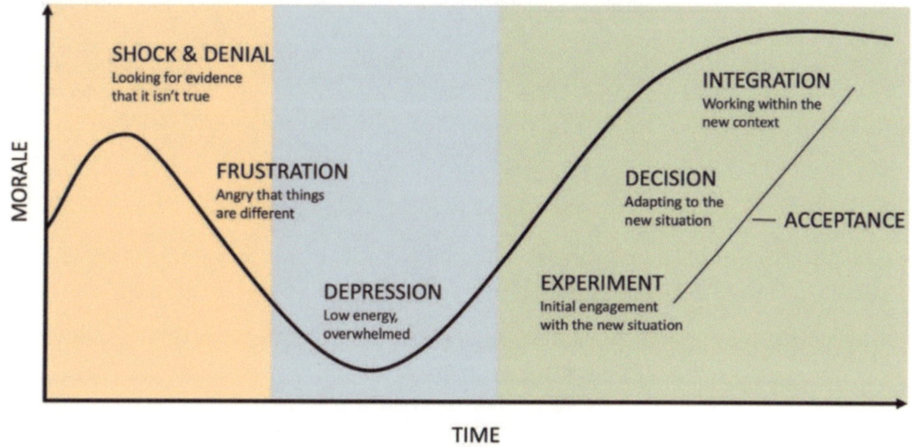

Figure 4.
Chaos of emotions of the grieving [4].

Since pain is a very subjective perception of signals emanating from different dimensions of the universe called human being, we can only understand it if we develop a broader view.

No less a figure than Cicely Saunders recognised this and contributed substantially to the understanding of the multidimensionality of chronic pain, coining the term "**Total Pain**". Cicely Saunders always stood for simplicity in explaining the phenomena and for a solution-oriented approach. The grande dame of palliative care implemented the ancient, empirical perception of pain and suffering (see "Altar of the Seven Sorrows", **Figure 5**) in her model of "Total Pain" (see **Figure 6**). This notion serves as the basis for the concept of "Total Care" which guides us, as caregivers, in our actions today [9].

With the help of this model, the necessity of a multi-professional approach to the treatment and care of patients with chronic pain becomes apparent.

Particularly in palliative care patients, who live under constant existential anxiety and are confronted with major problems in all dimensions of human existence, we often observe that pain chronification develops much faster, triggered by the mechanisms mentioned above.

This is particularly true for very old patients and those suffering from dementia. In advanced age, pain chronifies much more frequently. Also, any pain can directly be perceived as "total pain" by a patient with significant cognitive impairment or disturbance of consciousness [10].

Pain in PCPs bears, among others, the following characteristics:

- It is one of the most common symptoms;

- Often described as the most distressing of all symptoms;

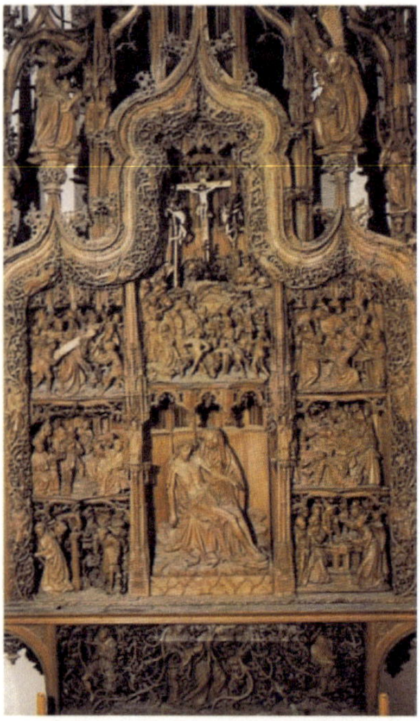

Figure 5.
Seven sorrows [6].

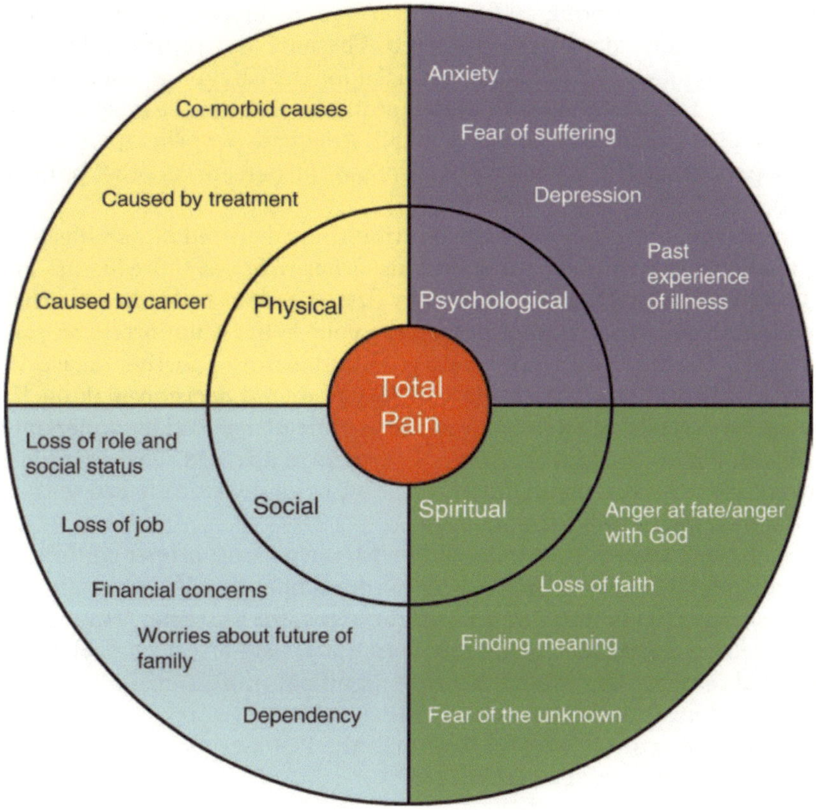

Figure 6.
Total pain [7, 8].

- Hence, the special status of pain within the realm of PCP symptoms:
    - the advanced illness patient associates pain with the underlying disease;
    - is linked to the progression of the disease;
    - tumour pain in particular occupies a particular psychological dimension;
- Pain influences other symptoms;
- Paint itself is influenced by other symptoms.

Thus, a vicious circle forms that carries a considerable negative impact on the quality of the patient's life [11]. Interrupting this vicious circle is one of the primary tasks in pain therapy for PCPs [12].

PCPs commonly exhibit several symptoms at the same time. On average, up to ten symptoms can be found in a palliative care patient that significantly impacts the quality of life. In addition to the symptoms that our patient report on a regular basis, such as pain, weakness, dyspnoea, nausea, vomiting, constipation, xerostomia, oedema, restlessness and sleep disturbances, our patients are also burdened by symptoms that occur less often and could therefore be more easily overlooked when the patient's clinical status is evaluated. These include pruritus, dysgeusia, dysphagia and singultus [13]. Thus, it is crucial for the caregiving team to utilise a checklist for the assessment of symptoms so that precise questions can be asked, examined and documented in detail. Adequate pain therapy takes into account the patient's entire symptom burden and the perception of all human dimensions.

In the treatment and support of the multimorbid advanced ill, establishing a working relationship with the patient and his or her relatives ("the Significant Others") is of utmost importance. Thus, our first questions towards the patient ought to be: "Who are you? What kind of person are you? What is important to you as a human being?" The discussion of therapy goals and planning further measures have to be performed alongside the patient on the basis of shared decision-making. Thus, the groundwork for establishing a successful therapeutic plan is laid by understanding the values, wishes, necessities and concerns of the person affected. This attitude is fundamental to palliative care. Only in grasping the situation holistically can we achieve meeting the patient at eye level.

In order to build a working relationship with the patient, proper communication is vital. An indispensable prerequisite for this is our ability to self-reflect. In doing so, one has to ask oneself a handful of critical questions, for example: "How do I, as a practitioner, affect my patient? And how does the patient affect me?" Here, the team is a substantial resource of support. Because dignified, professional care at eye level can only succeed in a multi-professional team.

By adopting this attitude, we can live up to the PCP's expectations and demands *vis-à-vis* his or her caregivers, notably:

- Having enough time for the patient;
- Being fair and holding a frank conversation;
- Being confident in our actions;
- Being flexible;
- Being able to make decisions together.

4. Pain assessment as a basis for decision-making in therapy

'No treatment of pain until the pain is well evaluated' – this motto is the key to successful pain therapy.

What does proper pain assessment mean? Cicely Saunders has been associated with having stated that the failure to assess pain is a critical barrier to good pain management.

Given the complexity and high subjectivity of experiencing pain, it is of utmost importance to let the patient talk freely about his sensations, to grant him enough space in order to describe the pain in as much detail as possible by himself. Thus, "patient self report"is the best tool for pain assessment. Therefore, the patient should lead an active role in the management of his own pain.

DOI: http://dx.doi.org/10.5772/intechopen.112325

There are additional preconditions for an ideal evaluation, diagnosis and continued monitoring of pain:

- Optimal pain evaluation and treatment can only be achieved within a team;
- Relatives of the patient should also be involved in pain evaluation. The perception of the patient's caregivers not only is able to reveal further details of pain analysis but also often shows important accompanying factors that can influence the entire experience of pain and the associated impairment;
- Each location of pain should be evaluated independently and separately;
- Reassessment should take place
    - At regular intervals;
    - After the initiation of therapy;
    - Whenever the intensity of pain escalates;
    - Whenever new localisations of pain occur.

Ideally, when evaluating pain, there should be a balance between self-observation and observation by others. In doing so, the patient should be allocated adequate space for his or her own pain assessment.

Pain assessment encompasses, on the one hand, the evaluation of all parameters of pain (see **Figure 7**). On the other hand, the precise analysis of the quality of pain is of particular importance for the preparation of an extended pain diagnosis as well (**Figure 8**).

PCPs often exhibit a "mixed pain" syndrome with components of both nociceptive and neuropathic pain [9]. This effect can be seen, that is, in the pathophysiological pain cascade of bone metastases (see **Figure 9**).

Furthermore, neuropathic pain in palliative therapy may also arise under the influence of specific mechanisms. Among those are:

Parameter of pain	Asking the patient!
Localisation	Where does it hurt?
Intensity	How strong is your pain?
Quality	How would you describe your pain?
Trigger	What actions intensify your pain?
Alleviating factor	What alleviates your pain?
Consequences	What troubles are associated with you feeling the pain?
Time course	Since when have you perceived the pain?
Daily dynamics	Do the characteristics of your pain symptoms change over the course of the day?

Figure 7.
Crucial parameters of pain evaluation. Source: Self-created.

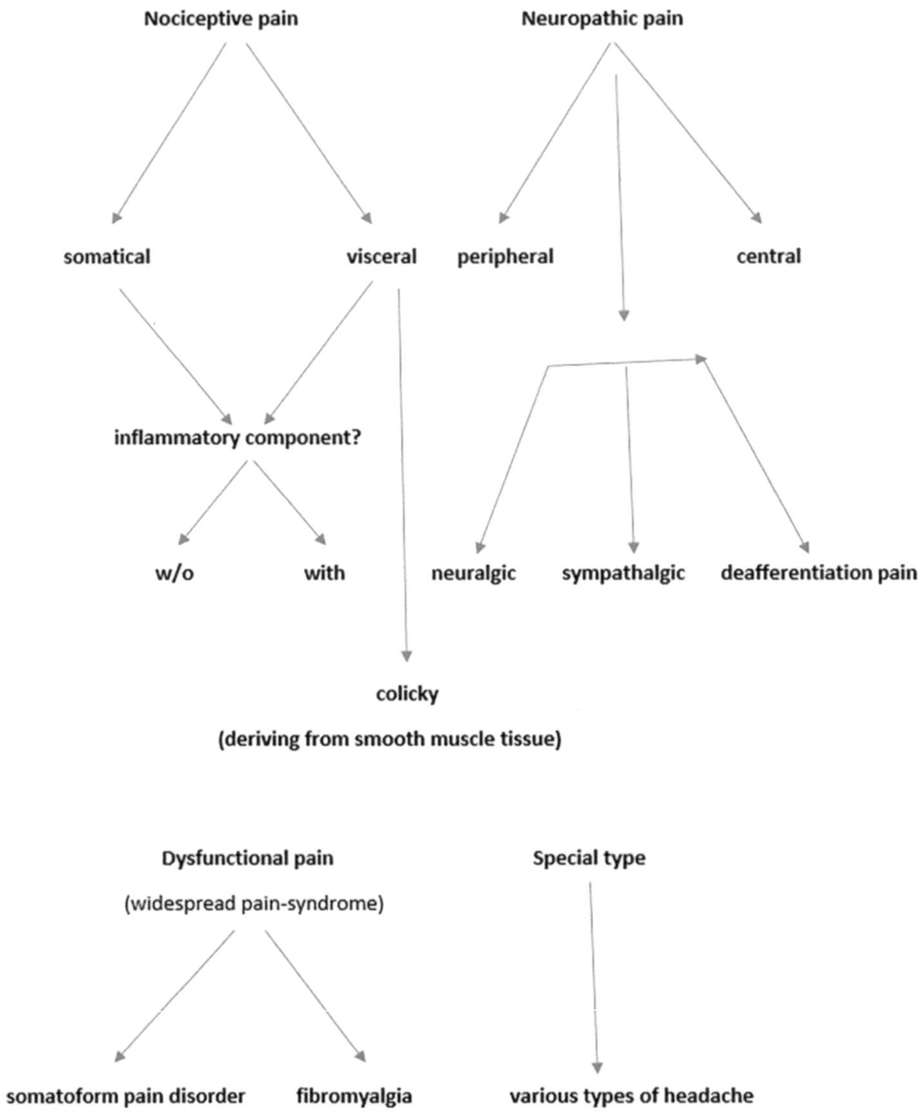

Figure 8.
Categorising pain based on pathophysiology (quality of pain). Source: Self-created.

- Tumour compression of nerves;
- Surgical resection of the tumour with iatrogenic impairment of nerval structures;
- Radiotherapy;
- Chemotherapy.

Among others, changes in mitochondrial function can facilitate the development of neuropathia [14, 15] as well as numerous cytostatic agents, for instance, Paclitaxel and Vincristine [16].

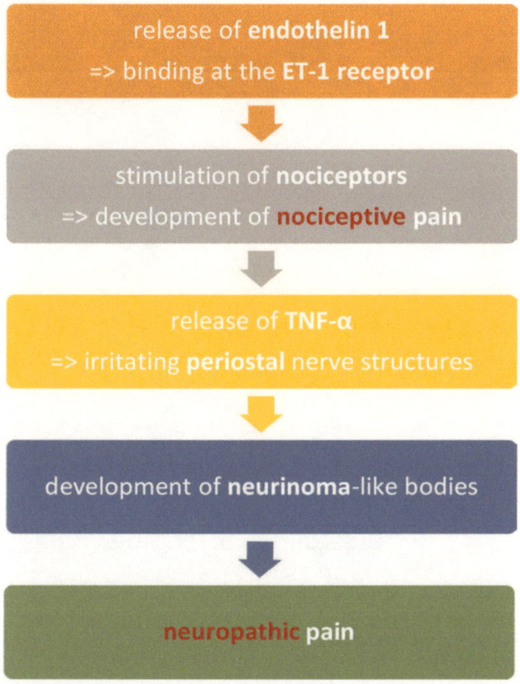

Figure 9.
Pathophysiology of pain in bone metastases. Source: Self-created.

The results of the pain analysis should be presented in a clear, simple and understandable manner with the help of suitable measuring instruments. Thus, transparency for the entire caregiving team is achieved and may serve as a basis for therapeutic action. The not purely physical mechanisms of pain development, which are rarely considered in classical pain evaluation forms, should be taken into particular account. In that way, the pain assessment is able to live up to the complexity and subjectivity of pain in patients with advanced chronic diseases.

For a proper cognitive-emotional diagnosis, tools such as the patient's self-esteem, self-efficacy, coping strategies as well as personal disease processing models, for example, externalisation, internalisation and catastrophising [17] may be taken into account.

For example, in Turk and Rudy's classification of patients with chronic pain (1988), the following is elaborated: [18].

Dysfunctional profile:

- High intensity of pain;
- High degree of interference between pain and activities;
- Low level of perceived control;
- High affective impairment;
- Low level of activity.

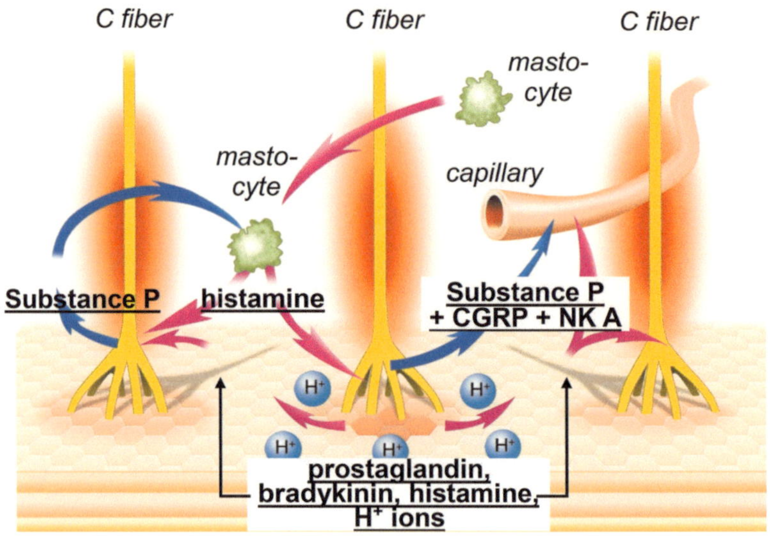

Figure 10.
Mechanisms of peripheral sensitisation: Nociceptive, inflammatory pain [19].

Interpersonal stress profile:

- Lack of social support.

Adaptive copers/minimisers:

- Low pain intensity;
- Low affective impairment;
- High level of perceived control;
- High activity profile.

After having conducted a proper pain analysis, classifying the patient's pain symptoms properly and adequately appears to bear tremendous significance for the success of pain therapy. Adding to that, understanding the mechanisms of peripheral and central sensitisation is indispensable for a differentiated targeted pain therapy (see **Figures 10** and **11**).

First, the noxious stimulation of afferent C fibres triggers the release of inflammatory neuropeptides such as Substance P, Calcitonin Gene-Related Peptide (CGRP) and Neurokinin A (NK A). The process of neurogenic inflammation is initiated. If the release of inflammatory mediators continues, pain chronification occurs. Adding to that, the ongoing neurogenic inflammation causes an awakening of dormant neurons leading to an increased emission of nociceptive stimuli. This pathophysiological cascade results in enhanced perception of pain—peripheral sensitisation emerges [21, 22].

In the case of central sensitisation (see **Figure 11**), chronic emission of nociceptive stimuli leads to an overactivity of the nociceptive system, which in turn can

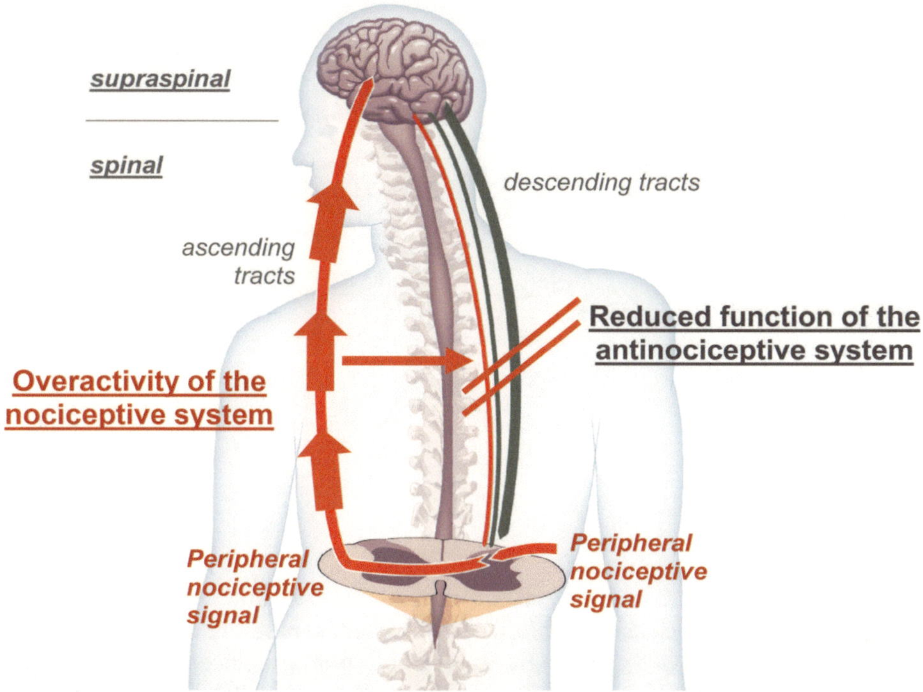

Figure 11.
Development of central sensitisation [20].

eventually result in a loss of function of the antinociceptive system. Thus, pain signals can be transmitted with less inhibition and the chronification of pain is further amplified. Furthermore, chronic pain also leads to morphological changes in the central nervous system [23].

In the advanced ill, the processes of pain chronification often arise quicker and with fewer preconditions. Even a small pain stimulus is able to trigger the image of "total pain".

5. Mechanisms-oriented pain therapy

A differentiated pain therapy can only succeed by taking into account the underlying mechanisms of pain. Accordingly, a proper pain analysis, including the precise description of pain characteristics (nociceptive, inflammatory, neuropathic, dysfunctional, mixed-pain), is a challenge within palliative care and a vital part of pain management.

Among other things, this statement is based on understanding the various main action sites for different analgesics (see **Figure 12**).

The fact that, on the one hand, different anatomical structures are activated at different levels during the development of different types of pain and, on the other hand, different analgesic substances exert their effect at different sites of action explains the importance of a targeted and varied approach in pain therapy. The principles of drug selection for pain therapy in chronic pain, in which different analgesic agents are combined, can be seen in **Figure 12**. Thus, in nociceptive pain,

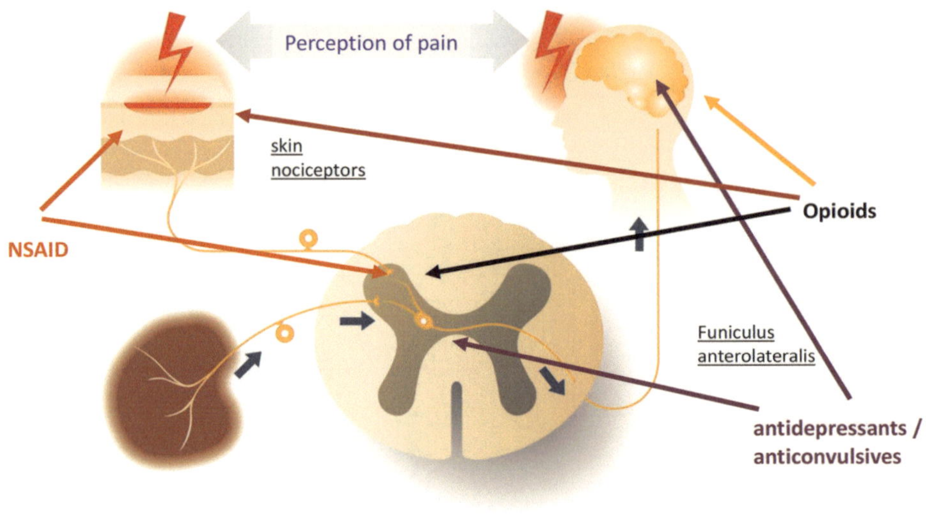

Figure 12.
Sites of action of analgesics.

both non-steroidal analgesics and opioids can be used, separately or in combination, since both substance classes exert their effect at peripheral nociceptors. At the same time, a combination of different analgesic classes allows the use of each substance's lowest dose. Particularly in geriatric patients or PCPs, it is vital to ensure that the dose of each individual analgesic substance is as low as reasonably achievable [10].

With regard to opioids, the research results of the last decades have revealed tremendous interindividual differences in opioid effectiveness [24]. This also applies to the side effects. In addition to pharmacokinetic factors, the genetic variability of opioid receptors due to numerous alternative splicing variants is discussed as a possible cause [25]. This variability can explain, among other things, different reactions to various opioids as well as deviating dose requirements and manifestations of side effects in patients [26].

For example, about one-eighth of the Caucasian population (10 to 14% of all patients) carrying the 118A > G single-nucleotide polymorphism in the MOR gene OPRM1 may require increased doses of opioids in order to achieve a similar analgetic effect in comparison to non-carriers [25, 27].

When treating PCPs, this practically means that special caution and flexibility is required in situations when:

- Consistent dose increases of an opioid do not lead to the desired analgesic effect;
- Severe and unusual side effects occur under opioid therapy;
- Signs of overdosing manifest even under low opioid doses.

6. Basics of pain management in PCPs

In general, adequate pain management in patients with cancer or other advanced chronic disease can be achieved through the following approaches:

- Primary (causal) measures;

- Systemic analgesic therapy;

- Drug-free measures, including psychological interventions, rehabilitative therapy, etc.

If adequate pain relief cannot be attained, other options should be discussed, including:

- Invasive pain therapy measures, such as blockades, catheter procedures;

- Palliative sedation therapy if symptoms are refractory in an end-of-life situation [28].

Causal measures must not be undervalued in the treatment of PCPs. For example, palliative radiotherapy of spinal metastases may help in achieving significant pain relief. However, as the chronic disease progresses, the patient's symptom burden increases and his general condition deteriorates. Thus, the options for causal therapy diminish and symptomatic pain therapy (systemic and also regional invasive measures) becomes more and more important.

As is known, the recommendations for the differentiated use of analgesic medication in patients with chronic pain are presented in the "WHO Analgesic Ladder" [29]. What practical significance does this scheme bear today, about 40 years after its first publication? And which aspects in patients with advanced illness and at the end of life do we have to pay particular attention to?

Are we meant to always adhere to the "WHO Analgesic Ladder"? Here are a few considerations along the way [30]:

- Particularly in the setting of palliative care, non-physical factors as well as all parameters evaluated in the assessment of pain play an important role in the decision-making process of prescribing pain medication. In contrast, the classical "WHO Analgesic Ladder", notably, takes into consideration only one single parameter-pain intensity, namely. Thus, the WHO scheme merely functions as an orientation guide!

- In the case of severe pain right at the onset of treating PCPs, not uncommonly, two stages of the WHO schemes are skipped, since:

    - 70% of all tumour patients end up needing level III drugs [31];

    - Strong stage III opioids can now also be dosed in very small quantities and thus carry less side effects.

- Significance of level II analgesics [32]:

    - **Tilidine**:

        a. Preferred in case of renal insufficiency;

        b. Tilidine is a prodrug that is probably activated by cytochrome isoenzyme (CYP) 3A4 to nortilidine;

c. In two successive phase I reactions (sequential metabolism), the analgesically active metabolite nortilidine is formed first, which is further degraded to the pharmacologically ineffective bisnortilidine. Both reaction steps are catalysed by CYP3A4;

d. Therefore, the AUC values (area under the blood-plasma-concentration vs. time curve) are of particular importance when considering the efficacy of this opioid. In one study, the combination of tilidine and the strong CYP3A4 inhibitor ritonavir led to altered pharmacokinetic parameters such as increased AUC values of nortilidine [33];

e. With regard to PCPs, on the one hand, a significant change in pharmacokinetics can lead to large variations of the AUC curve and thus to significant interindividual differences in the effectiveness of tilidine. But on the other hand, according to one study, adverse drug effects caused by this were of a merely moderate and transient nature due to the further degradation into the pharmacologically ineffective bisnortilidine [33];

f. The elimination of nortilidine is hardly changed in terminal renal failure, which means that a dose adjustment is not necessary. Thus, a reduction of the dose of tilidine in patients with severely impaired kidney function appears not to be required. Tilidine and its metabolites cannot be removed from the body by dialysis [34];

g. Neither Tilidine has serotonergic properties, nor does it lower the seizure threshold, a fact that renders it a favourable drug in advanced illness patients.

- **Codeine**:

  a. Its use in PCPs is evaluated as critical;

  b. Codeine is a prodrug and is only converted to active morphine by CYP2D6 through O-demethylation;

  c. Thus, the substance is subject to high individual variations depending on the metabolisation activity of the CYP2D6 enzymatic system;

  d. That is, patients who are "CYP2D6 ultrarapid metabolisers" will produce much higher amounts of morphine derived from codeine in a shorter period of time, whereas "CYP2D6 poor metabolisers" may hardly activate any codeine at all [35];

  e. In renal insufficiency, morphine-6-glucuronide and morphine-3-glucuronide accumulate as active metabolites of morphine, which can lead to a rapid overdosing [36, 37].

- **Dihydrocodeine (DHC)** [35]:

  a. A semi-synthetic derivative of codeine with a low bioavailability when administered orally (approx. 20%). This is due to poor gastrointestinal absorption;

b. Metabolised in the liver by CYP2D6 to an active metabolite, dihydromorphine, and by CY3A4 to a secondary primary metabolite, nordihydrocodeine;

c. The CYP2D6-catalysed metabolite dihydromorphine (DHM) has a 100-fold higher affinity for μ-opioid receptors than DHC but contributes only marginally to the analgesic effect of DHC, meaning:

1. clinical response independent of the patient's individual CYP2D6 metabolising phenotype;

2. Thus, with regard to the analgesic effect of DHC, clinically relevant interactions with CYP2D6 inhibiting substances are scarcely to be expected [38];

3. Among others, this is due to the fact that the parent substance DHC, in contrast to codeine, already unfolds an analgesic effect before entering biotransformation.

d. Nevertheless, drugs that either are degraded by or induce the CYP2D6 enzyme can significantly influence the plasma level of DHM and lead to severe side effects [35].

- **Tramadol:**

a. It is a prodrug: via CYP2D6, the active metabolite O-desmethyltramadol is formed;

b. Limited analgesic effect of tramadol expected in patients with poor metaboliser (PM) or intermediate metaboliser (IM) status;

c. Comedication with CYP2D6 inhibiting drugs reduces the formation of O-desmethyltramadol;

d. Belongs to the group of so-called dual opioids. This substance blocks the neuronal reuptake of serotonin and has the potential to induce serotonin syndrome when administered alone or in combination with other serotonergic drugs;

e. Notably, comedication of tramadol and selective serotonin reuptake inhibitors (SSRI) fluoxetine and paroxetine bears a serious risk. These SSRIs are potent inhibitors of CYP2D6, leading to a decreased formation of active analgesic tramadol metabolites when co-administered. This may result in failure of effective pain management, prompting the caregiver to increase the dose of tramadol while in doing so, as a consequence, increasing the likelihood of developing serotonin syndrome;

f. Particularly in advanced illness patients, this grave risk increases if elevated levels of the substances mentioned above are to be expected, for instance, in the case of deteriorating renal function.

- Potent opioids—what substance to select for the use in advanced illness patients [32]?
    - **Morphine**:
        a. Morphine is hepatically degraded by glucuronidation to morphine-3-glucuronide and morphine-6-glucuronide. Morphine-6-glucuronide is the pharmacologically active metabolite binding to the μ-opioid receptor (MOR) and is eliminated renally;

        b. One of the advantages of morphine in advanced illness patients is the possibility of using this substance, which has been known for almost 200 years, in all possible forms of administration:

            1. oral as tablets or drops;

            2. rectal;

            3. parenteral: subcutaneous, intravenous, epidural, intrathecal and also local application in the form of morphine-gel 0.1 or 0.2%, in order to also use the effect on MOR in the skin, for example, in treating exulcerating wounds.

        c. In the context of renal insufficiency, morphine-6-glucuronide accumulates in the plasma with not only an increased analgesic effect but also a consequential risk of overdosing, leading to sedation and respiratory depression;

        d. Morphine-3-glucuronide can also accumulate amid kidney impairment and bears a possible neuroexcitatory effect [39];

        e. In patients with a glomerular filtration rate (GFR) <30 mL/min, the dose of morphine should therefore be reduced or, preferably, avoided entirely [37, 40].

    - **Oxycodone**:
        a. Oxycodone is degraded by CYP3A4 to the inactive metabolite noroxycodone and metabolised by CYP2D6 to the active metabolite oxymorphone;

        b. CYP3A4 inhibitors, such as ciprofloxacin, clarithromycin, levomepromazine or ketoconazole, increase the plasma concentration of oxycodone and oxymorphone and thus enhance the analgesic effect and potentiate side effects. A daily intake of ca. 300 mL or more of grapefruit juice, also a known CYP3A4 inhibitor, can also become pharmacologically relevant;

        c. CYP2D6 inhibitors, including many substances such as celecoxib, dimenhydrinate, duloxetine, fluoxetine, levomepromazine, melperone and methadone, do not lead to clinically significant interactions with oxycodone;

d. In uraemic patients, the elimination of oxycodone is significantly reduced [41];

e. However, the half-life is significantly prolonged in patients on an individual basis, especially in advanced illness patients;

f. Oxycodone and its metabolites are dialysable. Thus, oxycodone should be administered after dialysis;

g. The same applies to the combination preparation of oxycodone/naloxone. Notably, liver insufficiency should be particularly taken into account in this case as well because naloxone, a potent MOR antagonist, is hepatically metabolised. Due to the naloxone not being adequately degraded amid liver insufficiency, its plasma level rises and it effectively binds to spinal MORs, partially cancelling out the analgesic effect of oxycodone;

h. Particularly in advanced illness patients, liver insufficiency among others has to be expected. We therefore consider the dosage of more than 40–50 mg of naloxone per day as critical for PCPs;

i. Furthermore, oxycodone has a non-negligible affinity to the ϰ-receptor (KOR).

- **Hydromorphone:**

a. Hydromorphone is absorbed in the gastrointestinal tract and is subject to presystemic elimination. The active substance has an oral bioavailability of about 32%. Hydromorphone is metabolised in the liver and eliminated renally predominantly in the form of conjugated hydromorphone, dihydroisomorphine and dihydromorphine [42];

b. The metabolisation leads to the formation of analgesically inactive substances that are known to be associated with various toxic side effects, for example, enhanced neuroexcitation [43, 44];

c. Haemodialysis reduces plasma concentration by about ½. This can result in failed symptom control regarding pain, eventually inducing withdrawal symptoms;

d. Nevertheless, hydromorphone is preferred by many caregivers as a substance that can be administered in renal insufficiency.

- **Fentanyl:**

  - Is a highly lipophilic molecule and thus bears significant plasma protein binding properties; [45]

  - As fentanyl binds to plasma proteins such as albumin and alpha-1-acid glycoprotein, hypoalbuminaemia (for example, due to cachexia or liver failure) may influence fentanyl pharmacokinetics [46, 47].

- Fentanyl is predominantly hepatically metabolised *via* CYP3A4 mediated *N*-dealkylation, resulting in the formation of inactive metabolites such as, among others, norfentanyl [48] (see **Figure 13**);

- Approximately 10% of the intact molecule as well as all inactive metabolites are excreted renally. Although this notion is widely accepted among scholars, a recent study has outlined that the hepatic *N*-dealkylation process may not be as important as formerly assumed. There may be various, yet unknown, metabolic processes involved for a significant part of fentanyl degradation;

- As fentanyl is mainly metabolised in the liver, the substance is suitable for use in patients with renal insufficiency [50, 51].

o **Buprenorphine**:

a. Binds with high affinity to MORs and, in doing so, acts as a partial agonist;

b. At the KOR, it bears partial agonistic and very effective antagonistic properties;

c. Is a highly lipophilic substance;

d. Carries only a moderate risk of respiratory depression at dosage increase compared to other opioids;

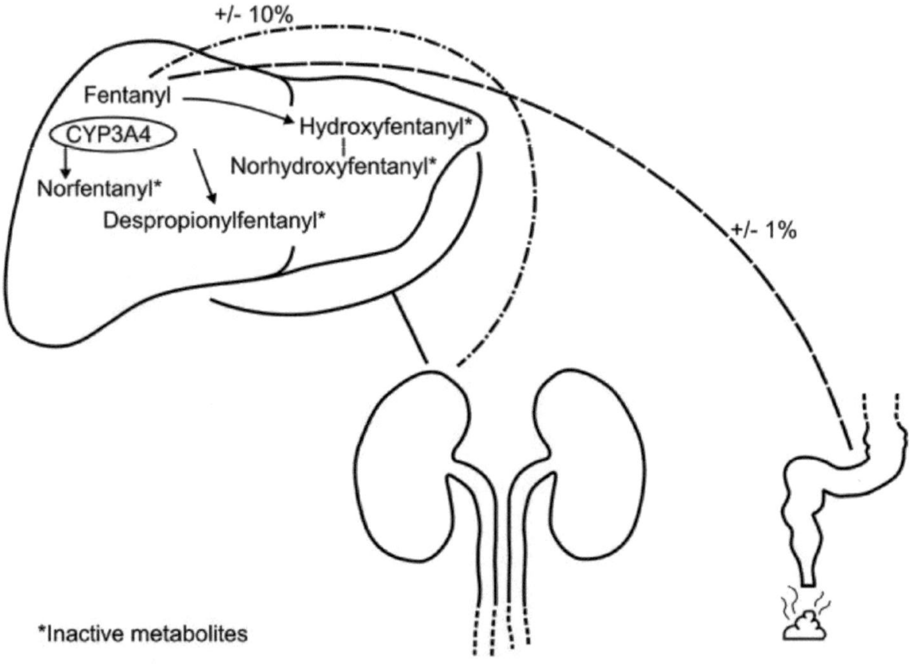

Figure 13.
Fentanyl metabolism and elimination [49].

e. Due to idle receptor kinetics, elimination progresses slower;

f. With an exceptionally high first-pass effect, the oral bioavailability is very low (approx. 6%). Therefore, oral administration appears not to be viable. Sublingual administration, however, results in a higher bioavailability, especially when administered in a liquid form [52];

g. CYP3A4 and CYP3A5 catalyse the formation of the active metabolite norbuprenorphine. However, its pharmacological efficacy is significantly lower compared to the initial substance. Buprenorphine itself inhibits CYP3A4;

h. Buprenorphine and norbuprenorphine are glucuronidated in the liver and excreted mainly *via* bile and faeces. Only 10 to 30% of the substance is excreted *via* the kidneys [53]. Therefore, the use of buprenorphine in patients with renal insufficiency is rational and applicable;

i. Due to the antagonistic effect on the KOR, a sedative effect is not expected to a significant extent. Thus, the patient's vigilance remains mostly unhampered by the medication, allowing the patient to be more active throughout the day. This phenomenon justifies the preferred use of buprenorphine in geriatric patients as well as in those with advanced illness, oftentimes being cachectic and therefore plagued by constant fatigue;

j. In addition, some authors point towards an antidepressant effect in patients with non-psychotic unipolar depression [54, 55]. Particularly, a PCP can benefit from this twice. This advantage is of substantial clinical significance given that some studies indicate that the antidepressant effect of buprenorphine takes maximum effect after a relatively short time (a few days), in contrast to conventional antidepressants (a few weeks).

- **Methadone**:

a. Is an opioid with dual effect as it binds at the MOR and partly also at the δ-opioid receptor (DOR), as an agonist, as well as at the NMDA receptor as an antagonist. Thus, methadone can be expected to be effective in both nociceptive and neuropathic pain, that is, in mixed-pain syndrome;

b. Is a racemate (R- and S- enantiomer);

c. Is a substrate of the CYP3A4 isoenzyme and is degraded into a few inactive metabolites. The interactions in biotransformation can lead, among others, to QT interval prolongation. Furthermore, MAO inhibitors should not be co-medicated with methadone because of the risk of a severe drop in blood pressure;

d. Adding to that, co-administering serotonergic agents can trigger serotonin syndrome [44, 56];

e. It has high oral bioavailability [57];

f. Renal and hepatic insufficiency does not have a significant effect on methadone clearance;

g. The relative equianalgesic ratio of oral morphine to oral methadone is estimated at 4:1 to 12:1 [58]. Due to the higher analgesic potency, changing opioid substances to methadone must be performed cautiously and gradually by titration;

h. Enhanced lipid solubility of methadone leads to a high volume of distribution: Topical forms of application are also conceivable. The fraction of plasma protein binding of the substance is 60–90%, almost twice as high as morphine's plasma protein binding property. These two qualities contribute to a relatively long plasma half-life and, consequently, to the risk of accumulation. Adding to that, plasma half-life of methadone is subject to extensive interindividual variations;

i. Therefore, in PCPs, we consider the use of methadone to be questionable as the plasma albumin levels in these patients are oftentimes significantly lowered—particularly in advanced stages of the disease. Due to this fact, it is particularly difficult to foresee and estimate the expected clinical effect in relation to the administered dose. The limited predictability bears the danger of rapid overdosing;

j. Among the potential side effects, neurotoxicity and myoclonia ought to be mentioned as these symptoms occur more frequently in PCPs when using methadone [43, 44].

- **Tapentadol:**

a. Like tramadol, tapentadol belongs to the group of opioids with a dual action mechanism, whereby analgesia is achieved, on the one hand, by agonising the MOR and, on the other hand, by an inhibition of noradrenaline reuptake;

b. Compared to other opioids, tapentadol has a better side effect profile which makes it a preferred choice in PCPs [59–62];

c. The dual action mechanism allows the substance to be used not only for chronic nociceptive pain but also for neuropathic pain;

d. Due to the first-pass effect, tapentadol has an oral bioavailability of slightly more than 30%;

e. Tapentadol is absorbed pretty quickly and, to a large extent, glucuronidated in the liver. Only about 20% of the substance remains bound to plasma proteins. The metabolites of tapentadol, including

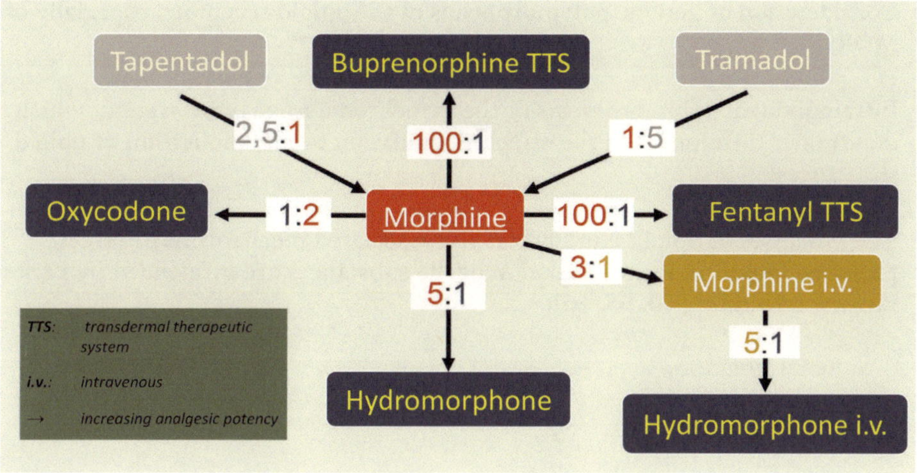

Figure 14.
Opioid conversion for morphine equivalent doses: "Cross of Sittl-Grießinger" [63].

tapentadol-O-glucuronide as the main metabolite and N-desmethyl tapentadol, are inactive;

f. Tapentadol itself has no influence on the activity of the CYP system, which significantly reduces the risk of pharmacological interactions. This is seen as a crucial advantage especially when being confronted with polypharmacy, a common sight in PCPs;

g. When comparing two dual action mechanism opioids—tapentadol and tramadol—the former is predominantly favoured:

1. Tapentadol bears a higher analgesic effectiveness;

2. The side effect profile of tapentadol is more beneficial;

3. The potential for pharmacological interactions is lower with tapentadol;

4. In contrast to tramadol, intraindividual genetic variations appear to hardly play a role with tapentadol, which facilitates the dosing and controllability of the substance and makes its use safer and its effects more predictable in PCPs.

- For recommendations of converting dosages of different opioids, see **Figure 14** [64].

7. What needs to be considered for differentiated opioid therapy in its practical implementation?

- Given the peculiarities of the various opioids at hand for the treatment of patients, numerous factors have to be taken into account before administering pain medication:

- Consideration of genetic polymorphisms of the opioid receptors, especially of the MOR;
- Intraindividual polymorphisms of the cytochrome isoenzyme system, which determines differences in the effect, degradation or metabolisation of opioid substances;
- The processes of opioid elimination and associated mechanisms of effect prolongation or toxic accumulation of the substances are influenced by various factors, including [40, 65, 66]:
    - Renal function;
    - Liver function;
    - Water solubility or lipophilicity of the substances;
    - Metabolites, possibly leading to increased plasma levels of active substances and to subsequent overdosing.
- In pain management for PCPs, pharmacological interactions often pose a challenge for the caregiver due to the even narrower therapeutic range of many substances and the high proportion of elderly patients with multiple concomitant diseases [67].

As an example, the serotonin syndrome, a feared possible outcome of medication interactions, should be mentioned (see **Figure 15**), especially when applying phenylpiperidine opioids, such as:

- Methadone;
- Fentanyl;
- Pethidine;
- Tramadol;

and morphine analogues, such as:

- Oxycodone;
- Codeine;

as co-medication together with:

- MAO inhibitors (rasagiline, moclobemide);
- SSNI, SNRI (venlafaxine, mirtazapine);
- Tricyclic antidepressants;

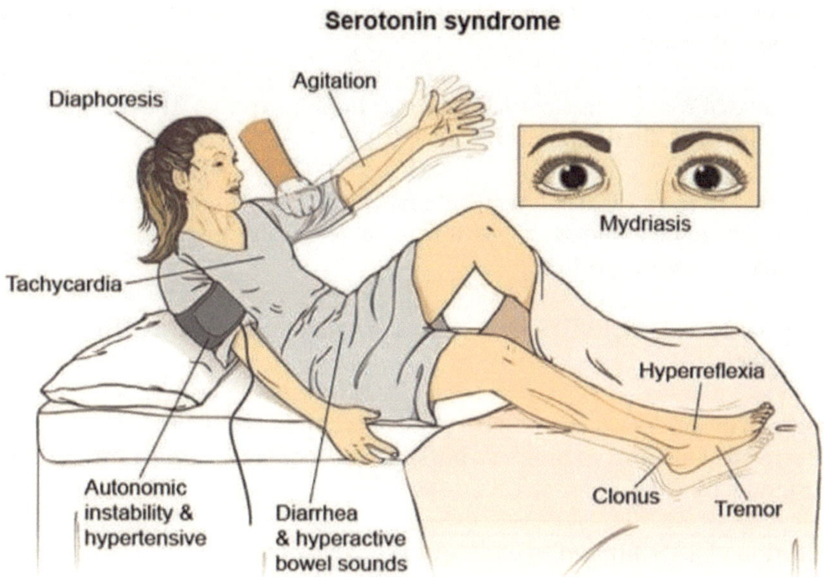

Figure 15.
Signs of serotonin syndrome.

- St. John's wort extract;
- Setrons (5-HT_3-receptor antagonists);
- Triptans;
- Levodopa.

Since the patient exhibits many serotonin-dependent effects—clinical symptoms that are, in itself, rather unspecific and generic—the clinical picture can often be overlooked, diagnosing is impeded and thus may ultimately lead to the death of the patient [68]. The neuroexcitatory triad of changes in consciousness, neuromuscular hyperactivity (such as tremor, hyperreflexia, myoclonia, rigidity) and autonomic instability is crucial in making the diagnosis, whereby—most notably—mydriasis and an increase in body temperature are indicative of the suspected pathology. Treating serotonin syndrome consists of the discontinuation of serotonergic pharmaceuticals and a symptomatic, if necessary, intensive medical therapy, as well as of using serotonin antagonists, such as cyproheptadine. Alternatively, atypical neuroleptics with antagonistic activity against the 5-hydroxytryptamine receptor 2A (5-HT_{2A} receptor), that is, olanzapine 10 mg sublingually, may be applied [69].

Side effects within the scope of differentiated opioid therapy often occur as a result of pharmacokinetic interactions, leading to changes in the concentration-time profiles of the simultaneously administered drugs. As a result, the effects on the body of at least one substance involved are altered.

In our practical work, we advocate opioid monotherapy, evading combinations of different opioid analgesics at the same time, if possible. Depending on the PCP's individual pain pattern and course of disease, we do not always succeed in adhering to this principle as we ought to combine two or even more different opioids when prescribing pro re nata medication (rescue substances).

Nowadays, morphine continues to retain its position as a drug of choice for differentiated opioid therapy, but:

- In the case of renal insufficiency, tilidine, buprenorphine, fentanyl or hydromorphone should be preferred [70];
- In the case of liver insufficiency, substances being predominately metabolised in the liver are to be avoided, if possible, or at least administered with a reduced dose, that is, buprenorphine.

In pain management of PCPs, transdermal therapeutic systems (TTS) bear particular significance:

- A main principle of palliative care states that oral opioid administration is preferred as long and as much as possible, in cooperation with the conscious and informed patient;
- Indication of TTS: limited to cases of dysphagia of various origins, otherwise only as alternative medication if other oral opioids have failed in alleviating the symptoms properly;
- However, the use of TTS can improve the quality of life or patient compliance, especially in advanced illness patients [63];
- The caregiver has to exercise caution regarding the application of TTS in the following circumstances:
    - Cachexia, which is a frequent concomitant feature in PCPs. This applies in particular to the fentanyl matrix patch [71]. Given the relatively high fat solubility of fentanyl, substance diffusion through the skin depends on the sufficient amount of fat tissue. It may also be difficult for the patch to stick firmly to the skin for the required three-day period in a cachectic patient. Thus, it is not uncommon for the patch to come off earlier;
    - Unstable pain syndrome (e.g., asymmetric pain curve);
    - Short life expectancy, as patients in an end-of-life (EoL) situation often show unstable pain curves. Yet flexibility in dosage is crucially important, most notably in opioid-naïve patients in an EoL situation. This can predominantly be achieved by using short-acting opioids. Consequently, when using TTS in opioid-naïve patients in the advanced phase of disease, adverse drug effects are more likely to occur as a result of changing absorption depending on the patient's skin condition and fluctuating body temperature. Hence, we can more frequently expect confusion, respiratory depression, nausea, vomiting, constipation and other side effects.
- Buprenorphine TTS:
    - Due to its high lipophilicity, this substance—like the fentanyl TTS [72]—needs enough fatty tissue in order to exhibit a stable and consistent effect

when applied as TTS. However, the adhesive matrix of this specific TTS generates more stable diffusion values and, due to the rear polyethylene cover sheeting, this TTS is less sensitive to, that is, mechanical and thermic interference [73];

- Can be applied in at low dosage, starting at 5 µg/h;

- Buprenorphine carries a relatively low risk for pharmacological interactions. Therefore, its use is of particular advantage in PCPs or patients of advanced age due to the frequent presence of numerous concomitant diseases and hence polypharmacy;

- Local allergic skin reactions appear to occur at a higher incidence when using transdermal buprenorphine in comparison with fentanyl patches.

8. Approach to the management of fluctuating pain dynamics: Asymmetrical pain, breakthrough pain, end-of-dose failure

In the course of the day, patients can experience a varying distribution of pain intensity. In order to register these intricacies as a caregiver in order to conduct proper targeted pain management, a detailed, extensive and standardised pain assessment is indispensable.

Given a consistent distribution of pain (see **Figure 16**, curve 1), it is comparably easy to alleviate the symptoms. Here, the aim is to achieve a consistent plasma level of the analgesic substance and hence pharmacologically "capturing" the consistent burden of pain symptoms. Unfortunately, when dealing with chronic persistent pain conditions in PCPs, this "simplest" form of pain distribution is hardly seen. Much more frequently, advanced illness patients report a varying, fluctuating intensity of pain over the course of the day (see **Figure 16**, curves 2 and 3).

A curve depicting an asymmetrical distribution of pain may correspondingly require an asymmetrical distribution of analgesic substances in the patient's blood plasma. For example, in the case of predominantly evening and nocturnal chronic pain, one third of the total daily dose is to be administered in the early and late morning, while two thirds are allocated to an afternoon and evening administration. Pain management results have to be closely and critically monitored and evaluated.

Apart from a varying intensity of the patient's baseline pain perception, pain management is additionally complicated by intermittent additional pain peaks known as breakthrough pain (BTP) [74]. BTP is comparably more common in PCPs.

Successful relief of breakthrough pain episodes depends on several factors, including: [75–77].

- Detailed and close analysis of breakthrough pain, for instance:
    - Predictability of BTP;
    - Initial development (relatively slow and building up vs. rapid, lightning-like onset);

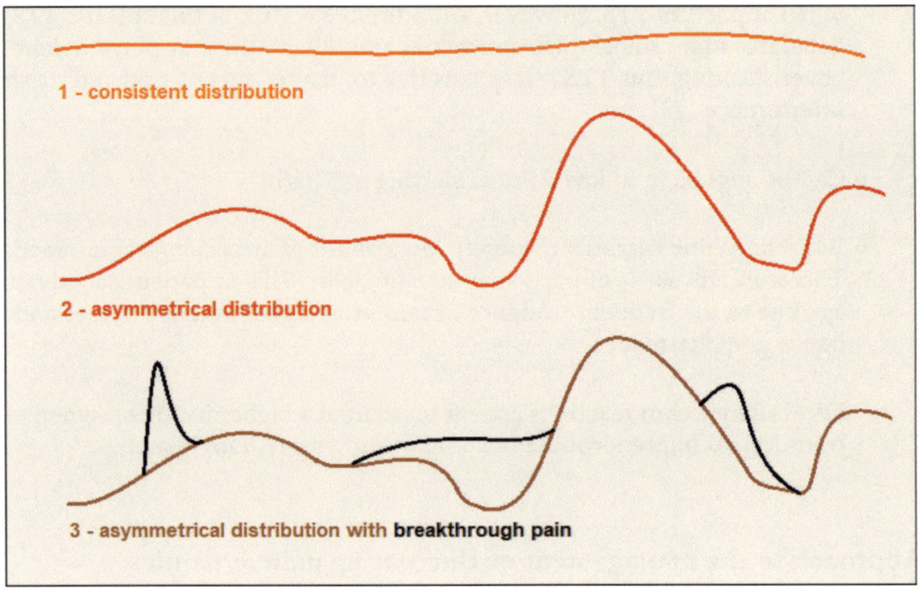

Figure 16.
Dynamic distribution of pain intensity over the course of the day. Source: Self-created.

- Duration of BTP episode;
- Frequency of episodes over the course of the day;
- Quality of BTP episodes:
  a. Nociceptive;
  b. Neuropathic;
  c. Mixed-pain.

- Usually, an adjustment to the baseline retard opioid medication is necessary [78].
- Crucially, a close dialogue within the interdisciplinary caregiving team has to be assured, that is, *via*:
  - Regular joint ward rounds at the patient's bedside (doctors/nurses);
  - Interdisciplinary meetings;
  - Standardised documentation within the team;
  - Raising the nursing staff's awareness to the topic of BTP;
  - Ensuring the patient's quick and unproblematic access to pro re nata (PRN) medication, that is, fast-acting analgesics;
  - Providing adequate training focussing on BTP to all professional groups involved.

The data available for patients with tumour disease points to the vital importance of addressing this topic thoroughly: [77].

- Prevalence of 40–80% of all tumour patients;
- Frequency of 1 to 6 episodes per day on average;
- Ca. 60% of patients suffer from 2 to 4 attacks per day;
- Poor predictability (only 25–30%);
- Short duration of <30 min in 75% of patients;
- High pain intensity at Numerical Rating Scale (NRS) 7–10;
- Mostly a mixed pain syndrome. Thus, BTP is commonly more difficult to treat.

As to our experience, ideal pain management, especially for BTP, can only be achieved within a well-functioning interdisciplinary team of caregivers. For example, in the case of a patient with osseous metastatic disease of prostate carcinoma, it is essential for the nursing staff to be briefed on the type of pain episodes, including the possibility of predictable BTP during movements or exercise. This empowers the caregivers to accordingly administer a PRN medication 20–30 minutes prior to, that is, morning care which constitutes a common reason for predictable pain episodes.

Retard formulation opioid analgesics are usually not applicable for disrupting BTP episodes. Here, fast-acting opioids and rapid onset opioids (ROO) are on hand. The decision, which of these substances to use, also depends on the results of the pain assessment. In the case of a BTP pain episode building up relatively slowly and longer lasting, the additional usage of fast-acting opioids is indicated [79]. In contrast, amid lightning-like pain peaks that could be described, that is, as an “electric shock”, usually lasting only a short time period, the use of ROOs is preferred.

ROO formulations are distinguishable by the administration form of its analgesic substance, fentanyl:

- Transmucosal;
- Buccal pill;
- Buccal film;
- Sublingual;
- Nasal spray.

The traditional recommendations of the “WHO Analgesic Ladder” with regard to PRN medication—$\frac{1}{10}$ to $\frac{1}{6}$ of the equivalent daily total dose of morphine at single administration—are substantially subject to individual variations and are only partially applicable, especially in advanced illness patients. Here, caution is especially required in patients whose daily dose, converted to morphine, exceeds 100 mg in total.

With regard to the dosage of ROOs, the following rule applies: Firstly, administer 100 µg of fentanyl sublingually, buccally or nasally. If the analgesic effect is insufficient, apply an additional equal dose after ca. 15 to 20 minutes. If there is a noticeable improvement in analgesia, administer 200 μg of fentanyl directly during the next episode of pain.

When facing a lack of therapeutic success with regard to BTP, consider the following pitfalls:

- Dosage too low of baseline therapy with slow-release, retard opioids;
- Dosage too low of PRN medication;
- Time intervals too long between dose administrations of baseline therapy ("end-of-dose failure", EoD). EoD "failure refers to medication wearing off before the next regular analgesic dose is due [...]" [80], leading to increasing pain perception in between dose applications.
    - The phenomenon of EoD failure is primarily due to individual differences in the pharmacokinetics of opioids, among others:
        a. Genetic polymorphisms of opioid receptors;
        b. Polymorphisms of hepatic enzyme systems given presence of several gene variants with different properties:
            1. rapid metabolisers;
            2. intermediate metabolisers;
            3. extensive metabolisers and
            4. poor metabolisers.
    - EoD failure is a not uncommonly seen trait of TTS, for example, with fentanyl patches.
- BTP episode of very short duration and very high intensity;
    - Conventional PRN medication is often administered in such cases, that is, fast-acting formulations of morphine, hydromorphone or oxycodone. These preparations only take effect after at least 20 to 30 minutes. Therefore, ROOs should be preferably considered;
    - The medication should be positioned within the patient's reach. No time should be wasted;
    - The nursing staff should be sensitised to the fact that the patient has to receive the medication immediately when pain is expressed.
- Delayed intake of PRN medication;
- Usage of slow-release retard formulations as PRN ("rescue medication").

9. Co-analgesics and topical application

In palliative care, classical co-analgesics are prescribed as well, but the usage frequency of these drugs is higher. This is due to the increased prevalence of difficult-to-treat neuropathic and atypical pain in advanced illness patients, especially in those with tumour pain. These pain syndromes cannot only be caused by the underlying tumorous disease but also occur as a consequence of treatment [81]. With regard to neuropathic pain, the fraction of pain caused by cancer treatment appears to be higher than the fraction of pain as a result of the disease itself [81].

It can further be inferred that neuropathic cancer pain leads to significantly greater impairment of the patient's daily life and quality of life and, consequently, to a higher need for analgesics than nociceptive cancer pain [82].

Here, too, evaluating pain quality plays a key role. In the treatment of neuropathic pain, a number of antidepressants and anticonvulsants are mainly recommended.

Antidepressants are mainly used for sympatalgia (e.g., for permanent burning pain accompanied by allodynia and tingling paraesthesia), while anticonvulsants like the calcium channel blockers pregabalin and gabapentin as well as the sodium channel blocker carbamazepine are primarily used for neuralgic pain.

- Recommended daily doses of common antidepressants in pain management:
    - **Amitriptyline** (TCA):
        a. 50–150 mg;
        b. Initial dosage (ID): 1 x 10 mg;
    - **Doxepin** (TCA):
        a. 25–150 mg;
        b. ID: 1 × 25 mg;
    - **Duloxetine** (SNRI):
        a. 30–60 mg;
        b. ID: 1 × 30 mg;
    - **Venlafaxine** (SNRI):
        a. 75–150 mg;
        b. ID: 1 × 75 mg;
    - **Mirtazapine** (NaSSA):
        a. 15–30 mg;
        b. ID: 1 × 7.5 mg.

In our experience, the usage of moderate doses of both antidepressants and anticonvulsants is recommended in PCPs. We rarely prescribe higher doses than 150 mg pregabalin or 300 mg gabapentin to minimise adverse drug effects.

Furthermore, analgesics are locally applied as well. On the one hand, topical formulations of morphine are used in exulcerating wounds, for instance, extensive ENT tumours, mammary carcinoma or decubital ulcers, applied as a 0.1% or 0.2% gel. On the other hand, the local anaesthetic lidocaine—approved for use in postherpetic neuralgia—can be applied as a 5% patch to many other local pain syndromes of neuropathic origin, too, according to our experience. A lidocaine patch is applied for 12 hours a day. It can be cut if necessary and thus adapted to the affected areas. The maximum daily dose is three patches.

In palliative care, the usage of capsaicin patches (i.e., 8% topical formulation) is rather limited due to its unpleasant irritating effect on the skin, especially at initial application.

Among all co-analgesics, ketamine comes to the fore as treatment in PCPs. The substance is often considered as ultima ratio for neuropathic pain control. As a highly lipophilic substance, this non-competitive N-methyl-D-aspartate (NMDA) receptor inhibitor leads to substantial analgesia in tumour-associated neuropathic pain as well as in ischaemic pain and in local pain syndromes when administered in subnarcotic doses. The substance can be applied variously: intravenous (0.5–1.5 mg/kg BW), subcutaneous, intramuscular, oral and topical [83]. Among others, a blockade of NMDA receptors is associated with reversal of opioid tolerance. Ketamine is metabolised *via* CYP3A4; interactions are hardly described. Ketamine is rightly classified by the WHO as an "essential drug for the management of refractory pain".

According to our experience, S-ketamine should be applied orally as follows:

- In combination with apple juice for the improvement of gustatory perception;
- Gradual titration over the course of several days, that is:
    - From **day 1** on: 3 × 5 mg
    - From **day 3** on: 3 × 10 mg
    - From **day 5** on: 3 × 15 mg
    - From **day 7** on: 3 × 25 mg
    - From **day 10** on: 3 × 50 mg

Case study 1:

- Female patient, 57 y.;
- Diagnosis: **metastasised cervix cancer**, encircling the entire pelvic area and lower abdomen;
- **Severe pain, NRS 8–10**: nociceptive and neuropathic (**mixed-pain**) in the entire lower abdomen/small pelvis;

- Initial treatment:
    - Opioids in increasing dosage, converted to up to 1000 mg morphine equivalents per day (in in opioid rotation technique) [84, 85]
    - Co-analgesics:
        a. Anticonvulsants, antidepressants;
        b. Dexamethasone;
        c. Bisphosphonates;
        d. Non-opioid analgesics.
    - No adequate pain relief!
- Thus, application of **S-ketamine**:
    - Orally, gradually titrated;
    - Starting at 3 × 5 mg/d to 4 × 250 mg/d (after 12 days);
    - Hereunder, **satisfying analgesia** with reduced pain intensity of NRS 2–3.

10. Problem area: opioid-induced hyperalgesia

When advanced illness patients receive opioid therapy, they de facto find themselves set in a field of tension between pain, analgesia, development of tolerance toward analgesics and opioid-induced hyperalgesia [86].

The phenomenon of opioid-induced hyperalgesia (OIH) is currently being described with increasing frequency [87, 88]. Among other things, it is associated with the fact that in the last two decades, more and more patients have been receiving permanent opioid treatment. Nowadays, many patients not suffering from a tumour disease as well as patients of advanced age and those living with dementia are also prescribed various opioid substances for the treatment of chronic pain and dyspnoea.

OIH describes a clinical situation when patients on long-term opioid therapy suddenly, or amid dose increase, begin to experience an uptick in pain intensity. This state is characterised by a hypersensitisation towards nociceptive stimuli, resulting in exacerbating pain in intensity and quality, exceeding the expected analgesic effect of dose increase (see **Figure 17**).

Risk factors for the occurrence of OIH constitute:

- Prolonged use of opioids;
- High doses of opioid analgesics;
- Frequent rotation of opioid classes;
- Frequent combinations of two or more different opioid substances;

Prognostic life expectancy	***Recommended measure of pain therapy***
< 3 months	Oral, transdermal, subcutaneous, epidural
3 to 6 months	Oral, transdermal, subcutaneous, intrathecal (external pump)
> 6 months	Oral, transdermal, subcutaneous, intrathecal (external or internally implanted pump)

Figure 17.
Pain therapy decision-making depending on PCP life expectancy.

- Abrupt discontinuation of opioids ("withdrawal syndrome"), especially if the last opioid substance has been taken for a long time;
- Administration of opioid antagonists amid long-term opioid therapy.

Adding to that, PCPs commonly exhibit several factors potentiating the above-mentioned risks, such as:

- Atypical pain patterns, more frequently;
- Higher prevalence of neuropathic pain or mixed-pain syndromes [81];
- Often "total pain" syndrome (**Figure 18**).

OIH is a well-known complication of opioid therapy [89]. The underlying mechanisms are not yet fully understood. Ultimately, imbalance of pronociceptive and antinociceptive systems seems to play a major role [90, 91]. According to the opponent-process theory, equilibrium is achieved by balancing the two opposing processes, pronociceptive and antinociceptive. A shift in balance by influencing one of the sides in particular can result in either opioid-induced analgesia or OIH.

Repeated opioid exposure leads to increasing activation of the pronociceptive systems and thus to a decrease in the analgesic effect of opioids. At the same time, an increase in the sensitivity of the nociceptors is observed as well as an activation of pain-modulating and pain-inhibiting systems alike. Thus, this is a pronociceptive process that is related to the processes of tolerance development to opioid substances but differs distinctly from opioid tolerance [92]. Via the process of OIH, opioids may enhance the sensibility towards nociceptive stimuli.

The following systems and mechanisms are pivotal to the development of OIH: [92].

- Central glutaminergic system;
- Spinal dynorphins may increase the levels of excitatory neuropeptides, enhancing the response to nociceptive stimuli;
- Activation of descending antinociceptive spinal pathways;
- Genetic mechanisms;
- Reuptake reduction of neuropeptides and amplification of the nociceptive response;
    - Possibly, morphine-3-glucuronide is involved in this process.

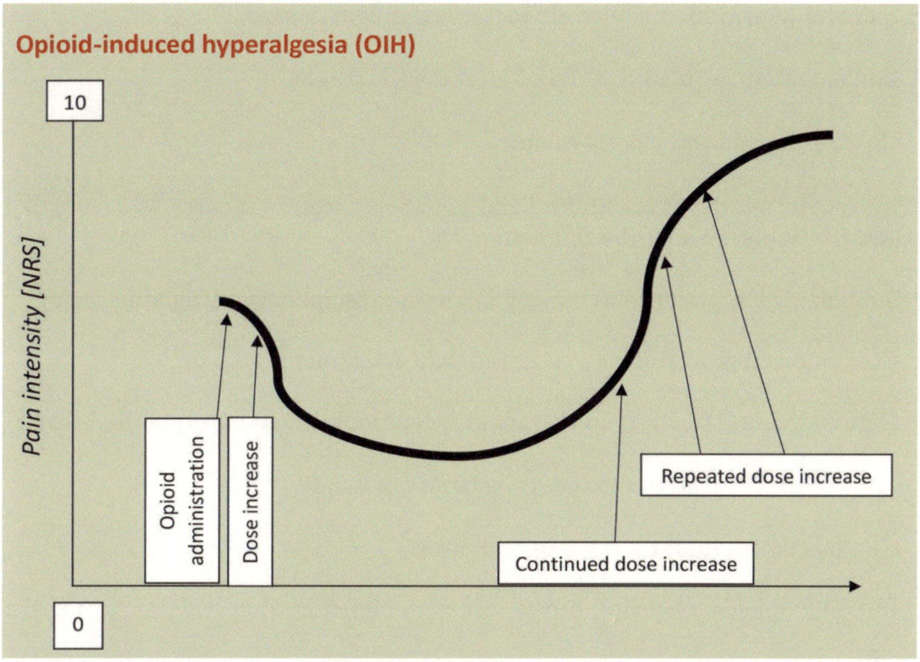

Figure 18.
Schematic depiction of OIH. Source: Self-created.

Changes in the activity of NMDA receptors are also associated with hypersensitivity of nociceptive structures. In 2009, Silverman described several factors linking the NMDA receptor to developing OIH: [86].

- NMDA receptors are found to be activated in OIH [93];
- Activation and inhibition of the glutamate transport system results in varying levels of glutamate available as a ligand for NMDA receptors;
- Long-term opioid therapy can lead to NMDA receptor-induced apoptotic cell death of spinal neurons in the dorsal horn;
- "Cross talk" between neural mechanisms of pain and tolerance may be at work.

Amid inhibition of the NMDA receptor, the development of OIH and opioid tolerance can be effectively prevented [86].

Unfortunately, the first possible signs of OIH are often overlooked in clinical routine. In addition, differentiating between OIH and opioid tolerance is de facto challenging. What can assist us in correctly diagnosing OIH in time? Telltale signs may include the following [86]:

- Unexplained increase in pain amid ongoing opioid therapy;
- Occurrence of diffuse allodynia unrelated to the original pain;

- Increase in pain intensity while increasing opioid dosage;
- Limited, short-termed pain relief after dose increase;
- Changes in pain intensity dynamics.

Therapeutic strategies are limited and not always lead to success. We have to consider the importance of the following:

- Supporting the patient intensively in an interdisciplinary caregiving team;
- Continuous monitoring and repeated pain assessment;
- High individual freedom in therapeutic decisions, made by a qualified team;
    - No prefabricated therapeutic schemes at hand!
- Careful reduction of the total opioid dose;
- Rotating opioids, choosing substances with higher antihyperalgesic properties:
    - Different opioids possess varying degrees of hyper- or antihyperalgesic qualities [90];
    - That is, fentanyl, sufentanil and alfentanil hold relatively high hyperalgesic qualities and are therefore considered to bear a significant risk for developing OIH;
    - Buprenorphine appears to have the highest antihyperalgesic activity among the most commonly used opioid substances. In particular, sublingual administration of buprenorphine seems to be an attractive option [86];
    - L-polamidone and methadone, as dual action mechanism opioids, can also be employed for opioid rotation [94] due to their antagonistic effect on the NMDA receptor;
    - In general, combining opioids with varying receptor selectivity is conceivable, thereby suppressing sensitisation processes and optimising pain therapy (**Figure 19**).
- COX inhibitors and, questionably, paracetamol reduce spinal release of excitatory neurotransmitters, which activate the pronociceptive and anti-opioid systems and thus show a synergistic effect together with NMDA receptor antagonists;
- NMDA antagonist ketamine is an excellent antihyperalgesic substance [83];
- $\alpha 2$-agonists, such as clonidine, moxonidine and methyldopa, may be beneficial [87];
- Tricyclic antidepressants (TCA) are said to play a role in treating OHI by inhibiting the release of acetylcholine;

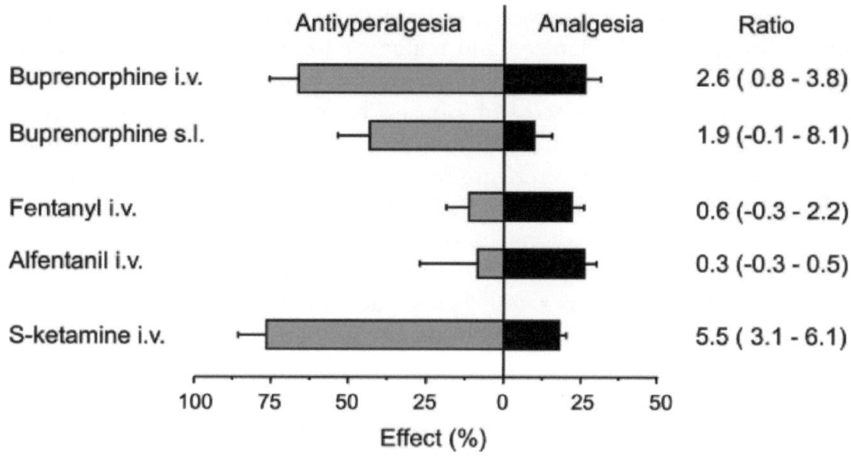

Figure 19.
Antinociceptive and antihyperalgesic effects [91].

- Memantine as a non-competitive antagonist of the NMDA receptor is applicable;
- Nitric oxide (NO) is assumed to have an effect on NMDA receptors as well [95];
- Interventional regional pain therapy procedures, including blockades (i.e., sympathetic blockade), catheter procedures:
    - Peripheral;
    - Epidural;
    - Intrathecal.
        a. When applying non-opioid analgesics intrathecally, a rapid and substantial reduction of opioid dosage is possible, and thus, an attenuation of hyperalgesic mechanisms is feasible.
- Ziconotide intrathecally. The preparation, first obtained from the venom of the Conus magus snail, is a highly potent non-opioid analgesic substance [96]. However, ziconotide can only be administered intrathecally and has an unfavourable side effect profile. Both factors justify the reluctant usage in palliative care and must therefore be considered merely as ultima ratio [97].

Our clinical observations have revealed that while opioid treatment remains a valid, effective and often the main therapeutic option in treating patients with chronic pain, we cannot consider it to be a panacea. Particularly in patients at advanced stages of disease, significant comorbidities and a high symptom burden, it is not uncommon for adverse drug effects, opioid tolerance or addiction to develop. Problems related to OIH have been capturing more and more attention in recent years as well. This prompts us to provide far-sighted, patient-centred support to our patients. Handling the prescribed medication is a very sensitive and decisive issue, especially given that polypharmacy is a common sight in PCPs. Furthermore, it is indispensable for the caregiving team to reflect extensively together with the patient and his relatives (the "Significant Others") on the aspired and realistic extent of therapeutic success. In doing so, talking frankly about possible side effects, complications and obstacles along the way as well is vital. This process of joint reflection shapes the therapeutic strategy and ultimately entitles us to make a mutual decision amid informed consent.

When facing a PCP in pain, there are myriads of various pharmacological and non-pharmacological treatment options, pathophysiological mechanisms and phenomena, obstacles and problem areas to consider along the way in order to establish effective pain management. We as caregivers have to broaden our horizon and not treat targeted pain therapy merely as a set of pharmaceuticals. "Differentiated pain therapy" requires a whole new philosophy in dealing with advanced illness patients [98].

11. Invasive pain therapy: a feasible option in palliative care?

Until the 1970s, invasive or neurodestructive methods dominated pain therapy for incurable (especially tumour) diseases. Invasive methods were used in ca. 85% of all tumour patients, whereas currently the share of invasive pain therapy measures is approx. 2–3% [99]. Given the advances in systemic pharmacotherapy, the proportion of non-invasive pharmacological management of patients with cancer-related pain has increased drastically. In 90 to 95% of cases, adequate pain control can be achieved *via* non-invasive pain therapy [100]. Nevertheless, 5–10% of patients continue to suffer from severe pain, even amid escalating combined systemic analgesic treatment [101].

In these situations, invasive pain management is one of the options to consider.

However, deciding on the use of aggressive pain management procedures in palliative care is often not straightforward. One of the most important principles of symptom control in PCPs is to alleviate discomfort without causing additional harm or adding new distress to the patient. Thus, in the decision-making process, it is imperative that we take into account the PCP's stage of the incurable disease and, accordingly, whether the invasive measures being considered are still appropriate.

Therefore, we see the option of invasive pain management in palliative care as an additive therapy rather than a substitute for pharmacological treatment. However, once the decision is made to go forward with invasive measures, the aim is twofold [102, 103]:

- Improving the analgesic effect of the preceding therapy;
- Dose reduction of conventional opioids and mitigation of side effects.

Close monitoring of the opioid dose after the application of invasive procedures is a top priority in order to avoid respiratory depression, especially in advanced phases of the disease.

Possible indications for invasive pain management in palliative care include: [104].

- Therapy-refractory pain, after having applied all feasible options according to the "WHO Analgesic Ladder";
- Unbearable side effects of conventional systemic pain therapy;
- Oral route of drug administration inapplicable;

- Tumour pain with a distinct neuropathic pain component, for example, plexopathy;

- Therapy-resistant, persistent and relapsing breakthrough pain whose intensity is significantly higher than the baseline pain.

The invasive procedures at hand may be categorised as either neuroablative and neurodestructive, causing irreversible damage to neural structures, or neuromodulative and neuroaugmentative, having a reversible influence on defined neural structures or systems.

Neurodestructive methods include: [99].

- Surgical sectioning or partial destruction of the nerve, for instance, using percutaneous catheter-assisted thermal lesion;

- Neurolytic methods utilising:

    - Alcohol 96%;

    - Phenol;

    - Glucose 40%.

Neuroaugmentative procedures modulate neuronal ionic currents or chemical information transmissions at the receptor or neuron of the spinal cord [99]. This also includes spinal (epidural or intrathecal) drug application and spinal cord stimulation (see **Figure 20**).

Reversible interruptions of stimuli with the help of local anaesthetics, such as peripheral nerve blocks and percutaneous intrathecal or peridural blocks, are an effective option for pain management in palliative care. However, invasive neuroablative methods, such as invasive neurolysis (i.e., percutaneous neurolysis of the celiac ganglion or plexus hypogastricus), percutaneous or open chordotomy as well as percutaneous rhizotomy, are hardly used in contemporary palliative care anymore [106–108].

Intrathecal analgesia has the following advantages: [109].

- Immediate effect of the substances at spinal receptors;

- Bypassing the hepatic first-pass metabolism;

Anatomical target structure	***Therapeutic measure***	***Practical significance****
Peripheral nerve	Transcutaneous nerve stimulation	+++
Funiculus posterior	SCS (Spinal Cord Stimulation)	+/-
Spinal receptors	Epidural / intrathecal drug administration	+++

**** significance:***
- no / + little / ++ medium / +++ substantial

Figure 20.
Neuroaugmentative measures in paint therapy [99, 105].

- Highest analgesic efficiency with relatively low toxicity in comparison with other administration forms;
- Neuroaugmentative measure with temporary effect, not neurodestructive;
- Intrathecally applied; analgesics bear a potency at least 100 times higher than orally and 10 times higher than epidurally applied; therefore:
    - Lower doses and volumes required for comparable analgesic effect;
    - Resulting in a more direct, local and targeted pain therapy;
    - While observing relatively little craniocaudal spread and hence evaluating the risk of serious respiratory or cardiovascular adverse drug effects as low and reasonable.

Among others, the following substances can be applied intrathecally:

- Opioids, blockage of opiate receptors in the substantia gelatinosa of the spinal cord:
    - Morphine;
    - Hydromorphone;
    - Fentanyl;
    - Sufentanil;
    - Buprenorphine;
- Local anaesthetics, blockage of Na^+ channels at Aδ and C fibres:
    - Ropivacaine;
    - Bupivacaine;
    - Lidocaine;
- And other non-opioid substances:
    - Ziconotide, blockage of N-type Ca^{2+} channels;
    - Clonidine, agonist at the α_2 receptor in the spinal cord;
    - Ketamine, blockage of NMDA receptors in the spinal cord.

For intrathecal or epidural use via continuous application, local anaesthetics can be combined with opioids, that is:

DOI: http://dx.doi.org/10.5772/intechopen.112325

- *Bupivacaine 0.2% + Hydromorphone 0.02 mg/mL*
    - Starting at 0.5 mL/h
    - Gradual increase, up to 1.5 mL/h

The following considerations are crucial for the practical implementation:

- The tip of the spinal catheter should be placed in the middle of the dermatome level of the required blockage area;
- The positioning of the catheter is vital, and therefore, it has to be X-ray-controlled;
- Substance spread within the spinal cord is limited to a few centimetres around the catheter tip, whereby differences arise depending on the substance's hydro- and lipophilicity:
    - Fentanyl, highly lipophilic: spread is oftentimes limited to area encompassing two vertebrae from the catheter tip
    - Morphine, highly hydrophilic: diffused spread and thus an effect similar to a systemic effect.

With regard to decisions on therapy options in palliative care, the selection criteria depend on the PCP's current situation and estimated prognostic life expectancy, which, among other things, can answer the question of the appropriateness of the measures being considered (see **Figure 17**) [110, 111].

If the patient has a short life expectancy and a high symptom burden, the decision would be made in favour of an epidural rather than a spinal catheter, with an external pump for drug application. If the patient has a longer life expectancy and is in an adequately good general state, an intrathecal (spinal) catheter may be justified, including the placement of an internal pump with subcutaneous catheter tunnelling.

Most usefully, the pumps should be operated in PCA (Patient Controlled Analgesia) mode. The following advantages apply to this procedure:

- Continuous administration allows for a constant level of analgesic substance to attained;
- Combinations of different drugs are possible as well;
- Bolus administration is feasible as PRN (or rescue) medication for breakthrough pain;
- Maximum amounts can be individually defined, facilitating good controllability and preventing overdosing;
- The patient remains mobile and flexible.

Case study 2:

- Female patient, 49 y.;
- Diagnosis: extensively cervically **metastasised mammary carcinoma**. Metastases are palpable subcutaneously, that is, at the interscalene triangle, non-exulcerating;
- Tumorous lesions encircling the right brachial plexus, resulting in plexopathy;
- **Severe pain of neuropathic origin**: peripheral, neuralgic and sympathalgic pain affecting the total upper right limb:
    - Shooting, "lightning strike"-like pain extending all the way down into the hand;
    - Burning pain attacks of the hand, **up to NRS 10**;
    - Tingling paraesthesia, numbness affecting the hand;
    - Allodynia;
    - Vegetative phenomena: thermal dysaesthesia, local diaphoresis;
    - Partial mono-palsy of the right arm and hand.
- Initial treatment:
    - Opioids:
        a. Initially, hydromorphone. Gradual dosage increase up to 2 × 64 mg;
        b. In addition: fentanyl patch. Gradual dosage increase up to 125 μg/h. Initially, changing patches every 72 h. Later, suspecting "end of dose failure", change at every 48 h;
        c. PRN medication:
            1. Hydromorphone acute 2.6 mg, max. 6× per day;
            2. Hydromorphone 2 mg s.c., max. 6× per day;
            3. Fentanyl sublingually (ROO), 100 to 400 μg, amid extreme pain spikes.
    - Co-analgesics, among others:
        a. Pregabalin, up to 300 mg per days;
        b. Amitriptyline, up to 100 mg per day;
        c. Dexamethasone, up to 24 mg per day.

- Non-opioid analgesics:

    a. Parecoxib 40 mg i.v., 1/d for 10 days;

    b. Metamizole 4–5 mg/d;

- Palliative radiotherapy of the region primarily affected.

- **Only marginal mitigation** of symptom burden (pain intensity fluctuating between NRS 5–10), **no adequate pain relief**!

- Notably, the burning pain attacks of the hand are perceived as unbearable and are not noticeably affected by the therapy. Due to the allodynia, the patient achieves **temporary limited pain relief by submerging her hand into boiling water**.

- Given the failure of the preceding pharmacological and radiotherapeutic pain management to sufficiently alleviate the PCP's symptom burden, a decision has been made to establish a **peripheral blockage of the right brachial plexus**:

    - Initially, a **diagnostical interscalene blockage** utilising 20 mL of ropivacaine 0.75% has been performed, resulting in almost complete anaesthesia of the upper limb and painlessness;

    - Given the difficulty of establishing a continuous blockage due to extensive subcutaneous metastases, the permanent measure *via* the interscalene triangle has been realised amid **CT guidance**;

    - **Successful blockage *via* the infraclavicular region**. Retrograde, CT-guided advance of the catheter tip towards the brachial plexus. Subsequently, 5-cm tunnelling of the catheter to reduce the risk of infection and catheter dislocation;

    - **Initiation of PCA analgesia *via* an external pump**, utilising ropivacaine 0.375% and buprenorphine 0.4 mg/d.

- **Substantial pain relief!** Currently, pain intensity amounts to NRS 3 and rare BTP episodes with reduced intensity of NRS 4. Subsequently, the **opioid dosage could be reduced** to less than 50 mg/d of morphine (converted), up to 2 × 4 mg of hydromorphone.

- **Permanent (> 3 months) satisfactory symptom control** (see **Figure 21**)!

12. Non-pharmaceutical aspects of pain management in palliative care

Preventive medicine and palliative care hold clinically relevant overlaps and are both classic, yet so far underdeveloped, cross-sectional areas of health care [112].

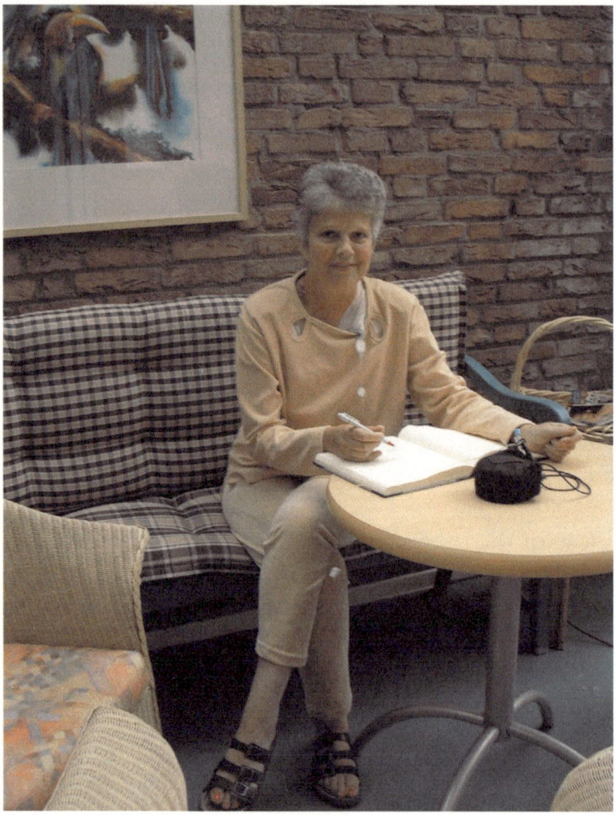

Figure 21.
PCP with infraclavicular catheter amid tumour lesions encircling the brachial plexus. Courtesy of Centre for Palliative Care, Unna, Germany. 2004.

Due the common presence of severe comorbidities, a poor general state and a lower resilience and endurance of the advanced ill, non-drug options of pain therapy are, unfortunately, frequently set aside. However, these methods can be an effective addition to drug treatment [113]. "Physiotherapy within the realms of palliative care is an exceptional means of preserving and improving quality of life and independence" [114].

Various methods can be considered as valid additive measures in pain therapy, [112, 115] including:

- General physical methods, that is:
    - Physiotherapy;
    - Stimulation methods (e.g., transcutaneous electrical nerve stimulation, TENS);
    - Massages;
    - Lymphatic drainage;
    - Positioning therapy;
    - Occupational therapy;

- Treatments with warmth and coldness;
- Vibrations and stimulation;
- Kinesiology tapes;

- Psychotherapeutic interventions, that is:
    - Psychotherapeutically oriented conversations;
    - Learning pain coping strategies
    - Relaxation techniques;
    - Stress management skills, biofeedback;

- Complementary measures, including:
    - Homoeopathy;
    - Aromatherapy;
    - Acupuncture;
    - Yoga, Qi-Gong;
    - Reiki therapy;
    - Rhythmic embrocation after Wegman and Hauschka;
    - Singing bowl massage;
    - Phytotherapy;
    - Music therapy;
    - Art therapy.

The significance and potential of rehabilitative measures in palliative care is substantial:

- It opens up the possibility of directing the patient's sight away from the illness and his frailty itself towards the proper use of the PCP's remaining resources. This in some cases new perspective aids in strengthening salutogenesis, a more positive attitude and resilience in general.

- In employing additional non-pharmaceutical approaches, the advanced ill feels his needs and sorrows being taken seriously. He feels understood, and even the slightest progress in addressing his symptom burden adds to his positivity. This may foster hope.

13. To ensure that pain management works well

What is the decisive factor for a good outcome of our efforts to ensure adequate pain management in palliative care?

Caring for an advanced illness patient constitutes a multidisciplinary challenge. Thus, when working together in a caregiving team of various professions, it is crucial to reflect on one's own actions and on those of the whole team with a critical look.

I asked my colleagues, especially the palliative care nurses: "What do you expect from us, the doctors, in the joint care of an advanced illness person in pain?"

The answers turned out to be telling:

- Openness and willingness to engage in interdisciplinary exchange and hence to share a preparedness to change perspectives;
- Focus on the patient's needs and sorrows;
- Flexibility and creativity in everyday work;
- Ensuring a continuity of patient care: asking questions on one's own initiative regularly, performing continuous pain and symptom control;
- When establishing a treatment regime for pain management, always include PRN or rescue medication;
- A close exchange of information between team members in the event of changes in therapy is indispensable;

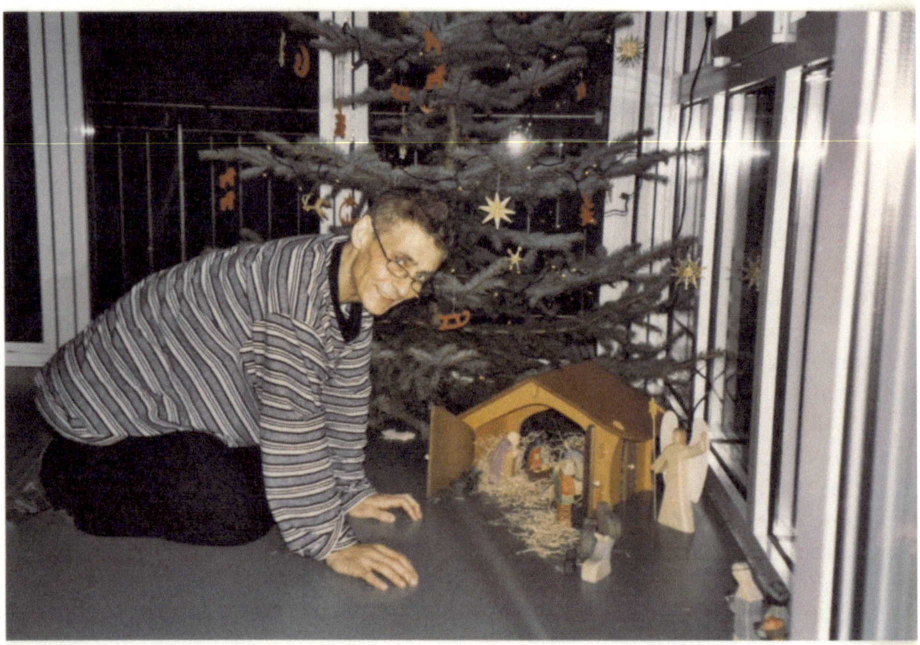

Figure 22.
When pain management succeeds. Courtesy of Centre for Palliative Care, Unna, Germany. 2006.

- Enabling the nursing staff, especially at outpatient care services, to make independent decisions on the administration of PRN medication within clearly communicated boundaries to ensure flexible, timely and goal-driven patient care. In order to do so, the colleagues have to be informed on, authorised for and entrusted with the application of the rescue medication and its limitations;

- Demanding and promoting additional training of nursing colleagues within the topics of palliative care and symptom control in particular.

The message for us doctors is to keep in mind seemingly simple notions—and to implement them into our work. And we will be rewarded for it. Because the greatest gift for us is our patients' satisfaction, their calm glance full of joy, hope and peace (**Figure 22**).

Acknowledgements

Translation: Robert Jonathan Hait.

Author details

Boris Hait
Centre for Palliative Care, Christliches Klinikum Unna-Mitte, Unna, Germany

*Address all correspondence to: b.hait@gmx.de

References

[1] World Health Organization. National Cancer Control Programmes. Policies and Managerial Guidelines. 2nd ed. Geneva: World Health Organization; 2002

[2] Boyd K, Murray SA. Recognizing and managing key transitions in EoL care. BMJ. 2010;**341**:c4863

[3] Trauern KV. Phasen Und Chancen Des Psychischen Prozesses. (Grieving: Phases and Chances of the Psychological Process). Freiburg im Breisgau, Germany: Kreuz; 2013. pp. 42-54.5

[4] Managing a Curriculum Innovation Process - Scientific Figure on ResearchGate. 2020. Available from: https://www.researchgate.net/figure/Kuebler-Ross-model-of-the-emotional-impact-of-change-based-on-their-grief-cycle-7_fig1_343844707 [Accessed: May 15, 2023].

[5] Kübler-Ross E. On Death and Dying. Toronto: Macmillan; 1969

[6] Douverman H. Altar of the Seven Sorrows. Kalkar, Germany: Church of St. Nicholas;

[7] Franklin AE, Lovell MR. Pain and Pain Management. Textbook of Palliative Care. Oxford, UK: Oxford University Press; 2018. pp. 1-29

[8] cf.Franklin AE, Lovell MR. Total pain, based on dame Cicely Saunders' model, pain and pain management. In: Textbook of Palliative Care. 2018. pp. 1-29

[9] Thöns M, Hait B. Schmerztherapie. In: Thöns M, Sitte T, editors. Hrsgb. Repetitorium Palliativmedizin. Vol. 3. Auflage. Berlin, Germany: Springer-Verlag; 2019. pp. 29-64

[10] Kojer M, Schmidl M. Demenz und Palliative Geriatrie in der Praxis. (Dementia and palliative geriatrics in practice). Vol. 2. Springer; 2016. pp. 39-65

[11] Saunders C, Baines M, Dunlop R. Living with Dying: A Guide to Palliative Care. Oxford, UK: Oxford University Press; 3rd ed. 1995

[12] Saunders C, Sykes N. The Management of Terminal Malignant Disease. 3rd ed. London: Edward Arnold; 1993

[13] Oestmann A. Vergessene Symptome bei Palliativpatienten. (forgotten symptoms in PCPs). Palliative-CH. 2011; **2**:5-7

[14] Finsterer J. Mitochondriopathies. European Journal of Neurology. 2004; **11-3**:163-186

[15] Flatters SJ, Bennet GJ. Studies of peripheral sensory nerves in paclitaxel-induced painful peripheral neuropathy: Evidence for mitochondrial disfunction. Pain. 2006;**122**(3):245-257

[16] Forsyth PA et al. Prospective study of paclitaxel-induced peripheral neuropathy with quantitative sensory testing. Journal of Neuro-Oncology. 1997;**35**(1):47-53

[17] Kröner-Herwig B, Frettlöh J, Klinger R. Schmerzpsychotherapie. In: Nilges P, editor. Psychotherapy in Pain Management. Berlin, Germany: Springer-Verlag; 2017. pp. 215-238

[18] Turk DC, Rudy TE. Toward an empirically derived taxonomy of chronic pain patients: Integration of psychological assessment data. Journal of Consulting and Clinical Psychology. 1988;**56**:233-238

[19] Von der Laage D, et al. Patientenatlas Schmerz ("Patient Atlas of Pain"). Aachen, Germany: Grünenthal; 2012

[20] Woolf CJ. American College of Physicians; American Physiological Society. Pain: Moving from symptom control toward mechanism-specific pharmacologic management. Annals of Internal Medicine. 2004;**140**(6):441-451. DOI: 10.7326/0003-4819-140-8-200404200-00010

[21] Reckinger K. Schmerztherapie in der Palliativmedizin. In: Koppert B, Willweber-Strumpf S, editors. Praktische Schmerzmedizin. Vol. 29. Berlin, Germany: Springer-Verlag; 2013. pp. 441-443

[22] Reckinger K et al. Der geriatrische Schmerzpatient. Aachen, Germany: Grünenthal; 2016

[23] Aprakian AV et al. Human brain mechanisms of pain perception and regulation in health and disease. European Journal of Pain. 2005;**9**:463-484

[24] Twycross R et al. Palliative Care Formulary. England: Palliativedrugs.com; 2015. pp. 291-458

[25] Lötsch J, Geisslinger G. Are μ-opioid receptor polymorphisms important for clinical opioid therapy? Trends in Molecular Medicine. 2005;**11**(2):82-89

[26] Galer BS, Coyle N, Pasternak GW, Portenoy RK. Individual variability in the response to different opioids: Report of five cases. Pain. 1992;**49**(1):87-91

[27] Klepstad P, Rakvag T, Kaasa S, et al. The 118 a>G polymorphism in the human μ-opioid receptor gene may increase morphine requirements in patients with pain caused by malignant disease. Acta Anaesthesiologica Scandinavica. 2004;**48**(10):1232-1239

[28] Cherny N. The management of cancer pain. CA: A Cancer Journal for Clinicians. 2000;**50**(70–116):79

[29] Caraceni A et al. Use of opioid analgesics in the treatment of cancer pain: Evidence-based recommendations from the EAPC. The Lancet Oncology. 2012;**13**:e58-e68

[30] Foley KM. Treatment of cancer-related pain. Journal of the National Cancer Institute Monographs. 2004;**32**: 103-104

[31] Vielhaber A, Portenoy RK. Advances in cancer pain management. Hematology/Oncology Clinics of North America. 2002;**16**(3):527-541

[32] Cherny NI, Fallon MT, Kaasa S, Portenoy RK, Currow DC. Oxford Textbook of Palliative Care. Vol. 9. Oxford, UK: Oxford University Press; Fifth ed. 2015. pp. 491-631

[33] Grün B et al. Contribution of CYP2C19 and CYP3A4 to the formation of the active nortilidine from the prodrug tilidine. British Journal of Clinical Pharmacology. 2012;**74**:854-863

[34] Seiler KU, Jähnchen E, Trenk D, Brennscheidt U, Heintz B. Pharmacokinetics of tilidine in terminal renal failure. Journal of Clinical Pharmacology. 2001;**41**:79-84

[35] Leppert W. CYP2D6 in the metabolism of opioids for mild to moderate pain. Pharmacology. 2011;**87**: 274-285

[36] Gl C, Matzke GR. Effects of renal insufficiency on the pharmacokinetics and pharmacodynamics of opioid

analgetics. Drug Intelligence & Clinical Pharmacy. 1987;**21**:773-783

[37] Liechti ME. Pharmakologie von Schmerzmitteln für die praxis. (pharmacology of analgesics for practical use). Schweiz Medical Forum. 2014;**14** (24):460-464

[38] Petri H. CYP450-Wechselwirkungen: Das Interaktionspotenzial der Antitussiva. (CYP450 interactions: Interaction potential of antitussives). Dtsch Arztebl. 2015;**112**(9):18

[39] Gelot S, Nakhla E. Opioid dosing in renal and hepatic impairment. US Pharm. 2014;**39**(8):34-38

[40] Rémi C et al. Arzneimitteltherapie in der Palliativmedizin. In: Pharmacotherapy in Palliative Care. 4. Auflage ed. Munich, Jena, Germany: Urban & Fischer München; 2022

[41] Foral P, Ineck JR, Nystrom KK. Oxycodone accumulation in a hemodialysis patient. Southern Medical Journal. 2007;**100**(2):212-214

[42] Freye E. Pharmakokinetik der Opioide: Bedeutung für den praktischen Einsatz. (pharmacokinetics of opioids: Significance for use in practice). In: Opioide in der Medizin. Berlin, Heidelberg: Springer; 2010. DOI: 10.1007/978-3-540-88797-3_20

[43] Sarhill N, Walsh D, Nelson KA. Hydromorphone: Pharmacology and clinical applications in cancer patients. Support Care Cancer. 2001;**9** (2):84-96

[44] Sarhill N et al. Methadone-induced myoclonus in advanced cancer. American Journal of Hospice and Palliative Medicine. 2001;**18**:51-53

[45] Davis MP. Fentanyl for breakthrough pain: A systematic review. Expert Review of Neurotherapeutics. 2011;**11**:1197-1216

[46] Tegeder I. Therapy with opioids in liver or renal failure. Der Schmerz. 1999; **13**:183-195

[47] Nomura M, Inoue K, Matsushita S, Takahari D, Kondoh C, Shitara K, et al. Serum concentration of fentanyl during conversion from intravenous to transdermal administration to patients with chronic cancer pain. The Clinical Journal of Pain. 2013;**29**:487-484

[48] Grond S, Radbruch L, Lehmann KA. Clinical pharmacokinetics of transdermal opioids: Focus on transdermal fentanyl. Clinical Pharmacokinetics. 2000;**38**:59-89

[49] Kuip EJM et al. Fentanyl metabolism and elimination. British Journal of Clinical Pharmacology. 2017;**83**(2): 294-313

[50] Smith H. Opioid metabolism. Mayo Clinic Proceedings. 2009;**84**(7):613-624

[51] Kuip EJM et al. A review of factors explaining variability in fentanyl pharmacokinetics; focus on implications for cancer patients. British Journal of Clinical Pharmacology. 2017;**83**(2): 294-313

[52] Strain EC, Moody DE, Stoller KB, Walsh SL, Bigelow GE: Relative bioavailability of different buprenorphine formulations under chronic dosing conditions. In: Drug and Alcohol Dependence Band 74, Nr. 1, 2004, S. 37–43

[53] Elkader A, Sproule B. Buprenorphine: Clinical pharmacokinetics in the treatment of opioid dependence. In: Clinical

Pharmacokinetics Band 44, Nr. 7, 2005, S. 661–680

[54] Bodkin JA, Zornberg GL, Lukas SE, Cole JO. Buprenorphine treatment of refractory depression. Journal of Clinical Psychopharmacology. 1995;**15**(1):49-57

[55] Nyhuis PW, Gastpar M. Opiate treatment in ECT-resistant depression. Pharmacopsychiatry. 2005;**38**:38-A175

[56] Nicholson AB, Watson GR, Derry S, Wiffen PJ. Methadone for cancer pain. Cochrane Database of Systematic Reviews. 2017;**2**:CD003971

[57] Bitar HN, Cipta AM, Lee KW, Woo WS. A unique case report on methadone used for treatment of opioid-induced hyperalgesia in a cancer patient at the end of life. Cureus. 2019;**11**:e5394

[58] Schuster M, Bayer O, Heid F, Laufenberg-Feldmann R. Opioid rotation in cancer pain treatment – A systematic review. Deutsches Ärzteblatt International. 2018;**115**:135-142. DOI: 10.3238/arztebl.2018.0135

[59] Singh DR et al. Tapentadol hydrochloride: A novel analgesic. Saudi Journal of Anaesthesia. 2013;**7**(3): 322-326

[60] Kneip C, Terlinden R, Beier H, Chen G. Investigations into drug-drug interaction potential of tapentadol in human liver microsomes and fresh human hepatocytes. Drug Metabolism Letters. 2008;**2**:67-75

[61] Etropolski MS, Okamoto A, Shapiro DY, Rauschkolb C. Dose conversion between tapentadol immediate and extended release for low back pain. Pain Physician. 2010;**13**:61-70

[62] Schwartz S, Etropolski M, Shapiro DY, Okamoto A, Lange R, Haeussler J, et al. Safety and efficacy of tapentadol ER in patients with painful diabetic peripheral neuropathy: Results of a randomized placebo controlled trial. Current Medical Research and Opinion. 2011;**27**:151-162

[63] Sittl R, Likar R, Poulsen NB. Equipotent doses of transdermal fentanyl and transdermal buprenorphine in patients with cancer and noncancer pain: Results of a retrospective cohort study. Clinical Therapeutics. 2005;**27**(2): 225-237

[64] Bernatzky G, Sittl R, Likar R. Schmerzbehandlung in der Palliativmedizin. Berlin, Germany: Springer-Verlag; 2012

[65] S3-Leitlinie Palliativmedizin 2.2. 2020. Available from: https://www.leitlinienprogramm-onkologie.de/leitlinien/palliativmedizin/September 2020 AWMF-Registernummer: 128/001OL

[66] Heyn J, Azad SC. Differential indications of opioids in pain therapy. Der Anaesthesist. 2017;**66**(11):829-839

[67] Petri H. Therapie mit Opioiden: Was es zu beachten gilt. (opioid therapy. What to keep in mind). Deutsches Ärzteblatt. 2014;**111**(41):12

[68] Schenk M, Wirz S. Serotoninsyndrom und medikamentöse Schmerztherapie: Was ist für die praxis relevant? [serotonin syndrome and pain medication: What is relevant for practice?]. Schmerz. 2015;**29**(2):229-251. German. DOI: 10.1007/s00482-015-1512-0

[69] Grotha AM et al. Das serotonin-Syndrom. (serotonin syndrome). Swiss Medical Forum. 2020;**20**(3134):463-465

[70] King S et al. A systematic revue of the use of opioid medication for those

with moderate to severe cancer pain and renal impairment. Palliative Medicine. 2011;**25**:525-552

[71] Margetts L, Sawyer R. Transdermal drug delivery: Principles and opioid therapy. Continuing Education in Anesthesia, Critical Care and Pain. 2007; **7**(5):171-176

[72] Heiskanen T, Matzke S, Haakana S, Gergov M, Vuori E, Kalso E. Transdermal fentanyl in cachectic cancer patients. Pain. 2009;**144**:218-222

[73] Budd K. Buprenorphine and the transdermal system: The ideal match in pain management. International Journal of Clinical Practice. Supplement. 2003; **133**:9-14

[74] Portenoy RK, Lesage P. Management of cancer pain. Lancet. 1999;**353**(9165): 1695-1700

[75] Porta-Sales J. Diagnosis and management of breakthrough cancer pain: Have all the questions been resolved? A Delphi-based consensus assessment (DOIRON). Clinical & Translational Oncology. 2016;**18**(9):945-954

[76] Davies AN et al. Breakthrough cancer pain (BTcP) management: A review of international and national guidelines. BMJ Supportive & Palliative Care. 2018;**8**(3):241-249

[77] Mercadante S, Portenoy RK. Breakthrough cancer pain: Twenty-five years of study. Pain. 2016;**157**(12): 2657-2663

[78] Portenoy RK. Breakthrough pain: Characteristics and impact in patients with cancer pain. Pain. 1999;**81**(1–2): 129-134

[79] Peter C, Watson N. Bonica's Management of Pain. 4th ed. New York, Ny: Lippincott Williams &Wilkins; 2010. pp. 13-23

[80] Doulton B. Pharmacologic management of adult breakthrough cancer pain. Canadian Family Physician. 2014;**60**(12):1111-1114 e585-9

[81] Bennett MI et al. Prevalence and aetiology of neuropathic pain in cancer patients: A systematic review. Pain. 2012;**153**(2):359-365

[82] Rayment C, Hjermstad MJ. Neuropathic cancer pain: Prevalence, severity, analgesics and impact from the European palliative care research collaborative–computerised symptom assessment study. Palliative Medicine. 2012;**27**(8):714-721

[83] Prommer EE. Ketamine for pain: An update of uses in palliative care. Journal of Palliative Medicine. 2012;**15**: 474-483

[84] Schnabel A, Rittner HL. Opioidrotation in der Praxis – Was, warum und wie? Arzneiverordnung in der Praxis (AVP). 2018;**45**:33-37

[85] Rost A. Schmerztherapie bei Tumorpatienten in der (fortgeschrittenen) Palliativsituation. In: Arzneiverordnung in der Praxis. 2020. pp. 1-11. Available from: https://www.akdae.de/fileadmin/user_upload/akdae/Arzneimitteltherapie/AVP/vorab/20200803-Tumorschmerztherapie.pdf

[86] Silverman SM. Opioid induced hyperalgesia: Clinical implications for the pain practitioner. Pain Physician. 2009;**12**(3):679-684

[87] Koppert W. Opioid-induzierte Hyperalgesie. (opioid-induced hyperalgesia). Der Anaesthesist. 2004; **53**:455-466

[88] Mercadante S. Opioid-induced tolerance and hyperalgesia. CNS Drugs. 2019;**33**(10):943-955

[89] Davis MP et al. When opioids cause pain. Journal of Clinical Oncology. 2007; **25**:4497-4498

[90] Koppert W. Opioidvermittelte Analgesie und Hyperalgesie. (opioid-induced analgesia and hyperalgesia). Der Schmerz. 2005;**19**:386-394

[91] Koppert W. Antinociceptive and antihyperalgic effects. Pain. 2005;**118**: 15-22

[92] Yi P, Pryzbylkowski P. Opioid induced hyperalgesia. Pain Medicine. 2015;**16**(Suppl 1):S32-S36

[93] Salpeter SR, Buckley JS, Bruera E. The use of very-low-dose methadone for palliative pain control and the prevention of opioid hyperalgesia. Journal of Palliative Medicine. 2013;**16** (6):616-622

[94] Mercadante S, Bruera E. Opioid switching: A systematic and critical review. Cancer Treatment Reviews. 2006;**32**(4):304-315

[95] Sorkin LS. NMDA evokes an L-NAME sensitive spinal release of glutamate and citrulline. Neuroreport. 1993;**4**(5):479-482

[96] Löschner D et al. Was wurde eigentlich aus Prialt®? Der Schmerz. 2021;**35**:343-348

[97] Jain KK. An evaluation of intrathecal ziconotide for the treatment of chronic pain. Expert Opinion on Investigational Drugs. 2000;**9**(10):2403-2410. DOI: 10.1517/13543784.9.10.2403

[98] Brush DE. Complications of long-term opioid therapy for management of chronic pain: The paradox of opioid-induced hyperalgesia. Journal of Medical Toxicology. 2012;**8**(4):387-392

[99] Willenbrink HJ. Schmerzbehandlung bei Tumorpatienten. In: 5. Bremer Palliativ Kongress. Aachen, Germany: Grünenthal; 2007. pp. 131-163

[100] de Leon-Casasola OA. Interventional procedures for cancer pain management: When are they indicated? Cancer Investigation. 2004;**22** (4):630-642. DOI: 10.1081/cnv-200027166

[101] Swarm RA et al. Interventional approaches for chronic pain. In: Oxford Textbook of Palliative Medicine. 5th ed. Vol. 9. Oxford, UK: Oxford University Press; 2015. pp. 589-631

[102] Bhatnagar S, Gupta M. Evidence-based clinical practice guidelines for interventional pain Management in Cancer Pain. Indian Journal of Palliative Care. 2015;**21**(2):137-147. DOI: 10.4103/0973-1075.156466

[103] Argoff CE, McCleane G. Interventional pain management. In: Pain Management Secrets Book. 3rd ed. Vol. 46. Amsterdam, Netherlands: Elsevier; 2009. pp. 357-363

[104] Lema MJ. Invasive analgesia techniques for advanced cancer pain. Surgical Oncology Clinics of North America. 2001;**10**(1):127-136

[105] Willenbrink HJ. Neuroaugmentative schmerztherapeutische Verfahren (Neuroaugmentative measures in paint therapy). In: Schmerzbehandlung bei Tumorpatienten, 5. Bremer Palliativ Kongress. Aachen, Germany: Grünenthal; 2007. pp. 131-163

[106] Smith H et al. The role of invasive pain management modalities in the

treatment of chronic pain. The Medical Clinics of North America. 2016;**100**(1): 103-115. DOI: 10.1016/j.mcna.2015.08.011

[107] Hankemeier U, Wagner T. Stellenwert der invasiven Maßnahmen in der Tumorschmerztherapie - aktuelle Bewertung. Zeitschrift für Palliativmedizin. 2003;**4**(2):55-58. DOI: 10.1055/s-2003-41382

[108] Eidelman A. Interventional therapies for cancer pain management: Important adjuvants to systemic analgesics. Journal of the National Comprehensive Cancer Network. 2007;**5** (8):753-760. DOI: 10.6004/jnccn.2007.0075

[109] Deer T, Hassenbusch SJ, et al. Recommendations for the management of pain by intrathecal drug delivery: Report of an interdisciplinary expert panel. Neuromodulation. 2007;**10**(4): 300-328

[110] Gehmacher O et al. Schmerztherapie in der Palliativmedizin. In: Klaschik E, Husebö S, editors. Palliativmedizin. Berlin, Germany: Springer-Verlag; 2017. pp. 159-213

[111] Gehmacher O, Likar R, et al. Schmerztherapie in der Palliativmedizin. In: Husebø S, Mathis G, editors. Palliativmedizin. Berlin, Germany: Springer-Verlag; 2017. pp. 159-213

[112] Schneider N, Walter U. Präventive Aspekte in der palliativen Versorgung (preventive aspects in palliative care). Prävention und Gesundheitsförderung. 2007;**2**:39-45

[113] Nieland P, Simader R. Physiotherapie in der Palliative Care – Rehabilitation am Lebensende. (Physiotherapy in Palliative Care – Rehabilitation at End of Life). Amsterdam, Netherlands: Elsevier; 2022. pp. 9-37

[114] Taylor J, Simader R, Nieland P. Potential and possibility: Rehabilitation at end of life. In: Physiotherapy in Palliative Care. Amsterdam, Netherlands: Elsevier; 2013

[115] Besendorfer A. Interdisziplinäres Schmerzmanagement. Praxisleitfaden zum Expertenstandart Schmerzmanagement in der Pflege. (Interdisciplinary pain management. Practical guidelines). Stuttgart: Kohlhammer; 2009. pp. 112-113

Chapter 9

Scrambler Therapy in Acute and Chronic Pain: A Review

James A. Tolley

Abstract

Scrambler therapy utilizes a device and technique that delivers a non-invasive electro-analgesic treatment regimen to patients in pain, both acute and chronic. It has been used in many patients suffering from neuropathic pain and other causes of pain that have been resistant to other treatment modalities, including oral analgesics, opioids, and nerve blocks. It operates using a specific protocol that requires training and experience but can be quite effective and lead to prolonged pain relief when administered appropriately. This chapter will review the relevant theory and mechanism of scrambler therapy and discuss the studies that have been conducted to evaluate its efficacy in a variety of pain disorders.

Keywords: scrambler therapy, chronic pain, acute pain, electroanalgesia, Calmare, neuropathic pain, neuropathy, non-invasive

1. Introduction

Chronic pain (CP) among adults is a common problem occurring in approximately 20% of the population in the United States and Canada [1, 2]. The prevalence of CP can increase with age with a recent survey of the elderly demonstrating a rate of 78% among respondents [3], many of whom had a neuropathic component to their pain. A total of 24% were taking opioids as part of their pain management regimen. Concerns with the use of opioids have led to the search for non-opioid alternatives of which gabapentin is one such option. However, the number needed to treat (NNT) neuropathic pain with gabapentin is relatively high at 6.6 [4]. Duloxetine has also been used to treat chronic back pain with a NNT of 10 [5]. As a group, serotonin-noradrenaline reuptake inhibitors have a NNT of 6.4 in a meta-analysis of pharmacologic therapy for neuropathic pain in adults [6]. Scrambler therapy has been touted as another alternative to treat neuropathic and other chronic pains with minimal side effects. This chapter will review scrambler therapy and its use to treat various chronic and acute pains.

2. Scrambler therapy history/mechanisms/theory

Scrambler therapy (ST) was developed in the early 1990s by Guiseppe Marineo in Italy [7]. It has been erroneously compared to transcutaneous electrical nerve stimulation (TENS), and although it is non-invasive and uses electrical stimulation, that is where the similarities end. TENS achieves its effects through several potential mechanisms, one of which involves the gate control theory of pain [8] as proposed by Melzack and Wall [9]. It is postulated that the peripheral stimulation of larger myelinated A-beta and A-delta fibers by the TENS device results in conduction blockade of the smaller pain transmitting C-fibers in the dorsal horn [8]. ST, alternatively, stimulates C-fibers directly and operates under the principles of information theory [10].

According to Claude E. Shannon's Information Theory [11], a communication system consists of five parts which are analogous to the components of the human nervous system, the purpose of which is to convey information about the environment to an individual. The information source produces the message, which in the case of pain, is the adverse stimulus that could cause potential harm to the organism. The transmitter alters the message and prepares it for transmission along the channel, which is what the nociceptor does in converting the stimulus into chemical information and then an electric action potential to transmit along the unmyelinated C-fiber. The receiver then restores the original message as intended for the ultimate destination which would be analogous to the somatosensory cortex and human consciousness, respectively [12].

Chronic pain is therefore a perturbation of an information system which ST seeks to correct. Guiseppe Marineo developed a device that acts as an artificial neuron to stimulate C-fiber receptors with "non-pain" information that the nervous system recognizes as "self" [10, 13, 14]. The commercially available version of the device contains five artificial neurons allowing for treatment of up to five areas of pain simultaneously [15]. Each artificial neuron can create 16 different synthetic action potentials which are then algorithmically combined into a total of 256 strings of "painless" information along with the "noise" that is necessarily present in information systems [10].

Testing to verify the safety and efficacy of the artificial neuron technology was performed at the University of Rome Tor Vergata for seven years from 1999 to 2006 on almost 2300 patients with severe neuropathic pain that had been refractory to other methods of treatment. Successful treatment was defined as more than 50% pain relief, and at 2-month follow-up, nearly 80% of patients had achieved this rate of success with essentially no side effects [10]. This data along with a few other clinical trials was used to obtain marketing approval in both Europe and ultimately from the United States Food and Drug Administration in 2009 [10, 16].

The inventor of the device has provided several recommendations and observations to improve outcomes of ST both in his own writings [10] and in response [17] to a multi-center study with a much lower rate of overall success at 38.1% [18] compared to the initial data with success rates near 80%.

- Patient selection: ST was developed for use in patients with neuropathic or cancer pain as opposed to nociceptive or mixed type pains [17].

- Protocol: The treatment consists of 10 applications over the course of 2 weeks [18, 19]. This number may be modified if the patient presents for a daily application and is pain-free or the patient may require more applications if taking a drug which can interfere with the response of the nervous system (see below).

- Provider: There is a learning curve associated with the use of the device [20], and it is recommended that electrocardiography electrodes with spongy contact surfaces are used along with a small amount of contact gel to optimize the stimulation of the C-fibers [10]. Stimulation should occur in an area adjacent to the pain, ideally in a dermatomal distribution and should not be painful.

- Pharmacology: Drugs that interfere with action potentials, such as anticonvulsants and local anesthetics will decrease the effectiveness of ST. Ketamine can have a similar effect, while muscle relaxants may increase the incidence of side effects such as muscle weakness or hypotension [10].

Considering the proposed role of information theory in the mechanism of ST, these recommendations would make sense. Neuropathic pain can be thought of as a disturbance in the normal homeostatic processes of the C-fibers and their receptors leading to chronic, neuropathic pain. Yet C-fibers also transmit pleasant tactile sensations [21] suggesting the lack of pain necessary during ST treatment for maximal efficacy has a biologic basis as does the interference found with certain drugs. During treatment, the changes that led to chronic, neuropathic pain are in effect being reversed, leading to a normalization of C-fiber activity that can persist over time.

However, one should note that the inventor does hold the patent to the device [22] and has had financial arrangements in place to benefit from its sale [23]. This is not to say that the device does not work precisely as described nor with the proposed efficacy, but one should evaluate the available information critically. The remainder of the chapter will review several of the available studies and case reports based upon indication and will allow the reader to come to their own conclusions.

3. Scrambler therapy for chemotherapy-induced peripheral neuropathy (CIPN)

As noted, ST was developed for use in patients with cancer pain or neuropathic pain [17], so it is not surprising that there are several studies looking at its use in patients who develop CIPN. In one of the first studies following FDA approval in 2009, Smith et al. [24] published, in 2010, a pilot trial reporting results on 16 patients with CIPN of three months to eight years duration with an average age of 58.6 years. The average reduction in pain at the completion of 10 days of 60-minute treatments was 59%. There was no difference in opioid usage and no adverse effects were noted.

At the 2013 meeting of the American Society for Clinical Oncology, Campbell et al. [25] presented an abstract comparing ST to an active sham device that delivered a barely perceptible electric sensation designed to be nontherapeutic. There were seven patients with painful CIPN that started in each arm of 10 daily sessions of 50 minutes. The authors state that there were no differences in the primary endpoint of pain reduction between groups but conclude that a sham is feasible and could be used for future controlled studies.

In 2013, Coyne and colleagues evaluated the effects of ST on 39 patients with cancer-related pain, 33 of which had CIPN [26]. The mean age of the patients was 56.5. ST treatments were 45 minutes in duration and performed for 10 daily sessions over a two-week period. Outcomes for pain and several quality-of-life measures were compared at baseline and days 14, 30, 60 and 90. Pain was significantly improved at all points following the conclusion of ST as were items on the Brief Pain Inventory (BPI) related to mood, sleep and relationships. Opioid usage did not change, however. There were no side effects noted. The authors felt that ST was effective in relieving CIPN and suggested that ST should be further investigated for other forms of pain also.

In 2015, Lee and colleagues published a pilot study on 20 patients with cancer-related neuropathic pain (CNP) of whom six had CIPN [27]. Patients had received conservative therapy for at least six months prior to enrollment in the study. The principal investigator had received training on the device from the inventor in Italy and in turn provided training to the others who would administer the ST treatments. Treatment consisted of ten daily 40-minute sessions with the possibility of skipping two days for weekends. The median age of these patients was 57.0. The endpoints were assessed at 2 weeks following conclusion of the ST compared to baseline. The decrease in pain score was statistically significant, but only six of the 20 patients reported more than 50% pain relief at the 2-week follow-up. Half the patients were satisfied with the treatment. Regular opioid usage did not decrease but rescue usage just achieved statistical significance at $P = 0.05$. None of the patients reported any significant adverse events. The authors mention in the discussion that their pain relief was decreased compared to other studies. They mention the heterogenicity of pain characteristics in their patients but do not state if the patients were continued on anticonvulsants which may have impacted the results.

Also in 2015, a study of 37 patients with CIPN was reported by Pachman et al. [20]. Patients had to have CIPN for greater than or equal to one month with a pain score of 4/10 or more. Patients were treated with up to 10 daily sessions of 30 minutes using ST. The average age was 58 with a range of 33 to 79 years. Patients were followed for 10 weeks. The study noted an average reduction in pain score of 53% following 10 days of treatment which seemed to persist throughout the follow-up period. However, the authors also note that later patients seemed to do better than earlier patients presumably as the study team gained more experience with the device and treatment protocol. Again, no adverse events were reported. The authors felt that this preliminary data showed ST may be effective for CIPN and called for additional studies.

In 2018, Tomasello et al. reported the results using ST for treating CIPN in 9 adolescents aged 12 to 17 [28]. The teens received 45-minute treatments over 10 consecutive days. At the end of the 10-day period, pain was significantly improved from an average of 9.22 to 2.33. Quality of life was improved in such metrics as generalized activity, walking, mood, sleep and relationships. Patients were on a variety of analgesic drugs which were tapered before or during ST. ST was tailored to each patient's needs with some requiring 14 days of treatment and one needing 21 days. In all but one patient, the pain score was 0 at the end of ST, and all patients were able to stop or decrease their analgesic drugs. Seven of the patients remained pain free at six months of follow-up. There were no reported adverse effects. The authors called for further studies with larger sample size but felt that ST could represent a good "first-line treatment" for CIPN given its efficacy and safety as well as the lasting effects.

In 2019, the results of a randomized phase II pilot study were published by Loprinzi et al. [29]. A total of 50 patients were randomized to receive either ST or TENS as a control group. The median ages were 61.5 for ST and 61.0 for TENS. ST sessions were for 30 minutes on 10 consecutive weekdays and TENS sessions were for 30 minutes per day for 14 days. Following the 2-week study period, patients were followed weekly for the next 8 weeks. A 50% or greater reduction in pain scores was seen in 40% of the ST patients and 20% of the TENS patients. At the end of the 8-week follow-up period, ST patients still had a 33% reduction in pain scores compared to baseline. One patient receiving ST noted minor ecchymosis at electrode placement sites and one noted contact dermatitis. Patients had to be willing to wean off gabapentin or pregabalin to participate in the study. The authors did not report other analgesic drugs that were being used nor the impact of the therapies on usage during the follow-up period. Patients receiving ST were more likely to recommend that treatment to others compared to the TENS group. There was an opportunity for the patients to crossover to the other treatment group following the 8-week follow-up period which is reported below in a separate publication by Childs et al. [30].

Of the 24 patients that had completed ST, 12 chose to crossover to the TENS group. Of the 22 patients completing the TENS arm in the first portion of the study, 10 chose to crossover and try ST. Again, treatments occurred over a 2-week period followed by 8 weeks of follow-up. The primary outcome of a 50% reduction in primary symptom score was achieved by 6 of the 10 patients undergoing ST and only 3 of the 12 patients treated with TENS ($P = 0.11$). Although not statistically significant, the trend was similar to the results of the initial phase and led the authors to conclude that larger studies on the efficacy of ST in treating CIPN are warranted [30].

In 2020, the results of a randomized trial of ST versus treatment with "sham" placement of electrodes was reported by Smith et al. [31]. A total of 35 patients were randomized with 17 in the ST group and 18 in the "sham" treatment arm. All patients were weaned off anticonvulsant medications. Treatments were for 30 minutes on 10 consecutive working days. Outcomes were recorded at baseline, day 10, and days 28, 60, and 90. The authors found no significant differences between the groups at any time point. Only 25% of patients in the ST group achieved a 33% reduction in pain at the 10-day mark compared to 17.6% in the "sham" group. Differences between the groups were not statistically significant. In the discussion, the authors offer several reasons as to why the results were not consistent with previous studies including placement of the electrodes such that the "nonpain" signal was ineffectively transmitted.

More recent publications have been systematic reviews of the literature looking at the treatment of CIPN with either pharmacologic or nonpharmacologic means and included ST. In a review of randomized controlled trials (RCTs) of both pharmacologic and nonpharmacologic management, Jones et al. [32] included three of the more recent studies mentioned above [29–31]. They point out the lack of statistical significance in these three RCTs and feel that ST for treatment of CIPN is not supported [32]. In another review, also published in 2022, Wang et al. [33] included the three RCTs [29–31] as well as four single arm studies [20, 24, 26, 27] concluding that ST was of limited or no efficacy in the treatment of CIPN and that the inconsistency between RCTs and the other studies suggested a placebo effect.

Finally in early 2023, Klafke et al. [34] published clinical recommendations for nonpharmacologic treatment of CIPN using a systematic review and an expert consensus process. Interestingly, the only studies included for ST were those by Coyne et al. [26] and Loprinzi et al. [29]. There were no specific conclusions nor recommendations for ST [34]. The authors felt that complimentary therapies should be considered in each individual case.

4. Scrambler therapy for cancer pain

The first reports of the use of ST involved patients with cancer pain and were published by the inventor of the technology. In 2003, Guiseppe Marineo reported on the use of ST in 11 terminal abdominal cancer patients [35], including pancreatic, gastric, and colon cancer. Nine of the 11 patients were able to stop oral analgesics in the midst of the ST sessions, and the other 2 were able to reduce dosages. The same year, Marineo et al. [13] published the results of an additional 33 terminal cancer patients treated with ST for their pain. All patients responded to the ST and 72% of them were able to stop oral analgesics completely while the rest were able to reduce the dosage considerably.

In 2013, Park et al. [36] reported a case series on three patients treated with ST that were not well managed with other modalities. All three patients were suffering from bony metastases and despite regional analgesic techniques in two of the patients and opioid usage in all three, pain scores ranged from 6 to 8 and severely impacted quality of life. The patients underwent 10 sessions of ST with a meaningful reduction in pain scores to 2–3.5/10 which lasted for two months. Two of the patients did have a worsening of pain at the two-month mark and underwent a second round of 10 ST sessions.

Two years later, a pilot study of ST for treating pain from bony and visceral metastases as well as primary tumors refractory to other therapies was published [37]. The study was a retrospective case series of 25 consecutive patients treated with ST who had failed standard treatments at the time. The average age of the patients was 62.0. All patients received at least 50% reduction in pain scores which lasted from 4 to 24 weeks. The average pain score was reduced from 8.4 at baseline to 2.9 following ST. Patients reported an increase in the average number of sleeping hours from 4.4 to 7.5. The authors state that patients reported a decrease in the usage of breakthrough opioids but do not quantify this information. They reported no adverse effects from ST.

In 2017, a series of three women with difficult to manage chronic post-mastectomy pain (cPMP) treated with ST was reported by Smith et al. [38]. ST sessions were 45 minutes in duration, but none of the patients required 10 consecutive treatments to obtain marked relief of over 75%. Quality of life improved for all three patients. One patient was able to wean off chronic opioids and another returned to work. Pain relief lasted for several months and treatments were repeated as necessary. There were no adverse effects noted.

The following year, another positive case report using ST for the treatment of pain due to breast cancer-related lymphedema was published [39]. The patient was 39 years old and had undergone a right mastectomy. Four years later, she underwent ST for a total of 10 sessions of 45 minutes each for treatment of pain. Her pain score was reduced from 8/10 to 2/10. No mention is made of other prior therapies for her pain nor is there any period of follow-up reported.

In 2020, a randomized controlled trial on the use of ST in pain due to head, neck and thoracic cancer was published by Kashyap et al. [40]. The study was specifically designed to determine the impact of ST on opioid usage in patients experiencing cancer pain. A total of 80 patients were enrolled into 2 arms, a control group and an intervention group receiving ST, which consisted of 40-minute treatment sessions over 10 consecutive weekdays, in addition to the usual analgesic therapy. One patient in the ST arm was lost to follow-up after the ninth day of ST because his pain had completely resolved and found further treatment unnecessary. Mean pain scores were similar at baseline between the two groups (6.57 for control and 6.65 for ST) and decreased during the trial period in both arms. However, the reduction in pain was greater in the ST group, and this difference was statistically significant from the third treatment onward. The total reduction in pain scores over the 10 days of treatment was 3.42 in the control arm and 5.91 for the ST group. There was no difference in the usage of tramadol, but a statistically significant reduction in the usage of morphine by the end of ST treatments. The authors suggested that being the "stronger" of the two opioids, morphine was reduced preferentially. There were no adverse effects reported with ST. The authors concluded that the use of ST for refractory head, neck and thoracic cancer pain is recommended.

This same group published the results of their quality of life (QOL) comparisons in a separate paper [41]. QOL assessments were conducted at baseline, at the end of the 10 days of ST, and at one week after the last ST session. Baseline QOL were similar between the two groups. Overall QOL worsened in the control group during the study, while it improved significantly for the ST intervention group. The authors felt that if QOL had been impacted solely by pain, there might be some improvement in the control group since there was pain reduction in both groups. It should be noted that morphine consumption did increase slightly in the control group which seemed to correspond with the changes in QOL. The authors felt that the benefits of ST could be explained by improved pain as well as decreased morphine intake and its related side effects.

Another case report on the use of ST for pain from bone metastases in a single patient was published in 2021 [42]. The 69-year-old patient with metastatic non-small cell lung cancer was severely limited in the ability to use his right arm due to scapular and humeral head involvement and the resultant pain. He had undergone radiation several months prior and cryoablation to the scapular mass one month prior to ST without benefit. He remained on his oral analgesic regimen but after six 30-minute sessions over 10 days, he was pain free and able to use his right arm to eat. He remained pain free for several weeks until his death.

Finally in 2020, Kashyap and Bhatnagar [43] published a systematic review on the use of ST for cancer pain. Their review included several of the studies mentioned in this section on cancer pain and the section on CIPN as well as some studies on chronic pain that contained mixed patient populations some of whom had noncancer pain. The reader is referred to the paper as it is a good source of references related to the topic of ST and cancer pain over the past 2 decades. They conclude that large RCTs are still needed but that ST may be an option for cancer pain unresponsive to other modalities.

The next section of this chapter will look at the available evidence for the use of scrambler therapy (ST) in other types of neuropathic pain unrelated to cancer or chemotherapy.

5. Scrambler therapy for peripheral neuropathic pain

Neuropathic pain occurs due to a disorder that affects the somatosensory nervous system and can have multiple etiologies affecting the peripheral or central nervous systems [44]. There is often a combination of loss of sensation and pain which can be spontaneous or evoked in the affected area. Examples would include post-herpetic neuralgia (PHN), diabetic neuropathy (DN), and central post-stroke pain to name a few. There is an excellent treatise on neuropathic pain published in 2021 by Finnerup et al. to which the reader is referred [44]. This section will discuss peripheral neuropathic pain while the next will discuss central neuropathic pain.

In 2012, the inventor of the ST technology along with several other authors [45] published a small RCT in which 52 patients were randomized to receive either standardized guideline-based drug management with amitriptyline, clonazepam, and oxycodone versus the same drug treatment with the addition of ST for 10 treatment sessions of 45 minutes each. There were 26 patients in each group with either PHN, post-surgical neuralgia, or spinal cord stenosis. Baseline pain scores were reduced from 8.1 to 5.8 in the control group and from 8.0 to 0.7 in the group receiving ST at one month and continued to be significantly reduced at three months. Furthermore, there was a significant reduction in the usage of pain medications in the ST group with more than half of those taking opioids and anticonvulsants able to eliminate them entirely. There were no adverse effects from the ST.

A series of 3 patients with PHN treated with ST was published in 2013 [46]. All 3 patients were elderly women who had failed other methods of treatment and despite daily analgesics suffered from pain scores ranging from 6 or 7 out of 10. Each underwent 10 ST sessions of 50 minutes each. By the end of the treatments, all patients had a pain score of 2 which only increased slightly to 3 or 4 at one month follow-up. There were no adverse effects reported.

Another case report of a 54-year-old woman was reported four years later [47]. There was no mention of prior or current analgesics. The patient underwent 10 ST sessions of 40 minutes. By the end of therapy, her pain score had decreased from 7 at baseline to 1, and QOL scores had increased. There were no reported adverse effects. There was no reported follow-up period, so it is unclear how long the effects lasted.

A more extensive case series of 10 patients with PHN was reported by Smith and Marineo in 2018 [48]. The patients consistently had pain scores greater than 5/10 and were part of a subgroup of two other studies, one of which was previously reported [45], that was analyzed separately. Patients were treated for 30 to 45 minutes with 10 weekday sessions of ST [48]. The average pain score decreased from an average of 7.64 at baseline to 0.42 at one month follow-up with continued marked improvement at three months. Five of the 10 patients had complete resolution of pain, and most were able to reduce or cease the use of oral analgesics. There were no adverse effects reported.

A prospective study of 45 patients with neuropathic pain of various etiologies treated with ST was published in 2018 [49]. Etiologies included lumbar radiculopathy, PHN, and trigeminal neuralgia to name a few. The primary endpoint was a decrease in the number of signs and symptoms of neuropathic pain according to the Neuropathic Pain Diagnostic Questionnaire (DN4) [50]. Patients underwent 45-minute sessions of ST on 10 consecutive weekdays [49]. Sessions were discontinued if the pain resolved or continued if the patient was continuing to receive benefit. Four of the patients had complete resolution of pain prior to completing 10 sessions. The median number of sessions was 10.5 with a range of 5–20. Of the 45 patients, 62.2% had a decrease in the DN4 score and 88.8% had a greater than 50% reduction in pain intensity.

Also in 2018, a case report on the treatment of DN using ST was published [51]. The patient was 45 years old and had been treated with insulin for five years. She developed bilateral plantar foot pain with subsequent electromyogram demonstrating peripheral polyneuropathy. Her pain score was 6/10. She did not respond to oral analgesics nor regional analgesia with injections of bilateral posterior tibial nerves and lumbar sympathetic ganglion blocks. She underwent 45-minute ST treatment sessions once per week for 10 weeks placing the electrodes around the ankles. Her pain score decreased to 2/10 by the end of treatment and one week later. It was decided that the patient would return when she felt it necessary and had not returned for six months.

Another case report using ST for the treatment of DN was published in 2021 [52]. An 80-year-old woman with longstanding severe DN in the hands and feet was treated with 3 sessions of ST of 40 minutes. She had no adverse effects attributed to ST but did develop recurrent atrial fibrillation which prevented further treatments. However, her pain score had been reduced from 8/10 to 0/10 which persisted at four- and 11-months post treatment.

In 2021, a prospective study analyzed subgroups of neuropathic pain phenotypes to determine if there was a differential response to ST based upon phenotype rather than etiology of the pain [53]. Twenty-five patients completed the study which consisted of a total of 10 ST treatments of 30 minutes each. The investigators divided the 25 patients into three clusters based upon responses to the Neuropathic Pain Symptom Inventory [54]. They found that patients with paroxysmal pain had more favorable outcomes than persistent pain [53]. The overall reduction in pain across the 25 patients was only 22%. The authors acknowledged that the ST operator's experience was limited and that 93% of the patients were taking anticonvulsants both of which have been suggested could have an impact upon outcomes [10]. The authors did feel that the more favorable response in paroxysmal pain could be due to damaged Aβ fibers [53], and since ST is felt to utilize C-fibers for transmission of the "non-pain" signals, the response to ST is preserved.

A narrative review of the four main neuromodulation modalities was published in 2022 [55], and evaluated spinal cord stimulation (SCS), peripheral nerve stimulation, TENS, and ST. Most of the literature that the authors were able to find related to SCS and TENS. They were only able to find the two case reports on ST treating DN noted in the above paragraphs. The authors concluded that SCS had the most data for efficacy, while data for TENS was mixed. There was simply not enough data available for ST and more studies are needed in treating DN.

In 2021, Abdi et al. published a focused review summarizing the history of ST, its mechanism of action, and the evidence at that time regarding the clinical effectiveness of ST in treating noncancer neuropathic pain [7]. Several of the studies have been mentioned in this section, but others have either mixed etiologies or include patients with cancer and noncancer pain that will be discussed in subsequent sections. The authors call for more clinical trials to confirm the positive findings reported thus far.

6. Scrambler therapy for central neuropathic pain

In 2018, D'Amato presented a case report in which a 52-year-old woman developed central neuropathic pain following resection and radiation of a brainstem medullary cavernoma [56]. She had suffered from a burning pain to her left leg for 12 years prior to ST. Oral analgesics including antidepressants, anticonvulsants, and opioids were of limited effectiveness, and her pain was 6/10 which would increase to 10/10 with activity. Pregabalin was discontinued prior to 10 ST sessions of 45 minutes each. By the completion of ST, her pain was 0–0.5/10 for almost two months when the pain returned. She underwent an additional 5 sessions of ST which reduced her pain to 2/10 for the next three months. She remained on duloxetine and only took occasional tramadol while enjoying improved physical functioning.

In 2019, there was case report using ST for the treatment of persistent central neuropathic pain following transverse myelitis [57]. The 65-year-old woman had tried multiple oral medications, including opioids, as well as meditation and acupuncture over the course of more than three years prior to ST which was administered in 45-minute sessions over 10 consecutive weekdays. Her pain was rated at 5/10 on the morning of her first session. Pain was in both lower extremities, her torso, and right arm. By the end of the 10 treatment sessions, her pain had essentially resolved and remained at low levels for 90 days. Her sleep and activity tolerance improved.

A year later, the same primary author published the results of a randomized single-blind, sham-controlled trial in patients with neuromyelitis optica spectrum disorder [58]. A total of 11 patients were assigned to the ST group and 11 to the sham group. Both ST and sham sessions were conducted for 10 consecutive weekdays for 35 minutes each. Baseline measures of pain severity, pain interference, sleep disturbance, anxiety and depression were obtained. These were reassessed at the end of treatment and at 30- and 60-day follow-up. The ST arm saw median pain scores decline from 5.0 at baseline to 1.5 which was statistically significant, whereas the sham group experienced a small, insignificant decline from 5.0 to 4.0. A reduction in depression was seen in the ST group, but scores related to anxiety, sleep and pain interference failed to reach statistical significance. Pain scores remained significantly decreased at 30 days ($p = 0.0195$) but not at 60 days ($p = 0.0518$). There were no serious adverse effects reported.

Also in 2020, a case report of a 56-year-old man with centralized post-stroke thalamic pain, or Dejerine-Roussy syndrome, treated with ST was published [59]. After six years of disabling pain, multiple daily 40-minute ST treatments followed by monthly booster treatments were able to nearly eradicate his pain allowing resumption of normal activity and cessation of all pain medications without any side effects.

In 2021, a case report treating centralized neuropathic pain associated with Parkinson's disease was published by Wang et al. [60]. A 63-year-old man suffered from constant shocking and burning pain in the lower extremities with severe nighttime pain flares in a "coat-hanger" distribution. The patient received a 35-minute ST treatment for his legs and the area of his nighttime flares during which his baseline pain of 5/10 decreased to 0/10 which lasted for three days. He was able to sleep through the night without any lower body or upper body pain or spasms. His second 35-minute treatment resulted in no pain for seven days. He then had a third and fourth treatment 24 hours apart with the result that his pain remained at 0/10 for six weeks. He reported markedly improved sleep and quality of life and wished to undergo booster treatments as necessary.

7. Other studies and case reports using scrambler therapy

This next section will discuss other uses for scrambler therapy. While some of the studies could have been included in the previous four sections on cancer-related pain and non-cancer neuropathies, they are included here either because they are larger studies including patients with both cancer and non-cancer pain, or they are somewhat unique, and it was felt that they should be included in their own section. This would include use of ST for treating pruritus in burn patients and the use of ST in acute pain or pediatric patients.

7.1 Larger studies with mixed groups of patients

In 2012, Sparadeo et al. [61] reported the results of 173 patients treated for chronic neuropathic pain. There were four groups including isolated spine pain, neuralgia, complex regional pain syndrome (CRPS), and multi-site pain patients. Patients underwent 10 treatment sessions of ST. The baseline pain score across all patients was 7.24 which had significantly decreased to 1 immediately following the final treatment. A total of 91 of the patients agreed to a 3–6-month follow-up survey with a mean follow-up period of 4.2 months. All seven variables of the Brief Pain Inventory (BPI) Score [62] were significantly reduced at follow-up. The authors concluded that ST is an effective treatment for chronic neuropathic pain [61].

In 2011, Ricci and colleagues [63] published the results of a prospective study of 73 patients with chronic pain, 41 of which had pain related to cancer and 32 with non-cancer pain. The etiologies and characteristics of the pain were quite varied with some having nociceptive pain, others with neuropathic pain, and others with mixed characteristics. The length of time the pain was present was variable as well as whether the pain was continuous or intermittent. ST treatments were for 30 minutes on 10 consecutive weekdays. The authors did report results for patients with and without cancer pain. The patients with cancer pain saw pain scores decrease from 5.4 to 1.4 and those with non-cancer pain from 7.0 to 1.8 by the end of treatment. At the 2-week follow-up period, pain scores remained significantly reduced at 2.6 and 3.4 respectively. At the end of the 4-week study, the authors reported that 81% of the overall group had achieved a response. There were no adverse events reported. The authors felt that further research might lead to possible explanations for the 20% of patients that exhibit no response to ST treatment.

Eight years later, Ricci et al. [64] published the results of an additional 219 patients using the same methodology as their 2011 study above. In this study, 83 patients had cancer pain, and 136 had non-cancer pain. Again, they analyzed the results of each individual group (cancer and non-cancer) as well as all patients together. As in the first study, pain etiologies were quite varied. The cancer patients saw pain scores decrease from 6.25 to 2.90 following ST treatment and 2.97 two weeks later. The non-cancer patients had a reduction of pain scores from 6.55 at baseline to 3.42 at the end of ST. These reductions were statistically significant. There were no adverse events reported. The authors do not provide the percentage of responders versus non-responders but do state that overall, 10.5% of the patients were pain free at the 2-week follow-up after completion of ST. There were 44 patients that repeated ST following successful treatment due to pain recurrence. The majority repeated treatment at two to five months following the first round of ST. Repeat treatments were able to reduce pain significantly from 6.27 at baseline to 2.94 at 4 weeks.

In 2015, there was a large multicenter retrospective analysis published on behalf of the Scrambler Therapy Group out of Italy [65]. There were 201 patients treated in one year with a variety of reasons for chronic pain, including PHN, low back pain, peripheral neuropathy, polyneuropathy, and other causes of chronic pain. The baseline pain score was 7.41 prior to the typical 10-day treatment course with 45-minute sessions. Following treatment, the mean pain score was 1.60. The success rate, defined as greater than 50% reduction in pain score, ranged from 82 to 93% when the four major types of chronic pain were analyzed separately. The authors note medication reductions among several oral analgesics and total elimination of opioids in 55 out of 77 patients. Three-month follow-up showed improvements in pain, sleep, and other quality of life metrics.

There was a prospective, double-blinded, randomized, sham controlled trial of military veterans suffering from chronic pain due to combat injury or repetitive use trauma published in 2020 [66]. The data from 47 patients were analyzed with 28 in the active ST group and 29 in the sham group. Pain scores were evaluated at baseline, at the conclusion of ten 30-minute sessions of treatment (ST or sham), and four weeks following the conclusion of the intervention. Most of the patients (97%) suffered from low back pain with radicular symptoms. Overall, 90% of patients responded to treatment regardless of the group assigned, and the authors found no difference in the reduction of pain, use of analgesics, and quality of life.

The inventor of the technology penned a letter to the editor [67] regarding the above study [66] stating that the protocol did not appear to comply with the methods of use presented to the FDA. He further states that because the proper use of ST requires operator and patient interaction for proper placement of the electrodes, it is essentially impossible to perform a true double-blinded study. He had submitted another letter [68] nearly a decade earlier in 2011 noting the same issues with the methodology of another study [63] and referenced many other methodological problems that existed [68]. As a result, a three-day training course on theory of ST and practical applications had been developed.

7.2 Burns

In 2016, there was a pilot study published on the use of ST in the management of burn scar pruritus [69]. Sixteen patients were treated with 10 weekday sessions of 40 minutes. The electrodes were placed on the skin surrounding the burn. If pruritus was not reduced at the beginning of treatment, electrodes were repositioned. The degree of pruritus was rated from 0 to 10, analogous to a pain scale. The degree of interference with daily activities was measured using the Leuven Itch Scale (LIS) [70]. Scores were recorded at baseline, following five treatments, and at the end of 10 treatments [69]. The degree of pruritus decreased significantly at both 5 and 10 days. Scores were 6.75 at baseline, 5.06 at day 5, and 4.13 at day 10. LIS scores also showed significant improvement. The authors concluded that ST was a feasible alternative for treatment of burn scar pruritus and further study was warranted.

In 2022, several of the same authors were part of a group that published the results from a prospective, double-blind RCT using a sham control [71]. Ten consecutive weekdays were used for treatment sessions of 45 minutes. The ST group received a stimulus that was the maximal amount tolerated without pain, whereas the sham group received a very low level of stimulus throughout the session. Measures of pain, depression and function were assessed at baseline and at the end of treatment. Furthermore, MRIs of the brain were obtained, and cerebral blood flow (CBV) was mapped at both time points. There was a total of 43 patients with 20 in the ST group and 23 in the sham group. Six of the 20 ST patients' pain improved such that they did not complete the two weeks of the study protocol and only data from 14 were included in the analysis. Both groups had a reduction in pain from baseline to the completion of treatment. The ST group median pain score decreased from 6 to 3, while the sham group decreased from 7 to 6. The publication stated that both changes were significant and that the p value for the sham decrease of 7 to 6 was actually more significant ($p = 0.001$) than the ST group ($p = 0.004$). There were also significant differences in CBV between the two groups, and the reader is referred to the study for a more detailed discussion [71].

7.3 Chronic post surgical pain

In 2019, Yarchoan et al. published a case report on two patients who received ST to treat post-surgical scar pain [72]. One of the patients was a 57-year-old woman with thoracotomy pain following surgery and chemoradiation for lung adenocarcinoma. Her pain was 9/10 which was reduced to zero 20 minutes into a 30-minute session. This relief lasted nearly six months. The other patient was 70 years old and underwent partial hepatectomy for cancer. Her pain prevented her from wearing a seat belt and a bra. It was constantly present and worsened significantly with movement. She underwent a 40-minute treatment session which eliminated her allodynia and pain, but the pain returned so on the eighth day, she underwent another treatment. At three months, her pain had remained at 2/10 or less.

In 2020, an additional two cases were published in a report by Kashyap et al. [73]. A 40-year-old male presented six months following adrenalectomy for cancer with 6/10 pain in the left lower back and iliac region. Oral analgesics escalated over the next six months to include 10 mg of morphine every 4 hours to maintain 6/10 pain. He underwent 10 sessions of ST of 35 minutes each after which his pain score had decreased to 1/10 and the morphine was no longer needed. The second patient was a 56-year-old male with carcinoma of the right buccal mucosa at the time of disease recurrence and reoperation. Subsequent pain of 6/10 on the right side of the face and chest despite tramadol prompted the use of ST as an alternative. Following 10 sessions of 35 minutes each, the patient's pain score was 0/10.

7.4 Other isolated case reports

Scrambler therapy has been used for several other chronic pain disorders for which isolated case reports are available including low back pain in which pain and depression was improved [74], arthritis of the knee with resulting improvement in pain and quality of life [75], and for paraneoplastic neuropathy and pruritus in which two patients were treated with very positive results [76].

One of the more impressive case reports involves the use of ST for treating HIV-related peripheral neuropathy [77]. In 2017, Smith et al. reported on a 52-year-old man suffering from neuropathy since 1998 who had been on long-acting morphine and oxycodone since 2012. In just four treatments of 45 minutes, his pain had decreased from an average of 8/10 to 1–2/10 on the right foot and 4/10 on the left. He was able to stop his opioids. Six months later, pain had returned in the toes such that he underwent only two treatments with one additional treatment four months later.

There are two case reports using ST to treat neuropathic pain associated with amyloidosis. In the first [78], a 58-year-old man with lower extremity neuropathy for a few years was diagnosed with amyloidosis and underwent chemotherapy. His pain spread to involve the trunk and upper extremities. The patient required methadone and oxycodone as part of his oral analgesic regimen. ST was effective in reducing his upper extremity pain by 40–50% but it only lasted for three weeks. He eventually underwent placement of an intrathecal drug delivery system. The second case report [79] describes a 70-year-old woman with 13 years of peripheral neuropathy from amyloidosis that was worsened by chemotherapy. She underwent four daily 40-minute treatments of ST for her upper extremities which declined to zero and lasted eight months. She did have worsening of lower extremity neuropathy and requested ST for that pain as well.

The first known case of ST used to treat pain from schwannomatosis was reported in 2022 [80]. A 48-year-old woman underwent five treatments to her right groin and anterior thigh during which her pain was reduced from 6/10 to 0/10 which had persisted for a minimum of three weeks.

Scrambler therapy has been used successfully in the treatment of radial and femoral nerve injuries following extracorporeal membrane oxygenation [81]. It is a brief report, but the pain score was reduced from 8/10 to 0.5/10 for two months following two days of treatment. In a letter to the editor [82], the use of ST to treat phantom limb pain is described. Following 10 weekday sessions of 30 minutes each, the patient remained pain free at two-month follow-up from a starting pain of 7/10.

Finally, there is a case report on the use of ST for pain and joint range of motion following arthroscopic rotator cuff repair [83]. It is unclear from the report how soon following surgery that ST was used for this patient and whether this was as part of the acute recovery process or as a result of chronic pain following surgery. The pain score was reduced from 8 to 1 following 10 sessions of ST and presumably physical therapy. Range of motion was likewise increased, but it is difficult to know how this would compare to ordinary post-operative progress.

7.5 Low back pain

In 2011, a small prospective study of eight patients with chronic low back pain was reported by Ghatak et al. [84]. Eight patients, half of whom were female, underwent six treatment sessions of 45 minutes each with pain scores and the Oswestry Disability Index (ODI) [85] compared at baseline and following the sixth treatment. Mean pain scores decreased from 8.1 to 3.6 and the ODI showed a significant improvement in functional status with the reduction from 49.9 to 18.4 being statistically significant.

An abstract on the use of ST for failed back surgery syndrome presented at the 2011 Annual Meeting of the American Society of Interventional Pain Physicians reported on 10 patients following 10 sessions of 60 minutes [86]. They reported a 28% reduction in pain without side effects.

In one of the more interesting studies published in 2015, Starkweather et al. [87] conducted a double-blind RCT dividing 30 patients into an active ST group and a sham group. Not only did the investigators compare pain scores and pain interference, but they also conducted quantitative sensory testing (QST) and drew blood to look at the mRNA expression of 84 genes involved in the pain pathway, i.e., transduction, maintenance, and modulation. The sham treatment was conducted with the same device at what was felt to be a subtherapeutic threshold for ten 30-minute sessions while the active group received ST. Each group was assessed at one and three weeks following the conclusion of treatment. The ST group showed a significant decrease in both pain and interference, whereas the sham group did not. There were differences between the groups on QST testing with the ST group experiencing less sensitivity to pain. There were 10 genes identified with differential expression in the ST group compared to the sham group at the three-week follow-up period when compared to baseline. In the discussion, the authors note that the levels of nerve growth factor and glial-derived growth factor were significantly lower in the ST group compared to the sham group at three weeks post treatment. Elevated levels of these proteins have been implicated in the process of peripheral sensitization [88], although it is unclear what role they might play in chronic low back pain.

8. Scrambler therapy for complex regional pain syndrome

There is one publication of four cases of adults with complex regional pain syndrome (CRPS) who have been treated with ST [89], although the report by Sparadeo et al. [61] mentioned previously did include 20 patients with CRPS. In the case report [89], the adults ranged from 41 to 70 years of age with a duration of CRPS symptoms from 4 to 38 months. The ST treatments were 45 minutes in duration and the required number to obtain complete pain relief ranged from 7 to 12 sessions. Baseline pain scores were 7/10 or above, and the pain free duration was 6 to 21 months without the need for medications. The authors felt that ST could be an effective treatment modality for patients with CRPS.

9. Scrambler therapy in pediatric patients

In addition to the nine adolescents who received ST for the treatment of CIPN reported by Tomasello et al. [28], there is a single case report of ST used to treat neuropathic pain related to leukemia in an 11-year-old [90] and one case report using ST to treat an episode of acute pain [91]. The patient with leukemia [90] was suffering from left groin and thigh pain. Lesions were discovered on pelvic MRI that were thought to involve the obturator nerve. Because the patient and caregiver were fearful of injections, rather than obturator nerve block, the patient underwent 45-minute ST sessions over three days during which pain was reduced from 8/10 to zero. Medications, including fentanyl patch, were weaned and discontinued. One month later, the patient remained pain free. In the other case report [91], a 12-year-old girl with a history of congenital myopathy and removal of osteoblastoma of the foot treated with surgery six years prior, developed acute right scapular pain without occurrence of trauma or any specific etiology. She continued to have 5/10 pain even after ketorolac and diazepam. She underwent four days of ST treatments of 45 minutes each after which she was pain free. She remained pain free for at least eight weeks following treatment.

10. Author's commentary

As a pediatric anesthesiologist and chronic pain physician, my interest in Scrambler Therapy began in 2013 when I had first learned about it while treating a pediatric patient with recalcitrant CRPS. The patient went to Dr. D'Amato in Rhode Island to undergo ST (aka Calmare). Although it did not change her pain, and she eventually required implantation of a spinal stimulator [92], I was intrigued by the concept. Since that initial exposure, I have sent several patients to New Jersey for ST, many of whom have had quite impressive results. Anecdotally, I felt that there was an "art" to the treatments and that experience played a role in outcomes. After the research for this chapter, I can see that my impressions were correct. CRPS has been called the "suicide disease" due to the unrelenting pain that patients experience and feel that suicide is the only means by which they can achieve relief. Almost half (49.3%) of adult patients with CRPS have contemplated ending their lives, and 15.1% have attempted suicide with average attempts of 2.1 [93]. It would be difficult to imagine the prospect of lifelong agony as a child or adolescent with CRPS. It is therefore my hope that more research into the effectiveness of ST for the treatment of pediatric CRPS can occur to add an additional modality in treating this disabling and excruciatingly painful disorder.

11. Conclusion

Scrambler therapy has been in use for more than 20 years and has been used to treat a wide variety of painful conditions especially those that are neuropathic in nature. It operates using a unique mechanism that is designed to recalibrate the nervous system and reverse changes that can theoretically occur with chronic pain. Although there are many studies and case reports that have examined its efficacy and have demonstrated the ability of scrambler therapy to decrease the use of opioids and other analgesics, it is still misunderstood and has yet to be widely adopted in the treatment of chronic and acute pain.

Conflict of interest

The author declares no conflict of interest.

Author details

James A. Tolley
Clinical Anesthesiology, Indiana University School of Medicine, Indianapolis, IN, USA

*Address all correspondence to: jtolley@iuhealth.org

References

[1] Yong RJ, Mullins PM, Bhattacharyya N. Prevalence of chronic pain among adults in the United States. Pain. 2021;**163**:e328-e332. DOI: 10.1097/jpain0000000000002291

[2] Shupler MS, Kramer JK, Cragg JJ, et al. Pan-Canadian estimates of chronic pain prevalence from 2000 to 2014: A repeated cross-sectional survey analysis. The Journal of Pain. 2019;**20**:557-565. DOI: 10.1016/j.jpain.2018.10.010

[3] Stompor M, Grodzicki T, Stompor T, et al. Prevalence of chronic pain, particularly with neuropathic component, and its effect on overall functioning of elderly patients. Medical Science Monitor. 2019;**25**:2695-2701. DOI: 10.12659/MSM.911260

[4] Wiffen PJ, Derry S, Bell RF, et al. Gabapentin for chronic neuropathic pain in adults. Cochrane Database of Systematic Reviews. 2017;**6**:CD007938. DOI: 10.1002/14651858.CD007938.pub4

[5] Kolber MR, Ton J, Thomas B, et al. PEER systematic review of randomized controlled trials: Management of chronic low back pain in primary care. Canadian Family Physician. 2021;**67**:e20-e30. DOI: 10.46747/cfp.6701e20

[6] Finnerup NB, Attal N, Haroutounian S, et al. Pharmacotherapy for neuropathic pain in adults: A systematic review and meta-analysis. Lancet Neurology. 2015;**14**:162-173. DOI: 10.1016/S1474-4422(14)70251-0

[7] Abdi S, Chung M, Marineo G. Scrambler therapy for noncancer neuropathic pain: A focused review. Current Opinion in Anesthesiology. 2021;**34**:768-773. DOI: 10.1097/ACO.0000000000001073

[8] Sluka KA, Walsh D. Transcutaneous electrical nerve stimulation: Basic science mechanisms and clinical effectiveness. The Journal of Pain. 2003;**4**:109-121. DOI: 10.1054/jpai.2003.434

[9] Melzack R, Wall PD. Pain mechanisms: A new theory. Science. 1965;**150**:971-979

[10] Marineo G. Inside the scrambler therapy, a noninvasive treatment of chronic neuropathic and cancer pain: From the gate control theory to the active principle of information. Integrative Cancer Therapies. 2019;**18**:1-17. DOI: 10.1177/1534735419845143

[11] Shannon CE. A mathematical theory of communication. The Bell System Technical Journal. 1948;**XXVII**:379-423

[12] Yam MF, Loh YC, Tan CS, et al. General pathways of pain sensation and the major neurotransmitters involved in pain regulation. International Journal of Molecular Sciences. 2018;**19**:2164. DOI: 10.3390/ijms19082164

[13] Marineo G, Spaziani S, Sabato AF, et al. Artificial neurons in oncological pain: The potential of scrambler therapy to modify a biological information. International Congress Series. 2003;**1255**:381-388. DOI: 10.1016/S0531-513(03)00661-7

[14] Scrambler therapy theory bases. [Internet]. Available from: https://www.scramblertherapy.org/scrambler-therapy-theory-bases.htm [Accessed: 10 April 2023]

[15] Sabato AF, Marineo G, Gatti A. Scrambler therapy. Minerva Anestesiologica. 2005;**71**:479-482

[16] 510(k) summary for the Competitive Technologies, Inc. Scrambler Therapy MC-5A TENS Device. [Internet]. Available from: https://www.accessdata.fda.gov/cdrh_docs/pdf8/K081255.pdf [Accessed: 15 April 2023]

[17] Abdi S, Smith TJ, Marineo G. Scrambler therapy for chronic pain. [letter]. The Clinical Journal of Pain. 2015;**31**:929. DOI: 10.1097/AJP0000000000000174

[18] Moon JY, Kurihara C, Beckles JP, et al. Predictive factors associated with success and failure for Calmare (scrambler) therapy: A multicenter analysis. The Clinical Journal of Pain. 2015;**31**:750-756. DOI: 10.1097/AJP0000000000000155

[19] Clinical practice area. [Internet]. Available from: https://www.scramblertherapy.org/clinical-practice.htm [Accessed: 10 April 2023]

[20] Pachman DR, Weisbrod BL, Seisler DK, et al. Pilot evaluation of scrambler therapy for the treatment of chemotherapy-induced peripheral neuropathy. Supportive Care in Cancer. 2015;**23**:943-951. DOI: 10.1007/s00520-014-2424-8

[21] Liljencrantz J, Olausson H. Tactile C fibers and their contributions to pleasant sensations and to tactile allodynia. Frontiers in Behavioral Neuroscience. 2014;**8**:1-6. DOI: 10.3389/fnbeh.2014.00037

[22] United States Patent Marineo. [Internet]. Available from: https://patentimages.storage.googleapis.com/32/22/5a/1492936230cf06/US8380317.pdf [Accessed: 15 April 2023]

[23] Calmare Therapeutics Inc Form 10-K. [Internet]. Available from: https://seekingalpha.com/filings/pdf/12185146 [Accessed: 15 April 2023]

[24] Smith TJ, Coyne PJ, Parker GL, et al. Pilot trial of a patient-specific cutaneous electrostimulation device (MC5-a Calmare) for chemotherapy-induced peripheral neuropathy. Journal of Pain and Symptom Management. 2010;**40**:883-891. DOI: 10.1016/j.jpainsymman.2010.03.022

[25] Campbell TC, Nimunkar AJ, Retseck J, et al. A randomized, double-blind study of "scrambler" therapy versus sham for painful chemotherapy-induced peripheral neuropathy (CIPN). Journal of Clinical Oncology. 2013;**31**:9635. DOI: 10.1200/jco.2013.31.15_suppl.9635

[26] Coyne PJ, Wan W, Dodson PA, et al. An expanded trial of scrambler therapy in the treatment of cancer pain syndromes and chronic chemotherapy-induced peripheral neuropathy. Journal of Pain & Palliative Care Pharmacotherapy. 2013;**27**:359-364. DOI: 10.3109/15360288.2013.847519

[27] Lee SC, Park KS, Moon JY, et al. An exploratory study on the effectiveness of "Calmare therapy" in patients with cancer-related neuropathic pain: A pilot study. European Journal of Oncology Nursing. 2016;**21**:1-7. DOI: 10.1016/j.ejon.2015.12.001

[28] Tomasello C, Pinto RM, Mennini C, et al. Scrambler therapy efficacy and safety for neuropathic pain correlated with chemotherapy-induced peripheral neuropathy in adolescents: A preliminary study. Pediatric Blood & Cancer. 2018;**65**:e27064. DOI: 10.1002/pbc.27064

[29] Loprinzi C, Le-Rademacher JG, Majithia N, et al. Scrambler therapy for chemotherapy neuropathy: A randomized phase II pilot trial. Supportive Care in Cancer. 2020;**28**:1183-1197. DOI: 10.1007/s00520-019-04881-3

[30] Childs DS, Le-Rademacher JG, McMurray R, et al. Randomized trial of scrambler therapy for chemotherapy-induced peripheral neuropathy: Crossover analysis. Journal of Pain and Symptom Management. 2021;**6**:1247-1253. DOI: 10.1016/j.jpainsymman.2020.11.025

[31] Smith TJ, Razzak AR, Blackford AL, et al. A pilot randomized sham-controlled trial of MC5-a scrambler therapy in the treatment of chronic chemotherapy-induced peripheral neuropathy (CIPN). Journal of Palliative Care. 2020;**35**:53-58. DOI: 10.1177/0825859719827589

[32] Jones KF, Wechsler S, Zulewski D, et al. Pharmacological and nonpharmacological management of chemotherapy-induced peripheral neuropathy: A scoping review of randomized controlled trials. Journal of Palliative Medicine. 2022;**25**:964-995. DOI: 10.1089/jpm.2021.0512

[33] Wang M, Yin Y, Yang H, et al. Evaluating the safety, feasibility, and efficacy of non-invasive neuromodulation techniques in chemotherapy-induced peripheral neuropathy: A systematic review. European Journal of Oncology Nursing. 2022;**58**:102124. DOI: 10.1016/j.ejon.2022.102124

[34] Klafke N, Bossert J, Kroger B, et al. Prevention and treatment of chemotherapy-induced peripheral neuropathy (CIPN) with non-pharmacological interventions: Clinical recommendations from a systematic scoping review and an expert consensus process. Medical Science. 2023;**15**:1-34. DOI: 10.3390/medsci11010015

[35] Marineo G. Untreatable pain resulting from abdominal cancer: New hope for biophysics? Journal of the Pancreas. 2003;**4**:1-10

[36] Park HS, Sin WK, Kim HY, et al. Scrambler therapy for patients with cancer pain: Case series. Korean J Pain. 2013;**26**:65-71. DOI: 10.3344/kjp.2013.26.1.65

[37] Notaro P, Dell'Agnola CA, Dell'Agnola AJ, et al. Pilot evaluation of scrambler therapy for pain induced by bone and visceral metastases and refractory to standard therapies. Supportive Care in Cancer. 2016;**24**:1649-1654. DOI: 10.1007/s00520-015-2952-x

[38] Smith T, Cheville AL, Loprinzi CL, et al. Scrambler therapy for the treatment of chronic post-mastectomy pain (cPMP). Cureus. 2017;**9**:e1378. DOI: 10.7759/cureus.1378

[39] Lee JS. Efficacy of scrambler therapy on breast cancer-related lymphedema. Journal of Physical Therapy Science. 2018;**30**:1370-1371

[40] Kashyap K, Singh V, Mishra S, et al. The efficacy of scrambler therapy for the management of head, neck and thoracic cancer pain: A randomized controlled trial. Pain Physician. 2020;**23**:495-506

[41] Kashyap K, Singh V, Dwivedi SN, et al. Scrambler therapy enhances quality of life in cancer patients in a palliative care setting: A randomised controlled trial. Indian Journal of Palliative Care. 2022;**28**:287-294. DOI: 10.25259/IJPC_94_2021

[42] Berninger LE, Smith TJ. Scrambler therapy for incident pain in bone metastases. Journal of Osteopathic Medicine. 2021;**121**:539-542. DOI: 10.1515/jom-2021-0027

[43] Kashyap K, Bhatnagar S. Evidence for the efficacy of scrambler therapy for cancer pain: A systematic review. Pain Physician. 2020;**23**:349-363

[44] Finnerup NB, Kuner R, Jensen TS. Neuropathic pain: From mechanisms to treatment. Physiological Reviews. 2021;**101**:259-301. DOI: 10.1152/physrev.00045.2019

[45] Marineo G, Iorno V, Gandini C, et al. Scrambler therapy may relieve chronic neuropathic pain more effectively than guideline-based drug management: Results of a pilot, randomized, controlled trial. Journal of Pain and Symptom Management. 2012;**43**:87-95. DOI: 10.1016/j.jpainsymman.2011.03.015

[46] Ko YK, Lee HY, Lee WY. Clinical experiences on the effect of scrambler therapy for patients with postherpetic neuralgia. The Korean Journal of Pain. 2013;**26**:98-101. DOI: 10.3344/kjp.2013.26.1.98

[47] Kim YN, Lee DK, Lee HJ. Effect of pain scrambler therapy on antineuralgic pain and quality of life after shingles. Journal of Physical Therapy Science. 2017;**29**:1113-1115

[48] Smith TJ, Marineo G. Treatment of postherpetic pain with scrambler therapy, a patient-specific neurocutaneous electrical stimulation device. American Journal of Hospice & Palliative Medicine. 2018;**35**:812-813. DOI: 10.1177/104990911394002

[49] Russo D, Zoratto F, Tirocchi G, et al. Scrambler therapy in the management of somatosensory signs and symptoms related to neuropathic pain: An exploratory and prospective analysis. Acta Bio-Medica. 2018;**89**:180-185. DOI: 10.23750/abm.v89i2.5704

[50] Bouhassira D, Attal N, Alchaar H, et al. Comparison of pain syndromes associated with nervous or somatic lesions and development of a new neuropathic questionnaire (DN4). Pain. 2005;**114**:29-36. DOI: 10.1016/j.pain.2004.12.010

[51] Lee YS, Park MK, Park HS, et al. Scrambler therapy for the treatment of diabetic peripheral neuropathy pain: A case report. Medicine. 2019;**98**:e15695. DOI: 10.1097/MD.0000000000015695

[52] Smith TJ. Successful treatment of diabetic neuropathy with scrambler therapy. [letter]. Journal of Palliative Medicine. 2021;**24**:320-321. DOI: 10.1089/jpm.2020.0658

[53] Min YG, Baek HS, Lee KM, et al. Differential response to scrambler therapy by neuropathic pain phenotypes. Scientific Reports. 2021;**11**:10148. DOI: 10.1038/s41598-021-89667-6

[54] Bouhassira D, Attal N, Fermanian J, et al. Development and validation of the neuropathic pain symptom inventory. Pain. 2004;**108**:248-257. DOI: 10.1016/j.pain.2003.12.024

[55] Wang EJ, Berninger LE, Komargodski O, et al. Painful diabetic neuropathy – Spinal cord stimulation, peripheral nerve stimulation, transcutaneous electrical nerve stimulation, and scrambler therapy: A narrative review. Pain Physician. 2022;**25**:E1163-E1173

[56] D'Amato SJ, Mealy MA, Erdek MA, et al. Scrambler therapy for the treatment of chronic central pain: A case report. A&A Practice. 2018;**10**:313-315. DOI: 10.1213.XAA.0000000000000695

[57] Mealy MA, Newsome SD, Kozachik SL, et al. Scrambler therapy for treatment-resistant central neuropathic pain in a patient with transverse myelitis. International Journal of MS Care. 2019;**21**:76-80. DOI: 10.7224/1537-2073.2017-083

[58] Mealy MA, Kozachik SL, Cook LJ, et al. Scrambler therapy improves pain in neuromyelitis optica: A randomized

controlled trial. Neurology. 2020;**94**:e1900-e1907. DOI: 10.1212/WNL.0000000000009370

[59] Christo PJ, Kamson DO, Smith TJ. Treatment of Dejerine-Roussy syndrome pain with scrambler therapy. Pain Management. 2020;**10**:141-145. DOI: 10.2217/pmt-2019-0065

[60] Wang EJ, Berninger LE, Pantelyat AY, et al. Scrambler therapy for the treatment of multiple system atrophy-parkinsonian subtype pain: A case report. A&A Practice. 2022;**16**:e01560. DOI: 10.1213/XAA.0000000000001560

[61] Sparadeo F, Kaufman C, D'Amato S. Scrambler therapy: An innovative and effective treatment for chronic neuropathic pain. Journal of Life Care Planning. 2012;**11**:3-15

[62] Cleeland CS, Ryan KM. Pain assessment: Global use of the brief pain inventory. Annals of the Academy of Medicine, Singapore. 1994;**23**:129-138

[63] Ricci M, Pirotti S, Scarpi E, et al. Managing chronic pain: Results from an open-label study using MC5-a Calmare device. Supportive Care in Cancer. 2012;**20**:405-412. DOI: 10.1007/s00520-011-1128-6

[64] Ricci M, Fabbri L, Pirotti S, et al. Scrambler therapy: what's new after 15 years? The results from 219 patients treated for chronic pain. Medicine. 2019;**98**:e13895. DOI: 10.1097/MD0000000000013895

[65] Compagnone C, Tagliaferri F. Chronic pain treatment and scrambler therapy: A multicenter retrospective analysis. Acta Bio-Medica. 2015;**86**:149-156

[66] Nayback-Beebe A, Panula T, Arzola S, et al. Scrambler therapy treatment: The importance of examining clinically meaningful improvements in chronic pain and quality of life. Military Medicine. 2020;**185**:143-147. DOI: 10.1093/milmed/usz253

[67] Marineo G. Inaccuracy in the article "scrambler therapy treatment: The importance of examining clinically meaningful improvements in chronic pain and quality of life." [letter]. Military Medicine. 2020;**185**:e1387. DOI: 10.1093/milmed/usaa089

[68] Marineo G. Inaccuracy in the article "managing chronic pain: Results from an open-label study using MC5-a Calmare device in support care Cancer." [letter]. Supportive Care in Cancer. 2011;**19**:1483-1484. DOI: 10.1007/s00520-011-1245-2

[69] Joo SY, Cho YS, Cho SR, et al. Effects of pain scrambler therapy for management of burn scar pruritus: A pilot study. Burns. 2017;**43**:514-519. DOI: 10.1016/j.burns.2016.09.028

[70] Haest C, Casaer MP, Daems A, et al. Measurement of itching: Validation of the Leuven itch scale. Burns. 2011;**37**:939-950. DOI: 10.1016/j.burns.2011.04.007

[71] Lee SY, Park C-h, Cho YS, et al. Scrambler therapy for chronic pain after burns and its effect on the cerebral pain network: A prospective, double-blinded, randomized controlled trial. Journal of Clinical Medicine. 2022;**11**:4255. DOI: 10.3390/jcm11154255

[72] Yarchoan M, Naidoo J, Smith TJ. Successful treatment of scar pain with scrambler therapy. Cureus. 2019;**11**:e5903. DOI: 10.7759/cureus.5903

[73] Kashyap K, Vig S, Bhan S, et al. Scrambler therapy – A novel treatment approach for chronic postoperative pain. [letter]. Journal of Anaesthesiology Clinical Pharmacology. 2020;**36**:276-278. DOI: 10.4103/joacp.JOACP_11_19

[74] Han JW, Lee DK. Effects of scrambler therapy on pain and depression of patients with chronic low back pain: Case study. Journal of Physical Therapy Science. 2018;**30**:913-914

[75] Jeong HJ, Lee DK, Kim YN, et al. The effects of pain scrambler therapy on the pain and quality of life of degenerative gonarthritis patients. Journal of Physical Therapy Science. 2018;**30**:479-480

[76] Murphy TK, Pardo CA, Roda RH, et al. Successful treatment of paraneoplastic neuropathy and pruritis with scrambler therapy: A case report. Cureus. 2022;**14**:e26861. DOI: 10.7759/cureus.26861

[77] Smith TJ, Auwaerter P, Knowlton A, et al. Treatment of human immunodeficiency virus-related peripheral neuropathy with scrambler therapy: A case report. International Journal of STD & AIDS. 2017;**28**:202-204. DOI: 10.1177/0956462416656688

[78] Warner NS, Watson JC, Bendel MA, et al. Refractory pain management in amyloid-associated peripheral neuropathy. Regional Anesthesia and Pain Medicine. 2018;**43**:434-437. DOI: 10.1097/AAP.0000000000000733

[79] Hunsberger JB, Rathee V, Smith TJ. Use of scrambler therapy in the treatment of amyloidosis neuropathic pain. Journal of Palliative Medicine. 2021;**24**:1579-1581. DOI: 10.1089/jpm.2020.0786

[80] Murphy T, Erdek M, Smith TJ. Scrambler therapy for the treatment of pain in schwannomatosis. Cureus. 2022;**14**:e23124. DOI: 10.7759/cureus.23124

[81] Smith TJ, Ferguson A, Baretti M, et al. Successful treatment with scrambler therapy for radial and femoral nerve injuries after extracorporeal membrane oxygenation. Mayo Clinic Proceedings. 2021;**96**:1374-1375. DOI: 10.1016/j.mayocp.2021.03.025

[82] Fabbri L, Pirotti SP, Rosati M, et al. Phantom limb pain successfully treated with scrambler therapy. [letter]. Minerva Anestesiologica. 2018;**84**:642-643. DOI: 10.23736/S0375-9393.18.12490-4

[83] Lee DK, Kim EK. Effect of pain scrambler therapy on shoulder joint pain and range of motion in patients who had undergone arthroscopic rotator cuff repair for the first time. Journal of Physical Therapy Science. 2016;**28**:2175-2177

[84] Ghatak RK, Nandi SN, Bhakta A, et al. Prospective study of application of biological communication (cybernatics) in management of chronic low back pain – A preliminary report. Nepal Medical College Journal. 2011;**13**:257-260

[85] Fairbank JC, Couper J, Davies JB, et al. The Oswestry low back pain disability questionnaire. Physiotherapy. 1980;**66**:271-273

[86] Abdi S, Lakkimsetty VM, Barrera J, et al. The use of "scrambler therapy" for failed back surgery syndrome. [abstract presentation]. 2011 13th annual meeting of the American Society of Interventional Pain Physicians. Pain Physician. 2011;**14**:E465-E491

[87] Starkweather AR, Coyne P, Lyon DE, et al. Decreased low back pain intensity and differential gene expression following Calmare: Results from a double-blinded randomized sham-controlled study. Research in Nursing & Health. 2015;**38**: 29-38. DOI: 10.1002/nur.21632

[88] Malin S, Molliver D, Koerber H, et al. Glial cell line-derived neurotrophic factor family members sensitize nociceptors in vitro and produce

thermal hyperalgesia in vivo. Journal of Neuroscience. 2006;**26**:8588-8599. DOI: 10.1523/JNEUROSCI.1726-06.2006

[89] Raucci U, Tomasello C, Marri M, et al. Scrambler therapy MC-5A for complex regional pain syndrome: Case reports. Pain Practice. 2016;**16**:E103-E109. DOI: 10.1111/papr.12474

[90] Park HS, Kim WJ, Kim HG, et al. Scrambler therapy for the treatment of neuropathic pain related to leukemia in a pediatric patient: A case report. Medicine. 2017;**96**(45):e8629. DOI: 10.1097/MD.0000000000008629

[91] Congedi S, Spadini S, Di Pede C, et al. Use of scrambler therapy in acute paediatric pain: A case report and review of the literature. Case Reports in Pediatrics. 2016;**2016**:ID2628919. DOI: 10.1155/2016/2628919

[92] Bakr SM, Knight J, Johnson SK, et al. Spinal cord stimulation improves functional outcomes in children with complex regional pain syndrome: Case presentation and review of the literature. Pain Practice. 2020;**20**:647-655. DOI: 10.1111/papr.12882

[93] Sharma A, Agarwal S, Broatch J, et al. A web-based cross-sectional epidemiological survey of complex regional pain syndrome. Regional Anesthesia and Pain Medicine. 2009;**34**:110-115. DOI: 10.1097/AAP.0b013e3181958f90

Chapter 10

Vestibular Migraine

Kristina Ryliškienė and Mantas Jokubaitis

Abstract

The consensus diagnostic criteria for vestibular migraine (VM) are used to specifically describe episodic vestibular symptoms associated with migraine. Because of an incomplete understanding of the etiology, a variety of clinical manifestations, and overlap with other vestibular disorders, the precise prevalence of VM is unknown. Clinical examination during vestibular episodes and vestibular laboratory tests interictally are more commonly abnormal in patients with VM than in controls, but none of the findings are specific for the diagnosis. The majority of information about VM treatment originates from case studies and retrospective reviews. In this chapter, the current epidemiology data, pathophysiology, significance of clinical and laboratory findings, and possible therapeutic approaches with existing and new medications or devices will be discussed.

Keywords: vestibular migraine, epidemiology, diagnostic criteria, pathophysiology, treatment

1. Introduction

Migraine and dizziness are frequently reported symptoms in clinical neurology. In a recent meta-analysis [1], it was found that the relative frequency of headache-associated vertigo in patients with migraine was 33.9%; however, there was significant heterogeneity between analyzed studies. Other researchers have reported episodic vertigo as a prodromal symptom in 3.3% of migraine patients [2], whereas headache phase-associated vertigo frequency varied between 6.4% and 44.7% [2–4]. Various names were interchangeably used to define a clinical entity that incorporates vestibular and migraine symptoms, including "migrainous vertigo, migraine-related vestibulopathy, migraine-associated vertigo, and migraine-associated dizziness" [5]. In 1999, Dieterich and Brandt coined the term vestibular migraine (VM), which is now used to describe vertigo or vestibular symptoms during a migraine attack [6]. Due to the heterogeneous clinical presentation, the lack of biological markers, and high comorbidity with other vertigo-causing diseases even in the presence of established diagnostic criteria [5, 7], diagnosis of VM might be challenging. VM is currently either underdiagnosed or misdiagnosed, and disabling vestibular symptoms still lack the approved management [8].

2. Vestibular migraine

2.1 Definition and diagnostic criteria

Currently, there are globally used International Headache Society and Barany Society consensus criteria for VM diagnosis (see **Table 1**) [5]. The diagnostic criteria are solely based on history taking. Only criterion D is based on the absence of physical examination or laboratory findings that might imply an alternative diagnosis.

Even though they are joint criteria of the two societies, in their respective classifications (the third edition of the International Classification of Headache Disorders [9] (ICHD-3) and International Classification of Vestibular Disorders (ICVD)), there are some differences. In ICHD-3, the criteria are more stringent, and VM is classified under the appendix, indicating that further research is needed and VM criteria have not yet been sufficiently validated to include in the main body. In contrast, ICVD includes additional criteria for probable VM in order to minimize the exclusion of patients affected by VM and to facilitate research. Despite the presence of official diagnostic criteria for VM, some researchers argue that they should be even expanded and potential subtypes of VM refined, as has been done for migraine headache [8, 10].

Although VM is considered an episodic vestibular disorder, the available literature indicates that a large proportion of patients experience symptoms between the attacks [5].

International Headache Society criteria for VM and Barany Society consensus criteria for definite VM (ICHD-3, 2018; ICVD, 2012, updated 2022)	Barany Society consensus criteria for probable VM (ICVD, 2012, updated 2022)
(A) At least 5 episodes with vestibular symptoms of moderate or severe intensity lasting 5 minutes to 72 hours	(A) At least 5 episodes with vestibular symptoms of moderate or severe intensity, lasting 5 minutes to 72 hours
(B) Current or previous history of migraine with or without aura according to the ICHD-3 criteria	(B) Only one of the criteria B and C for vestibular migraine is fulfilled (migraine history or migraine features during the episode)
(C) One or more migraine features with at least 50% of the vestibular episodes: 1. Headache with at least two of the following characteristics: a. One-sided location b. Pulsating quality c. Moderate or severe pain intensity d. Aggravation by routine physical activity 2. Photophobia and phonophobia 3. Visual aura	(C) Not better accounted for by another vestibular or ICHD diagnosis
(D) Not better accounted for by another vestibular or ICHD diagnosis	

ICHD-3—the third edition of the International Classification of Headache Disorders; ICVD—the International Classification of Vestibular Disorders; VM—vestibular migraine.

Table 1.
Criteria for vestibular migraine by the international headache society and for definite and probable vestibular migraine by the Barany society [5, 7, 9].

ICVD discusses chronic VM, which may be associated with interictal visually induced, head motion-induced, or persistent dizziness. Because these symptoms are reported by a significant number of patients, upon further research, chronic VM may be included in a revised version of ICVD [5]. However, it may be more appropriate to make a coexisting diagnosis of persistent-postural perceptual dizziness (PPPD) if criteria for that condition are met [5, 7].

Additionally, there are other disorders closely related to VM. Migraine with brainstem aura (previously called basilar migraine) may also manifest with headache and vertigo; however, this diagnosis requires at least two focal neurologic brainstem symptoms in addition to visual, sensory, or dysphasic aura, and these criteria are met

Benign paroxysmal vertigo (of childhood) (ICHD-3, 2018)	**Vestibular migraine of childhood (ICVD, 2021)**	**Recurrent vertigo of childhood (ICVD, 2021)**
(A) At least five attacks fulfilling criteria B and C	(A) At least five episodes with vestibular symptoms of moderate or severe intensity lasting between five minutes and 72 hours	(A) At least three episodes with vestibular symptoms of moderate or severe intensity, lasting between 1 minute and 72 hours
(B) Vertigo occurring without warning, maximal at onset, and resolving spontaneously after minutes to hours without loss of consciousness	(B) A current or past history of migraine with or without aura	(B) None of the criteria B and C for vestibular migraine of childhood
(C) At least one of the following five associated symptoms or signs: 1. nystagmus 2. ataxia 3. vomiting 4. pallor 5. fearfulness	(C) At least half of the episodes are associated with at least one of the following three migraine features: 1. Headache with at least two of the following four characteristics: a. One-sided location b. Pulsating quality c. Moderate or severe pain intensity d. Aggravation by routine physical activity 2. Photophobia and phonophobia 3. Visual aura	(C) Age < 18 years
(D) Normal neurological examination and audiometric and vestibular functions between attacks	(D) Age < 18 years	(D) Not better accounted for by another headache disorder, vestibular disorder, or other conditions
(E) Not attributed to another disorder	(E) Not better accounted for by another headache disorder, vestibular disorder, or other conditions	

ICHD-3—the third edition of the International Classification of Headache Disorders; ICVD—the International Classification of Vestibular Disorders.

Table 2.
Criteria of benign paroxysmal vertigo, vestibular migraine of childhood, and recurrent vertigo of childhood by the international headache society and Barany society [9, 11].

by less than 10% of VM patients [9]. Therefore, while a subset of patients may fit the diagnostic criteria for both disorders, they are recognized as distinct entities.

ICHD-3 defines benign paroxysmal vertigo as an episodic syndrome that may be associated with migraine, which occurs primarily (but not exclusively) in healthy children. In 2021, the Barany Society proposed a new consensus document [11] with an aim to change the terminology from "benign paroxysmal vertigo" to definite and probable "VM of childhood" and "recurrent vertigo of childhood." Contrary to the ICHD-3 criteria, which do not specify an age limit, the ICVD criteria do (see **Table 2**). One of the reasons for the change of terminology was confusion about the term "paroxysmal," which is designated for vestibular symptoms lasting less than one minute. Additionally, while being thought to be a migraine precursor, the diagnosis of benign paroxysmal vertigo does not include any migrainous characteristics [11]. Migraine diagnosis is commonly absent due to a short clinical history of headaches and difficulties distinguishing children's symptoms [12]. However, a substantial proportion of children with episodic vertigo also display migraine features. New criteria distinguish these groups by employing a continuum ranging from probable and definite VM to recurrent vertigo of childhood, allowing for more precise research [11].

2.2 Epidemiology and comorbidity

The precise prevalence of VM is unknown; however, it is thought to be a very common condition, with an estimated prevalence of 1% to 2.7% in the general population [13, 14] and 11–13% in specialized dizziness and headache centers [15, 16]. Probable and definite VM was the most frequent episodic non-positional non-ischemic vestibular syndrome in primary care [17]. In both familial and non-familial cases of VM, there was a female predominance in most of the studies included in systematic review [13]. The mean age of onset of VM in patients with concurrent migraine and vertigo manifestation was found to be 22.7 ± 10.4 years, whereas patients with a non-simultaneous presentation of symptoms were somewhat older, with a mean age of onset for vertigo of 35.6 ± 12.4 years and 24 ± 8.9 years for migraine [18].

The frequent comorbidity of migraine with other vertigo-causing diseases complicates diagnosis and undoubtedly distorts data on VM prevalence. Comorbid conditions and disorders associated with VM include benign paroxysmal positional vertigo (BPPV), Ménière's disease (MD), motion sickness, Mal de Debarquement syndrome (MdDS), PPPD, and anxiety disorder [19, 20].

BPPV is one of the most common causes for short episodic dizziness and vertigo [21]. Migraine patients have a 2.5-fold increased risk of BPPV recurrence, whereas BPPV patients have an increased risk of migraine [22–24].

MD and VM share many similar clinical features. Patients with MD present with migraine twice as often as the control group [25, 26].

Motion sickness, visually induced motion sickness (VIMS), and corresponding disorders may co-occur, and the severity of symptoms may be increased by a variety of vestibular disorders, including VM [27].

MdDS is a syndrome defined by non-spinning vertigo with an oscillatory perception that occurs within 48 hours of the end of passive motion. The symptoms last for at least 48 hours and are temporarily alleviated by recurrence of passive motion [28]. Migraine headaches may develop alongside the onset of MdDS and worsen as the disease progresses [29].

PPPD is characterized by one or more symptoms of dizziness, unsteadiness, or non-spinning vertigo, which are present on most days for three months or more and are exacerbated by upright posture, active or passive movement, and exposure to moving or complex visual stimuli. VM attacks are one of the most common precipitating conditions leading to the development of comorbid PPPD [30].

Cross-sectional studies conducted in specialized vertigo and dizziness centers revealed that nearly half of the dizzy patients had a psychiatric disorder compared to 20% of the general population [31–33]. Nevertheless, psychiatric comorbidities were not consistent across different vestibular disorders. VM had one of the highest rates for psychiatric comorbidity (49%). In addition, anxiety and phobic disorders were the most common among VM patients (32.6%) [31].

It must be highlighted that any vestibular disorder might be complicated by migraine. Therefore, the nonspecific co-occurrence of migraine and vestibular symptoms necessitates the consideration of differential diagnoses (see Chapter 2.5).

2.3 Pathophysiology

The pathophysiology of VM is multifactorial and not fully understood, as evidenced by the multitude of hypotheses proposed to explain VM. Suggested central mechanisms include a cortical spreading depression induced by an unknown trigger impacting the vestibular cortex and, as a result, affecting brainstem vestibular nuclei via vestibular-thalamic cortical pathways or a brainstem aura directly affecting these nuclei [34, 35]. Yet only 2–30% of individuals fulfill the migraine aura criteria, that is, vertigo lasting 5 to 60 minutes prior to the onset of the headache [36].

In addition, altered sensory processing and integration have been proposed as one of the contributing mechanisms for VM [24]. In order to maintain spatial orientation when the head position is changed, the brain must integrate vestibular and visual inputs. Inaccuracies in this process have been described in VM patients with spatial perception errors consistent with overestimation of the head position [24, 37]. Consequently, VM patients predominantly report dizziness when their heads are tilted in the same direction, which causes greater spatial orientation error, indicating that altered sensory processing and integration may be a cause of visuospatial symptoms in VM [24].

Alternatively, activation of the trigeminovascular system represents a peripheral mechanism. The inner ear, cochlear nucleus, and superior olivary complex are innervated by neurons of the trigeminal ganglion [38, 39]. It has been previously shown in experimental studies that chemical and electrical stimulations of the trigeminal ganglion cause a considerable increase in inner ear blood flow and alterations of vascular permeability, causing plasma protein extravasation and disruption of inner ear metabolism [40, 41]. The chemical stimulation in VM occurs by substances released during the cortical spreading depression (potassium, glutamic, and arachidonic acid), which activate the trigeminal pain receptors and neurons of the trigeminal nucleus [42]. Moreover, this notion is supported by painful electrical stimulation to the trigeminal nerve, triggering peripheral spontaneous nystagmus or enhancing pre-existing spontaneous nystagmus in migraine patients [43]. In addition, calcitonin gene-related peptide (CGRP) has been identified in sensory fibers that innervate vestibular nuclei and the inner ear, explaining the possible role of CGRP inhibitors in the treatment of VM [44].

There has been research associating migraine and vertigo to ovarian hormones, particularly estrogen and progesterone [45]. Vestibular symptoms in women can become more severe or begin around menopause, which may be explained by the modulating action of ovarian hormones on monoaminergic systems in various cerebral structures, including the vestibular and trigeminal nuclei.

VM has been documented in families with an autosomal dominant pattern and reduced penetrance in men [46]. Additionally, VM is related to familial hemiplegic migraine (FHM) and episodic ataxia type 2 (EA-2) in that both conditions frequently present with vertigo and migraine. Furthermore, VM is associated with mutations of CACNA1A (coding for neuronal calcium channel), ATP1A2 (coding for Na/K ATPase), and SCN1A (coding for voltage-gated sodium channel), which may occur in FHM and EA-2 [47].

2.4 Clinical characteristics

VM patients frequently experience vestibular symptoms following headache; fewer patients have vestibular symptoms right before headache, whereas some individuals never experience headache and vestibular symptoms simultaneously [24].

The most common vestibular symptoms include spontaneous vertigo, positional vertigo, head motion-induced vertigo, and visually induced vertigo [13, 24]. However, patients frequently employ a variety of different terminologies to describe these symptoms, reflecting the diverse internally perceived experiences. The majority of VM patients experience more than one vestibular symptom during an acute attack, with the most common being spinning vertigo (72%), disequilibrium and/or Mal de Debarquement (58%), and rocking/tilting sensation (43%), whereas most common migraine symptoms include headache (81%), visual aura (26%), and photophobia (23%) [48]. Vertigo is frequently triggered by head motion (44%), visual stimuli (41%), or positional change in the supine position (25%) followed by spontaneous vertigo [49]. Nausea is also common (55%), with almost 20% of all patients progressing to vomiting [48]. The duration of vestibular symptoms varies greatly, with approximately 30% of patients estimating that the symptoms continue for minutes, 30% for hours, and 30% for days. The remainder 10% describe fluctuating daily symptoms [24]. Additionally, one study found that visually induced dizziness (89%) and head motion-induced dizziness (66%) were extremely common during the interictal period [19].

Along with vestibular symptoms and migrainous headache, VM patients frequently experience unilateral or bilateral auditory symptoms such as tinnitus (52%), aural fullness (41%), mild and easily reversible low-frequency hearing loss (21%), and even otalgia (8.4%) [50]. However, because of their great incidence in other vestibular disorders, it was decided that auditory symptoms should not be included in the VM diagnostic criteria [5].

2.5 Differential diagnosis

Differential diagnoses for VM include MD, BPPV, vertebrobasilar transient ischemic attacks (TIAs), vestibular paroxysmia (VP), and episodic ataxia type 2 (EA2).

MD is characterized by recurrent spontaneous vertigo lasting 20 minutes to 12 hours and cochlear signs: sensorineural hearing loss, fluctuating tinnitus, and aural fullness [51]. VM and MD are the most difficult diagnoses to differentiate between, usually necessitating several follow-up visits to a specialist in order to make a clear distinction [52]. Patients meeting both definite VM and definite MD criteria have been described repeatedly in the literature, suggesting the possibility of an overlap syndrome and a shared pathophysiology [53]. Signs and symptoms such as aural pressure, tinnitus, migrainous headache, auras, and endolymphatic hydrops can occur in both of these disorders. Nevertheless, a low-frequency hearing loss is the key finding that differentiates MD from VM [52]. Hearing loss in VM typically is bilateral and down sloping as opposed to unilateral or asymmetric and flat in MD [5]. The Barany Society recommends diagnosing MD even if migraine symptoms occur during episodes of vertigo. Additionally, only patients with different types of attacks who meet the diagnostic criteria for VM and MD (in respect to different attack types) should be diagnosed with both disorders [7].

BPPV is a common cause of paroxysmal (less than 1 minute) dizziness and vertigo, which occurs due to abnormal stimulation of the semicircular canals by otoliths [21]. The primary distinction between BPPV and VM is the duration of the vertigo episode: an acute episode of BPPV lasts less than one minute, whereas a typical episode of VM lasts 5 minutes to 72 hours [5]. Although residual dizziness and associated symptoms in BPPV may be misinterpreted as an active continuation of the vertigo episode, a thorough history taking and the use of repositioning maneuvers that result in semicircular canal-specific nystagmus with latency, as opposed to persistent nystagmus of moderate velocity in VM, may help in differential diagnosis [5, 54].

Although rare, vertebrobasilar TIAs can occur as isolated episodes of vertigo, lasting minutes to hours without additional brainstem symptoms; however, TIAs are not associated with headache and usually follow a course of increasing frequency (if evident cardiovascular risk factors are not corrected) rather than weeks or months of vertigo-free periods as in the case of VM [36, 55]. In suspected stroke cases, HINTS (head impulse test, nystagmus, and skew test) examination may be beneficial [54].

VP is distinguished by brief (less than a minute, usually a few seconds) episodes of transient vertigo that are unrelated to migraine attacks. Successful treatment with carbamazepine or oxcarbazepine may also aid in diagnosis [5, 54].

EA2 is a genetic autosomal dominant disorder that typically manifests at the age of 20 [55]. EA2 is characterized by a sudden onset of vertigo and associated with headache and ataxia [52, 55]. Vertigo episodes can last from hours to days and are usually brought on by emotional stress, physical exertion, and alcohol consumption [55]. The time between episodes can range from a few days to several years. As a result of the clinical similarities, the vertigo caused by EA2 cannot be reliably distinguished from VM [52, 55]. Additional changes in MRI consist of cerebellar atrophy of anterior vermis, and treatment with acetazolamide may attenuate or prevent attacks in up to 50 percent of patients [55]. The combination of these clues, together with typical triggers and a positive family history, may help in diagnosis.

2.6 Clinical and laboratory findings

The heterogenic nature of VM is reflected by great variation of vestibular and audiological findings between different investigators and even across patients. The neurologic examination is usually normal between acute attacks. Some studies have reported various oculomotor abnormalities interictally in up to 55% of individuals such as spontaneous, gaze evoked, central positional nystagmus, or smooth pursuit deficits; however, they were nonspecific [6, 56–59].

During vertigo episodes, up to 71% of patients had spontaneous nystagmus, with horizontal direction in 50%, down-beat in 12%, and up-beat in 10% [56]. In addition, it was found that the use of a visual fixation block can reveal low-velocity positional nystagmus, which is either horizontal, vertical, or torsional [36]. Furthermore, spontaneous horizontal nystagmus can be provoked by the headshaking test in 35% of VM patients during an attack [36]. Interestingly, one study found that severe spontaneous horizontal nystagmus with a speed greater than 12 degrees per second was more sensitive and specific for MD, whereas spontaneous vertical nystagmus was more specific for VM [60]. A majority of VM patients show unidirectional nystagmus during repeated attacks, with only a small fraction displaying nystagmus direction reversal [56]. Additionally, an abnormal head impulse test may accompany spontaneous horizontal nystagmus in VM, indicating a unilateral deficit in the vestibuloocular reflex [36]. During episodes of VM, most patients have impaired stance and gait, with difficulties performing the Romberg test, tandem gait, or even standard gait [36].

There are no conclusive tests to confirm VM. The diagnosis is based on consensus criteria, and VM should be regarded as a diagnosis of exclusion. Nevertheless, due to a variety of phenotypes, VM may mimic other vestibular disorders, in which case additional testing might be beneficial; thus, instrumental findings will be further discussed. The absence of any structural lesions supports the diagnosis of VM and can reduce patients' anxiety.

Video head impulse testing (vHIT) performed interictally may demonstrate reduced gain of lateral semicircular canals; however, gain changes in addition to saccade frequency, amplitude, and duration are insignificant compared to normal controls [56]. In contrast, a majority of VM patients during acute vertigo display vHIT results consistent with peripheral dysfunction [56, 61].

Caloric testing is rarely useful in distinguishing VM patients from those with other causes of vertigo [20, 36]. Bithermal caloric testing is abnormal in approximately 15–20% of patients, with the most common deficits being a reduced unilateral response, directional preponderance, and, in some cases, a reduced bilateral response [36, 56].

On a firm surface, posturography findings do not differ between VM patients and control groups; however, on a foam surface, the mean center of gravity sway velocity with eyes open and closed is increased in VM patients [58]. Nonetheless, posturography results are insufficient to diagnose VM and must be interpreted in conjunction with other vestibular tests.

Vestibular-evoked myogenic potentials (VEMPs) have recently received additional attention in the differential diagnoses of VM and MD [62]. By testing for cervical VEMPs, it is possible to selectively measure the function of saccule, while ocular VEMPs reflect the function of utricle [63]. In a recent study, it has been found that the decrease in saccular function is greater than the decrease in utricular function in MD, whereas the degree and asymmetry of saccular and utricular dysfunctions in VM are low and tend to be equal in both labyrinths. As a result, different patterns of saccular and utricular dysfunctions may help differentiate VM from other causes of dizziness over time [62]. However, several other studies measuring VEMPs have yielded contradictory results [49, 64, 65]. Although the rate of VEMP abnormalities is higher in patients with vestibular disorders than in controls, there are as yet insufficient data to confirm that VEMPs can confidently distinguish between VM and MD [20, 36].

Even though many VM patients have mild auditory symptoms, audiometry results show that the majority of individuals have normal symmetric function or age-related symmetric high-frequency hearing loss, whereas only less than 8% of patients display asymmetry or loss of hearing in more than one frequency [56]. On the other hand, audiometric testing should be performed in patients who exhibit any auditory symptoms during or between attacks to confirm the subclinical or evident hearing loss, which is characteristic of MD. It should be noted that while initial testing may be negative, in the case of unknown diagnosis, follow-up audiometry could add additional value [66].

Endolymphatic hydrops, a characteristic finding of MD classically described in the literature, may also occur in VM. According to studies performing high-resolution

MRI of the inner ear, the presence of endolymphatic hydrops was found to be the most common in MD (79%), the least common in VM (12%), and intermediate in the VM-MD overlap syndrome (25%; i.e., when both criteria of VM and MD are met) [48]. Moreover, studies report a relatively high prevalence of endolymphatic hydrops in healthy controls [10]. As a result, while the rate of endolymphatic hydrops in VM is lower than that in MD, there is still controversy about the utility of distinguishing these two diseases based on the presence of hydrops. Alternatively, in cases of suspected VM, the main indication for neuroimaging is a new onset of isolated vertigo lasting minutes in those with additional vascular risk factors to exclude vertebrobasilar transient ischemic attacks [36].

2.7 Treatment of vestibular migraine

There are currently no evidence-based treatment guidelines for VM [67]. Furthermore, randomized controlled trials are scarce, and most treatment recommendations are based on either case series, individual case reports, or retrospective studies with no control groups. In addition, patient documentation of headache and vestibular symptoms could significantly improve the rate of correct diagnosis and be used to assess treatment efficacy in everyday practice; nevertheless, it is still underused.

2.7.1 Non-pharmacologic treatment

Education in VM is one of the most important aspects of disease management. Reassuring patients that the episodes are only temporarily disabling and not related to stroke and not associated with permanent hearing or vestibular function loss may significantly help to relieve VM-associated anxiety. Although follow-up studies show that as many as 90% of patients still suffer from VM after 9 years of initial diagnosis, the frequency of vertigo decreases in over 50% of patients [68]. As a result, cautious positive expectation formation is reasonable.

Identifying modifiable lifestyle factors that contribute to VM (e.g., sleep disturbances, stress, insufficient physical activity, food triggers) and encouraging patients to take an active role in their disease management is another key intervention during consultation. In addition, vestibular rehabilitation should be recommended as it may increase the threshold of a VM attack to some extent [54]. Vestibular rehabilitation typically consists of four groups of exercises (gaze stability exercises, habituation exercises, gait and balance training, and walking to improve endurance), and some studies, albeit with low-quality evidence, suggest that it may be more effective than pharmacologic intervention [54, 69]. Furthermore, some randomized controlled trials concerning alternative non-pharmacologic prophylaxis (e.g., acupuncture) are underway [70].

Lastly, studies with external trigeminal nerve stimulation (eTNS) and non-invasive vagus nerve stimulation (nVNS) for acute VM symptoms (including both vertigo and headache) have shown promising results, with no intolerable side effects and mean vertigo reduction of 61.3% with eTNS and 46.9% with nVNS [71, 72].

2.7.2 Treatment of acute attack

In the case of short, infrequent, and mild episodes of VM, it should be discussed with the patient whether pharmacologic treatment is indicated. On the other hand, if significant vertigo and/or nausea lasts longer than the time required for the drug to

Drug	Dosage	Notes
Dimenhydrinate [73]	25–50 mg, may be repeated every 6 h	May cause sedation, vision impairment, urinary retention
Diphenhydramine [73]	50–100 mg, may be repeated every 6 h	As above
Meclizine [73]	25–50 mg, may be repeated every 6 h	As above
Metoclopramide [74]	10 mg, may be repeated every 4 h	May cause QT prolongation, extrapyramidal effects
Almotriptan [75]	12.5 mg	May cause nausea, xerostomia, paraesthesia
Rizatriptan [76]	10 mg	As above
Zolmitriptan [77]	2.5 mg	As above
Methylprednisolone [78]	1000 mg i/v	Primarily used to decrease the severity of unusually long episodes

Table 3.
Treatment of acute symptoms in vestibular migraine.

start working (usually more than 30 minutes), pharmacologic intervention should be initiated [36]. Despite the lack of high-quality evidence on efficacy, acute VM treatment mainly consists of antivertiginous and antiemetic medications [36, 54, 55, 73]; see **Table 3**. In addition, benzodiazepines may be used to suppress vestibular system and consequently reduce the symptoms of acute VM. Triptans have been reported to reduce vertigo; however, most studies investigating triptans in the treatment of acute VM provide low-quality evidence [75–77]. The combination of different classes of aforementioned drugs may be used if nausea and/or vomiting is particularly severe. Additionally, analgesics should be added if headache is present. Finally, in treatment-resistant cases, intravenous methylprednisolone has been shown to be successful in some case reports [78].

2.7.3 Preventive treatment

Most medications for VM treatment are targeted at prophylaxis. Prophylaxis may be appropriate for patients who have long, frequent, and severe episodes or in cases of acute treatment failure. In addition, combining pharmacologic and non-pharmacologic treatment (e.g., vestibular rehabilitation) may be more effective than either treatment alone [73].

Due to a lack of trials focusing specifically on VM, treatment approaches are based on migraine research with the goal of reducing the frequency and severity of VM attacks. In practice, medication selection is based on side effects and comorbidities rather than on data of efficacy see **Table 4** [36, 54, 79]. Nonetheless, a recent meta-analysis has found that propranolol, followed by venlafaxine, resulted in the greatest short-term improvement in the dizziness handicap index [67].

To date, there have been only two randomized controlled trials in VM prophylaxis. One study found that flunarizine reduced the frequency and severity of vertigo without reduction in headache [81], while the other showed that vertigo and dizziness were significantly reduced in patients treated with propranolol or venlafaxine [80]. In addition, venlafaxine was superior to propranolol in the treatment of comorbid mood

Drug	Dosage	Notes
Propranolol [80]	40–160 mg/d	Useful in cases of hypertension, tachycardia, anxiety. May cause bronchial constriction, impotence. May worsen depression. RCT available.
Venlafaxine [80]	37.5–150 mg/d	Useful in cases of obesity, mood disorders. May cause fatigue, insomnia. RCT available.
Flunarizine [81]	10 mg/d	May cause weight gain, somnolence, nausea. RCT available.
Topiramate [73]	50–100 mg/d	Useful in cases of obesity and fatigue. May cause cognitive dysfunction, somnolence, paresthesia. Teratogenic.
Valproic acid [54]	500–1000 mg/d	May cause weight gain, somnolence, thrombocytopenia, hepatotoxicity. Teratogenic.
Amitriptyline [73]	25–75 mg/d	Useful in cases of insomnia. May cause constipation, sedation, weight gain, conduction block.

RCT—randomized-controlled trial.

Table 4.
Prophylactic treatment typically used in vestibular migraine.

disorders and is believed to be a preferred choice when VM coexists with persistent postural-perceptual dizziness, depression, or anxiety [80, 82].

New treatment strategies, for example, anti-CGRP medications or onabotulinumtoxin A injections, have been also employed in small studies. Anti-CGRP medications (monoclonal antibodies and gepants) have demonstrated moderate to significant VM improvement in 60% (n = 15) of patients [83]. Onabotulinumtoxin A injections have been shown to be effective in reducing vertigo and headaches in resistant VM cases, as reflected by improvements in the Headache Impact Test, Migraine Disability Assessment, Dizziness Handicap Inventory, Vertigo Symptom Scale, and even changes in functional brain connectivity [84].

Many patients prefer non-pharmacologic treatment to taking medications on a daily basis. In those cases, alternative methods such as relaxation training, biofeedback training, and cognitive behavioral therapy that have shown significant improvements could be suggested [73].

3. Conclusions

VM is a disorder characterized by migrainous headaches and associated vestibular symptoms. VM is believed to be a very common condition affecting up to 2.7% of the general population, whereas probable and definite VMs are reported to be the most frequent episodic non-ischemic vestibular syndrome in primary care. Furthermore, VM is frequently comorbid, with other vertigo-causing disorders. The diagnosis of VM is based on the consensus diagnostic criteria and the exclusion of other vestibular disorders. There is no single instrumental or laboratory test that can reliably confirm or reject the diagnosis of VM. Although no evidence-based guidelines exist for the treatment of VM, in clinical practice, a combination of painkiller and vestibular suppressant for acute VM attacks is commonly used.

Similarly, personalized prevention of migraine headaches has been shown to reduce the frequency of VM episodes.

Conflict of interest

The authors declare no conflict of interest.

Author details

Kristina Ryliškienė and Mantas Jokubaitis*
Faculty of Medicine, Centre of Neurology, Institute of Clinical Medicine, Vilnius University, Vilnius, Lithuania

*Address all correspondence to: mantas.jokubaitis1@gmail.com

References

[1] Iljazi A, Ashina H, Lipton RB, et al. Dizziness and vertigo during the prodromal phase and headache phase of migraine: A systematic review and meta-analysis. Cephalalgia. 2020;**40**:1095-1103. DOI: 10.1177/0333102420921855

[2] Lampl C, Rapoport A, Levin M, et al. Migraine and episodic vertigo: A cohort survey study of their relationship. Journal of Headache and Pain. 2019;**20**: 1-5. DOI: 10.1186/s10194-019-0991-2

[3] Akdal G, Özge A, Ergör G. The prevalence of vestibular symptoms in migraine or tension-type headache. Journal of Vestibular Research. 2013;**23**:101-106. DOI: 10.3233/VES-130477

[4] Carvalho GF, Vianna-Bell FH, Florencio LL, et al. Presence of vestibular symptoms and related disability in migraine with and without aura and chronic migraine. Cephalalgia. 2019;**39**:29-37. DOI: 10.1177/0333102418769948

[5] Lempert T, Olesen J, Furman J, et al. Vestibular migraine: Diagnostic criteria. Journal of Vestibular Research. 2022;**32**: 1-6. DOI: 10.3233/VES-201644

[6] Dieterich M, Brandt T. Episodic vertigo related to migraine (90 cases): Vestibular migraine? Journal of Neurology. 1999;**246**:883-892. DOI: 10.1007/S004150050478

[7] Lempert T, Olesen J, Furman J, et al. Vestibular migraine: Diagnostic criteria. Journal of Vestibular Research. 2012;**22**:167-172. DOI: 10.3233/VES-2012-0453

[8] Mallampalli MP, Rizk HG, Kheradmand A, et al. Care gaps and recommendations in vestibular migraine: An expert panel summit. Frontiers in Neurology. 2022;**12**:2371. DOI: 10.3389/fneur.2021.812678

[9] Olesen J. Headache classification Committee of the International Headache Society (IHS) the international classification of headache disorders, Cephalalgia, 3rd edition. 2018;38, 1-211. DOI:10.1177/0333102417738202.

[10] Perez-Carpena P, Lopez-Escamez JA. Do we need to reconsider the classification of vestibular migraine? Expert Review of Neurotherapeutics. 2021;**21**:503-516. DOI: 10.1080/14737175.2021.1908129

[11] van de Berg R, Widdershoven J, Bisdorff A, et al. Vestibular migraine of childhood and recurrent vertigo of childhood: Diagnostic criteria consensus document of the Committee for the Classification of vestibular disorders of the Bárány society and the international headache society. Journal of Vestibular Research. 2021;**31**:61-67. DOI: 10.3233/VES-200003

[12] Langhagen T, Landgraf MN, Huppert D, et al. Vestibular migraine in children and adolescents. Current Pain and Headache Reports. 2016;**20**:1-10. DOI: 10.1007/S11916-016-0600-X

[13] Neuhauser HK, Radtke A, von Brevern M, et al. Migrainous vertigo: Prevalence and impact on quality of life. Neurology. 2006;**67**:1028-1033. DOI: 10.1212/01.WNL.0000237539.09942.06

[14] Formeister EJ, Rizk HG, Kohn MA, et al. The epidemiology of vestibular migraine: A population-based survey study. Otology and Neurotology.

2018;**39**:1037-1044. DOI: 10.1097/MAO.0000000000001900

[15] Neuhauser H, Leopold M, Von Brevern M, et al. The interrelations of migraine, vertigo, and migrainous vertigo. Neurology. 2001;**56**:436-441. DOI: 10.1212/WNL.56.4.436

[16] Cho SJ, Kim BK, Kim BS, et al. Vestibular migraine in multicenter neurology clinics according to the appendix criteria in the third beta edition of the international classification of headache disorders. Cephalalgia. 2016;**36**:454-462. DOI: 10.1177/0333102415597890

[17] Domínguez-Durán E, Moreno-de-Jesús C, Prieto-Sánchez-de-Puerta L, et al. Identifying training, diagnostic and therapeutic needs from a comparison in the distribution of vestibular disorders in primary care and in a Neurotology unit. Frontiers in Neurology. 2020;**11**:1554. DOI: 10.3389/fneur.2020.605613

[18] Paz-Tamayo A, Perez-Carpena P, Lopez-Escamez JA. Systematic review of prevalence studies and familial aggregation in vestibular migraine. Frontiers in Genetics. 2020;**11**:954. DOI: 10.3389/fgene.2020.00954

[19] Beh SC, Masrour S, Smith S v., et al. The Spectrum of vestibular migraine: Clinical features, triggers, and examination findings. Headache 2019;59, 727-740. DOI:10.1111/head.13484.

[20] Zaleski-King A, Monfared A. Vestibular migraine and its comorbidities. Otolaryngologic Clinics of North America. 2021;**54**:949-958. DOI: 10.1016/j.otc.2021.05.014

[21] von Brevern M, Bertholon P, Brandt T, et al. Benign paroxysmal positional vertigo: Diagnostic criteria. Journal of Vestibular Research. 2015;**25**:105-117. DOI: 10.3233/VES-150553

[22] Zhu CT, Zhao XQ, Ju Y, et al. Clinical characteristics and risk factors for the recurrence of benign paroxysmal positional vertigo. Frontiers in Neurology. 2019;**10**:1190. DOI: 10.3389/fneur.2019.01190

[23] Kim SK, Hong SM, Park IS, et al. Association between migraine and benign paroxysmal positional vertigo among adults in South Korea. JAMA Otolaryngology. Head & Neck Surgery. 2019;**145**:307-312. DOI: 10.1001/jamaoto.2018.4016

[24] Huang TC, Wang SJ, Kheradmand A. Vestibular migraine: An update on current understanding and future directions. Cephalalgia. 2020;**40**:107-121. DOI: 10.1177/0333102419869317

[25] Radtke A, Lempert T, Gresty MA, et al. Migraine and Ménière's disease: Is there a link? Neurology. 2002;**59**:1700-1704. DOI: 10.1212/01.WNL.0000036903.22461.39

[26] Swaminathan A, Smith JH. Migraine and vertigo. Current Neurology and Neuroscience Reports. 2015;**15**:515

[27] Cha YH, Golding JF, Keshavarz B, et al. Motion sickness diagnostic criteria: Consensus document of the classification Committee of the Bárány Society. Journal of Vestibular Research. 2021;**31**:327-344. DOI: 10.3233/VES-200005

[28] Cha YH, Baloh RW, Cho C, et al. Mal de débarquement syndrome diagnostic criteria: Consensus document of the classification Committee of the Bárány Society. Journal of Vestibular Research. 2020;**30**:285-293. DOI: 10.3233/VES-200714

[29] Cha YH, Cui Y. Rocking dizziness and headache: A two-way street.

Cephalalgia. 2013;**33**:1160-1169. DOI: 10.1177/0333102413487999

[30] Staab JP, Eckhardt-Henn A, Horii A, et al. Diagnostic criteria for persistent postural-perceptual dizziness (PPPD): Consensus document of the committee for the classification of vestibular disorders of the Bárány society. Journal of Vestibular Research. 2017;**27**:191-208. DOI: 10.3233/VES-170622

[31] Lahmann C, Henningsen P, Brandt T, et al. Psychiatric comorbidity and psychosocial impairment among patients with vertigo and dizziness. Journal of Neurology, Neurosurgery, and Psychiatry. 2015;**86**:302-308. DOI: 10.1136/JNNP-2014-307601

[32] Best C, Eckhardt-Henn A, Tschan R, et al. Psychiatric morbidity and comorbidity in different vestibular vertigo syndromes. Results of a prospective longitudinal study over one year. Journal of Neurology. 2009;**256**:58-65. DOI: 10.1007/S00415-009-0038-8

[33] Kessler RC, Wai TC, Demler O, et al. Prevalence, severity, and comorbidity of twelve-month DSM-IV disorders in the National Comorbidity Survey Replication (NCS-R). Archives of General Psychiatry. 2005;**62**:617. DOI: 10.1001/ARCHPSYC.62.6.617

[34] Furman JM, Marcus DA, Balaban CD. Migrainous vertigo: Development of a pathogenetic model and structured diagnostic interview. Current Opinion in Neurology. 2003;**16**:5-13. DOI: 10.1097/01.WCO.0000053582.70044.E2

[35] Shin JH, Kim YK, Kim HJ, et al. Altered brain metabolism in vestibular migraine: Comparison of interictal and ictal findings. Cephalalgia. 2014;**34**:58-67. DOI: 10.1177/0333102413498940

[36] Eggers SDZ. Episodic Spontaneous Dizziness. Continuum Lifelong Learning in Neurology. 2021;**27**:369-401. DOI: 10.1212/CON.0000000000000931

[37] Li ZY, Si LH, Shen B, et al. Altered brain network functional connectivity patterns in patients with vestibular migraine diagnosed according to the diagnostic criteria of the Bárány society and the international headache society. Journal of Neurology. 2022;**269**:3026-3036. DOI: 10.1007/s00415-021-10868-0

[38] Vass Z, Shore SE, Nuttall AL, et al. Direct evidence of trigeminal innervation of the cochlear blood vessels. Neuroscience. 1998;**84**:559-567. DOI: 10.1016/S0306-4522(97)00503-4

[39] Shore SE, Vass Z, Wys NL, et al. Trigeminal ganglion innervates the auditory brainstem. Journal of Comparative Neurology. 2000;**419**:271-285. DOI: 10.1002/(SICI)1096-9861(20000410)419:3<271::AID-CNE1>3.0.CO;2-M

[40] Vass Z, Steyger PS, Hordichok AJ, et al. Capsaicin stimulation of the cochlea and electric stimulation of the trigeminal ganglion mediate vascular permeability in cochlear and vertebro-basilar arteries: A potential cause of inner ear dysfunction in headache. Neuroscience. 2001;**103**:189-201. DOI: 10.1016/S0306-4522(00)00521-2

[41] Koo JW, Balaban CD. Serotonin-induced plasma extravasation in the murine inner ear: Possible mechanism of migraine-associated inner ear dysfunction. Cephalalgia. 2006;**26**:1310-1319. DOI: 10.1111/j.1468-2982.2006.01208.x

[42] Zhang X, Levy D, Kainz V, et al. Activation of central trigeminovascular neurons by cortical spreading depression.

Annals of Neurology. 2011;**69**:855-865. DOI: 10.1002/ANA.22329

[43] Marano E, Marcelli V, Di Stasio E, et al. Trigeminal stimulation elicits a peripheral vestibular imbalance in migraine patients. Headache: The Journal of Head and Face Pain. 2005;**45**:325-331. DOI: 10.1111/J.1526-4610.2005.05069.X

[44] Ahn SK, Khalmuratova R, Jeon SY, et al. Colocalization of 5-HT1F receptor and calcitonin gene-related peptide in rat vestibular nuclei. Neuroscience Letters. 2009;**465**:151-156. DOI: 10.1016/J.NEULET.2009.09.008

[45] Park JH, Viirre E. Vestibular migraine may be an important cause of dizziness/vertigo in perimenopausal period. Medical Hypotheses. 2010;**75**:409-414. DOI: 10.1016/J.MEHY.2009.04.054

[46] Lee H, Jen JC, Cha YH, et al. Phenotypic and genetic analysis of a large family with migraine-associated vertigo. Headache. 2008;**48**:1460-1467. DOI: 10.1111/J.1526-4610.2007.01002.X

[47] Von Brevern M, Ta N, Shankar A, et al. Migrainous vertigo: Mutation analysis of the candidate genes CACNA1A, ATP1A2, SCN1A, and CACNB4. Headache: The Journal of Head and Face Pain. 2006;**46**:1136-1141. DOI: 10.1111/J.1526-4610.2006.00504.X

[48] Oh SY, Dieterich M, Lee BN, et al. Endolymphatic hydrops in patients with vestibular migraine and concurrent Meniere's disease. Frontiers in Neurology. 2021;**12**:270. DOI: 10.3389/fneur.2021.594481

[49] Roceanu A, Allena M, de Pasqua V, et al. Abnormalities of the vestibulo-collic reflex are similar in migraineurs with and without vertigo. Cephalalgia. 2008;**28**:988-990. DOI: 10.1111/j.1468-2982.2008.01641.x

[50] Shi S, Wang D, Ren T, et al. Auditory manifestations of vestibular migraine. Frontiers in Neurology. 2022;**35**:1433. DOI: 10.3389/FNEUR.2022.944001

[51] Lopez-Escamez JA, Carey J, Chung WH, et al. Diagnostic criteria for Menière's disease. Journal of Vestibular Research. 2015;**25**:1-7. DOI: 10.3233/VES-150549

[52] Stolte B, Holle D, Naegel S, et al. Vestibular migraine. Cephalalgia. 2015;**35**:262-270. DOI: 10.1177/0333102414535113

[53] Murofushi T, Tsubota M, Kitao K, et al. Simultaneous presentation of definite vestibular migraine and definite Ménière's disease: Overlapping syndrome of two diseases. Frontiers in Neurology. 2018;**9**:749. DOI: 10.3389/fneur.2018.00749

[54] Li M, Xu X, Qi W, et al. Vestibular migraine: The chameleon in vestibular disease. Neurological Sciences. 2021;**42**:1719-1731. DOI: 10.1007/s10072-021-05133-1

[55] Beh SC. Vestibular migraine: How to Sort it out and what to do about it. Journal of Neuro-Ophthalmology. 2019;**39**:208-219. DOI: 10.1097/WNO.0000000000000791

[56] Young AS, Nham B, Bradshaw AP, et al. Clinical, oculographic, and vestibular test characteristics of vestibular migraine. Cephalalgia. 2021;**41**:1039-1052. DOI: 10.1177/03331024211006042

[57] von Brevern M. Vestibular migraine: Vestibular testing and pathophysiology. Vestibular Migraine and Related Syndromes. 2014;**12**:83-90. DOI: 10.1007/978-3-319-07022-3_7/COVER

[58] Çelebisoy N, Gökçay F, Şirin H, et al. Migrainous vertigo: Clinical,

oculographic and posturographic findings. Cephalalgia. 2008;**28**:72-77. DOI: 10.1111/j.1468-2982.2007.01474.x

[59] Boldingh MI, Ljøstad U, Mygland Å, et al. Comparison of Interictal vestibular function in vestibular migraine vs migraine without vertigo. Headache: The Journal of Head and Face Pain. 2013;**53**:1123-1133. DOI: 10.1111/HEAD.12129

[60] Young AS, Lechner C, Bradshaw AP, et al. Capturing acute vertigo: A vestibular event monitor. Neurology. 2019;**92**:E2743-E2753. DOI: 10.1212/WNL.0000000000007644

[61] ElSherif M, Reda MI, Saadallah H, et al. Video head impulse test (vHIT) in migraine dizziness. Journal of Otology. 2018;**13**:65. DOI: 10.1016/J.JOTO.2017.12.002

[62] Dlugaiczyk J, Habs M, Dieterich M. Vestibular evoked myogenic potentials in vestibular migraine and Menière's disease: cVEMPs make the difference. Journal of Neurology. 2020;**267**:169-180. DOI: 10.1007/s00415-020-09902-4

[63] Rosengren SM, Welgampola MS, Colebatch JG. Vestibular evoked myogenic potentials: Past, present and future. Clinical Neurophysiology. 2010;**121**:636-651. DOI: 10.1016/J.CLINPH.2009.10.016

[64] Zaleski A, Bogle J, Starling A, et al. Vestibular evoked myogenic potentials in patients with vestibular migraine. Otology & Neurotology. 2015;**36**:295-302. DOI: 10.1097/MAO.0000000000000665

[65] Makowiec KF, Piker EG, Jacobson GP, et al. Ocular and cervical vestibular evoked myogenic potentials in patients with vestibular migraine. Otology and Neurotology. 2018;**39**:e561-e567. DOI: 10.1097/MAO.0000000000001880

[66] Radtke A, Neuhauser H, von Brevern M, et al. Vestibular migraine--validity of clinical diagnostic criteria. Cephalalgia. 2011;**31**:906-913. DOI: 10.1177/0333102411405228

[67] Byun YJ, Levy DA, Nguyen SA, et al. Treatment of vestibular migraine: A systematic review and meta-analysis. The Laryngoscope. 2021;**131**:186-194. DOI: 10.1002/lary.28546

[68] Radtke A, von Brevern M, Neuhauser H, et al. Vestibular migraine: Long-term follow-up of clinical symptoms and vestibulo-cochlear findings. Neurology. 2012;**79**:1607-1614. DOI: 10.1212/WNL.0B013E31826E264F

[69] Alghadir AH, Anwer S. Effects of vestibular rehabilitation in the management of a vestibular migraine: A review. Frontiers in Neurology. 2018;**9**:440. DOI: 10.3389/fneur.2018.00440

[70] Hu T, Hu H, Chen F, et al. The efficacy and safety of acupuncture for prophylaxis of vestibular migraine: A study protocol for a randomized controlled trial. Frontiers in Neurology. 2021;**12**:1081. DOI: 10.3389/fneur.2021.709803

[71] Beh SC. External trigeminal nerve stimulation: Potential rescue treatment for acute vestibular migraine. Journal of the Neurological Sciences. 2020;**408**:116550. DOI: 10.1016/j.jns.2019.116550

[72] Beh SC, Friedman DI. Acute vestibular migraine treatment with noninvasive vagus nerve stimulation. Neurology. 2019;**93**:E1715-E1719. DOI: 10.1212/WNL.0000000000008388

[73] von Brevern M, Lempert T. Vestibular migraine: Treatment and prognosis. Seminars in Neurology. 2020;**40**:83-86. DOI: 10.1055/s-0039-3402067

[74] Kirthi V, Derry S, Moore RA, et al. Aspirin with or without an antiemetic for acute migraine headaches in adults. Cochrane Database of Systematic Reviews. 2010;**89**:CD008041. DOI: 10.1002/14651858.CD008041.PUB2

[75] Cassano D, Pizza V, Busillo V. P074. Almotriptan in the acute treatment of vestibular migraine: A retrospective study. The Journal of Headache and Pain. 2015;**16**:1-2. DOI: 10.1186/1129-2377-16-S1-A114/METRICS

[76] Furman JM, Marcus DA, Balaban CD. Rizatriptan reduces vestibular-induced motion sickness in migraineurs. Journal of Headache and Pain. 2011;**12**:81-88. DOI: 10.1007/S10194-010-0250-Z/FIGURES/3

[77] Neuhauser H, Radtke A, von Brevern M, et al. Zolmitriptan for treatment of migrainous vertigo: A pilot randomized placebo-controlled trial. Neurology. 2003;**60**:882-883. DOI: 10.1212/01.WNL.0000049476.40047.A3

[78] Prakash S, Shah ND. Migrainous vertigo responsive to intravenous methylprednisolone: Case reports. Headache. 2009;**49**:1235-1239. DOI: 10.1111/J.1526-4610.2009.01474.X

[79] Robbins MS, Burch R. Preventive migraine treatment. Continuum (Minneap Minn). 2021;**27**:613-632. DOI: 10.1212/CON.0000000000000957

[80] Salviz M, Yuce T, Acar H, et al. Propranolol and venlafaxine for vestibular migraine prophylaxis: A randomized controlled trial. The Laryngoscope. 2016;**126**:169-174. DOI: 10.1002/LARY.25445

[81] Lepcha A, Amalanathan S, Augustine AM, et al. Flunarizine in the prophylaxis of migrainous vertigo: A randomized controlled trial. European Archives of Oto-Rhino-Laryngology. 2014;**271**:2931-2936. DOI: 10.1007/S00405-013-2786-4

[82] Wang F, Wang J, Cao Y, et al. Serotonin-norepinephrine reuptake inhibitors for the prevention of migraine and vestibular migraine: A systematic review and meta-analysis. Regional Anesthesia and Pain Medicine. 2020;**45**:323-330. DOI: 10.1136/RAPM-2019-101207

[83] Hoskin JL, Fife TD. New anti-CGRP medications in the treatment of vestibular migraine. Frontiers in Neurology. 2022;**12**:2598. DOI: 10.3389/fneur.2021.799002

[84] Oh S-Y, Kang J-J, Kim S, et al. A preliminary trial of botulinum toxin type a in patients with vestibular migraine: A longitudinal fMRI study. Frontiers in Neurology;**13**:955158. DOI: 10.3389/FNEUR.2022.955158

Chapter 11

Nociplastic Pain in Gynecology: Understanding This Painful Experience in Women

Lucia Merlino, Alba Crognale, Maria Grazia Piccioni, Maria Grazia Porpora, Roberto Senatori, Luca Titi and Carlo Della Rocca

Abstract

The term "nociplastic pain" was introduced in 2017 by the International Association for the Study of Pain (IASP) to describe pain that results from impaired nociception despite no clear evidence of actual or potential tissue damage causing activation of peripheral nociceptors or evidence of disease or lesion of the somatosensory system causing the pain. It is a definition born from the need to recognize early the presence of central sensitization of the nervous system in patients with chronic pain; we can find ourselves in the co-presence of nociceptive or neuropathic pain and nociplastic pain. In gynecological pathology, nociplastic pain plays an important role characterizing some important pathologies that can be associated with chronic pelvic pain in women. It is essential to understand the mechanisms of pathogenesis and maintenance of nociplastic pain in order to undertake a multidisciplinary path for the treatment of these patients.

Keywords: pain, gynecology, vulvar pain, pelvic chronic pain, nociplastic pain

1. Introduction

The term "nociplastic pain" was introduced in 2017 by the International Association for the Study of Pain (IASP) to describe pain that results from impaired nociception despite no clear evidence of actual or potential tissue damage causing activation of peripheral nociceptors or evidence of disease or lesion of the somatosensory system causing the pain. The term was first proposed in 2016, as a mechanistic descriptor for chronic pain states not characterized by obvious activation of nociceptors or neuropathy, but in whom clinical and psychophysical findings suggest altered nociceptive function [1]. Nociplastic pain refers to a physiologically based category that is particularly applicable to chronic primary pain conditions outlined in the new International Classification of Diseases, 11th edition, published by WHO.

The IASP has subdivided chronic primary pain conditions into the following five categories [2]:

1. chronic widespread pain;

2. complex regional pain syndrome;

3. chronic primary headache and orofacial pain;

4. chronic primary visceral pain;

5. chronic primary musculoskeletal pain.

Nociplastic pain can be mechanistically defined as pain arising from the altered function of pain-related sensory pathways in the periphery and central nervous system, causing increased sensitivity. It can occur in isolation or as a comorbidity in individuals with chronic pain conditions that are primarily nociceptive or neuropathic. Nociplastic pain is often associated with other symptoms, such as fatigue, sleep, memory, and mood problems, leading experts to propose expansive terminology to include the term "syndrome," namely nociplastic pain syndrome. Caring for patients with nociplastic pain is challenging; the pain complaint is often difficult to describe. There are associated subjective symptoms and pathognomonic clinical findings, or biomarkers are absent. Nociplastic pain conditions are frustrating for both healthcare professionals and patients, with physicians uncertain regarding diagnosis and patients resentful that their symptoms are doubted [3].

2. Physiopathologic mechanisms of nociplastic pain

Nociplastic pain is a phenotypic expression of multifactorial processes. It represents a dynamic interplay of various mechanisms causing or amplifying pain, arising de novo or triggered by pain generators. It originates from different inputs, which could be either a bottom-up response to a peripheral nociceptive or a neuropathic trigger, or a top-down central nervous system-driven response [4].

The mechanistic common denominator of nociplastic pain is the amplified processing of and/or decreased inhibition of pain stimuli at multiple levels in the nervous system. The amplified processing of a noxious stimulus is called "wind-up" and it occurs, for example, when there is an enhanced spinal neuron response after C-fiber or, less commonly, A-δ stimulation [5]. Diminished descending modulation, instead, might manifest as hyperalgesia—increased pain in response to painful stimuli—and allodynia—pain in response to normally nonpainful stimuli [6].

There are probably numerous initiating routes that lead to a final common pathway of the amplification of nociceptive perception, transduction, and transmission, and a lot of these mechanisms have yet to be discovered [7].

When a traumatic noxious stimulus occurs, pain hypersensitivity can arise, mediated by both peripheral and central nervous system changes. This phenomenon is called "central sensitization," and it is strictly associated with chronic pain such as fibromyalgia, irritable bowel syndrome (IBS), and interstitial cystitis [8]. The involvement of central nervous system and the widespread of pain signals is the reason why these diseases are often characterized by an emotive component and symptoms such as fatigue, sleep, mood alterations, and memory difficulties, and sensitivity to non-nociceptive sensory stimuli such as light and sound.

Central sensitization is the phenomenon by which a neural signaling undergoes an amplification in the central nervous system that spurs pain hypersensitivity outside the primary area of tissue injury or damage. It represents the major underlying mechanism of nociplastic pain syndrome [9]. Chronic pain can often be found in the absence of a peripheral pathology or because of a discrepancy between the tissue damage and the magnitude of the resulting pain and disability [10].

Behind this process, there are mechanisms of central sensitization, which consist of altered sensory processing in the brain, malfunctioning of descending pain inhibitory mechanisms, increased activity of pain facilitatory pathways, and temporal summation of second pain or wind-up [11]. When a noxious stimulus occurs, there is an activation of peripheral C-fibers axons with the transmission of the signal to the spinal cord and the central nervous system. This mechanism causing a "first pain," that is the immediate painful sensation, and a "second pain," that is a painful sensation that starts a few seconds after and lasts longer, even when the stimulus ceases. Low-frequency repetitive stimulation of unmyelinated C-fibers is called "wind-up." The "wind-up" occurs when dorsal spinal horn neurons receive stimulations with a frequency higher or equal to 0.33 Hz [12]. This process results in a progressive increase of pain intensity when noxious stimulation remains constant or disappears: a phenomenon called temporal summation of "second pain" [13]. Neziri et al. showed how spinal cord hypersensitivity and temporal summation second pain are greater in patients with chronic pelvic pain than controls. They used spinal withdrawal reflex to assess the extension of receptive fields in patients with endometriosis and chronic pelvic pain and patients without a pain syndrome, showing larger fields and lower threshold to induce pain in patients with chronic pelvic pain [14].

Involvement of the central nervous system has also been demonstrated in voxel-based morphology studies, showing changes in gray matter density and volume in patients having chronic pelvic pain. Studies reported greater decreases in gray matter volume in regions of the pain system including thalamus, cingulate cortex, putamen, insular cortex, and areas involved in pain modulation, such as the prefrontal cortex. Regional increase in gray matter volume was found in right inferior and middle frontal gyrus, left amygdala, and mesencephalon, which are all pain modulatory-related areas [15].

Both top-down and bottom-up mechanisms play an important role in the pathophysiology of nociplastic pain, and accumulating evidence suggests that it is also driven by neuroinflammation in the peripheral and central nervous system. For example, peripheral injury or other stressors trigger the release of proinflammatory cytokines, with the consequent activation of spinal cord glia with cyclooxygenase-2 and prostaglandin E2 expression in the central nervous system [16]. Neuroinflammation is a form of inflammation that occurs in both the peripheral and central nervous systems, characterized by four features: vasculature changes that result in increased vascular permeability, infiltration of leukocytes and macrophages, activation of glial cells, and production of inflammatory mediators [17].

Pain was one of the four cardinal signs of inflammation, as recorded by Celso in the first century AD. As previously mentioned, peripheral axons of nociceptors carry the painful stimulus into the dorsal root ganglia and then into the spinal cord. They are pseudounipolar neurons with their distal axonal branches innervating a peripheral organ and their proximal axonal branches innervating the dorsal horn of the spinal cord. The repetitive stimulation of these fibers not only provokes a sensory hypersensitivity, but also the release of neuropeptides which increase inflammatory processes, such as calcitonin gene-related peptide (CGRP) and substance P (SP). These peptides are released from both the distal and proximal axons. The last one innervates the dorsal horn of the spinal cord, where afferent neurons of other peripheral organs arrive. The cross-activation of afferent neurons coming from other tissues that are not primarily damaged causes a release of neuropeptides

Spinal mechanisms	Supraspinal mechanisms	Peripheral features
• Regional clustering and convergence of signals from different pain loci • Spinal cord reorganization • Amplified spinal reflex transmission • Diminished spinal inhibition • Wind-up and temporal summation • Glial cell activation	• Hyper-responsiveness to pain stimuli • Hyperactivity and connectivity in and between brain regions involved in pain • Decreased activity of brain regions involved in pain inhibition (e.g., descending inhibitory pathways) • Elevated cerebrospinal fluid substance P and glutamate concentrations, decreased GABAergic transmission • Changes in the size and shape of gray and white matter regions involved in pain processing • Glial cell activation	• Minor local muscle pathology • Peripheral sensitization (e.g., expansion of receptivefields, elevated cytokine, and chemokine concentrations) • Hyperalgesia, dysesthesia, and allodynia • Localized or diffuse tenderness, or both

Ref. [3].

Table 1.
Mechanisms of nociplastic pain.

into the uninjured peripheral organs, provoking neurogenic inflammation and diffuse pain [18]. That is the reason why in chronic pain syndromes there are often viscero-visceral and viscero-somatic sensitization, for example, colon-to-bladder cross-sensitization in patients affected by irritable bowel syndrome [19]. A recent review summarizes a list of chemicals that are released from the soma of neurons within dorsal root ganglia in inflammatory and visceral sensitization processes (ATP, CGRP, SP, glutamate, GABA, galanine, NO, and BDNF) [20]. Soma of nociceptors in ganglia do not contract synapses with each other, but they are connected by satellite glial cells (SGCs). The nearness between neurons and SGCs implements a paracrine mechanism, according to which SGCs are stimulated by neuropeptides (e.g., BDNF that binds TrkB on the surface of the glia) and in response, they produce "gliotransmitters" (e.g., interleukines, NO, and TNF-alpha) that are sent back to the neurons. Pseudounipolar neurons also produce colony stimulating factor-1 (CSF-1) that attracts and spurs proliferation of macrophages in the nearby axons [21]. Macrophages produce proinflammatory factors. The persistent upregulation of production of proinflammatory factors is a crucial mediator in the development of chronic pain syndromes (**Table 1**).

3. Nociplastic pain in gynecology

In gynecological pathology, nociplastic pain plays an important role characterizing some important pathologies that can be associated with chronic pelvic pain in women. It is essential to better understand the basis of these kinds of conditions and to undertake a multidisciplinary path for the treatment of these patients.

Chronic pelvic pain is estimated to affect 26% of the world's female population [22].

Chronic pelvic pain is a pain that originates from the pelvis, noncyclic or cyclic or related to menstruation (dysmenorrhea) and intercourse (dyspareunia), typically lasting more than 6 months. It is often associated with negative cognitive, behavioral, sexual, and emotional consequences and symptoms suggestive of lower urinary tract, sexual, bowel, myofascial, or gynecologic dysfunction. The 6-month cut-off is not a requirement if central sensitization pain and nociplastic mechanisms (with cognitive, behavioral, and emotional impairment) are documented [23].

There is an interconnection between visceral and somatic structures in the female pelvis, known as viscero-visceral cross-sensitization, in which activity in one organ (e.g., uterus) can hypersensitize another organ (e.g., bowel or bladder). Cross-sensitization among pelvic structures may contribute to chronic pelvic pain of unknown etiology and involves convergent neural pathways of noxious stimulus transmission from two or more organs. Besides the viscera, somatic areas may also be involved. Given enough time, trigger points can develop in peripheral somatic tissue in response to increased nociceptive visceral input: This is called viscero-somatic sensitization [24]. Persistent input from malfunctioning pelvic muscles, injury, or surgery can lead to visceral dysfunction characterized by bowel symptoms such as constipation and bladder symptoms such as urgency, frequency, and incomplete emptying. The viscero-visceral cross-sensitization can enhance nociplastic pain mechanisms by amplifying central nervous system responsiveness and decreasing pain inhibition descending pathways, resulting in overall pain hypersensitivity and central sensitization presenting as widespread pain (outside the pelvic area), sleep disturbance, and deterioration in mood and coping [25, 26].

3.1 Fibromyalgia

An example of a chronic pain condition, which represents a struggle for gynecologists because it often occurs in a female population, is fibromyalgia. According to the latest guidelines elaborated by Fibromyalgia Working Group members, fibromyalgia is defined as a chronic pain disorder: In other words, all patients would be required to have chronic pain to be diagnosed with fibromyalgia. Fibromyalgia was defined as a "widespread" pain syndrome, and it is still counted in this category according to the IASP. The American College of Rheumatology (ACR) redefined the diagnostic criteria in 2010 by renaming it as a "multisite" pain syndrome [27]. In fact, when a patient has pain in a self-reported number of sites distributed throughout the body, including joint sites, this is sufficient for defining fibromyalgia. The number of pain sites needed to define "multisite" pain in fibromyalgia is found to be ≥8. Furthermore, fibromyalgia is associated with sleep disturbance, fatigue, and other cognitive and somatic features that are now considered core symptoms of this condition [28].

3.2 Vulvodynia

Although no epidemiological study of prevalence has been carried out worldwide, it is estimated that vulvodynia affects 8–10% of women of all ages [29]. Vulvodynia is defined as vulvar pain lasting at least 3 months, without a clear identifiable cause, which may have potential associated factors that contribute to the development and perpetuation of this clinical condition [30]. These associated factors include (i) psychosocial factors, such as anxiety, depression, posttraumatic stress, and sexual problems; (ii) chronic pain conditions in the pelvic area, such as urological or coloproctological pain syndromes or irritable bowel syndrome; and (iii) chronic pain conditions in other areas of the body, such as fibromyalgia [31]. It suggests that there could be the same neurophysiological substrate underlying these chronic pain syndromes. Vulvodynia has been always defined as a neuropathic pain due to its burning nature and because of the hypersensitivity of the vulvar mucosa. This can be justified by a greater nerve fiber proliferation in the vulvar vestibule; indeed, some studies have found an increase in the density of C nociceptor endings [32]. However, it is reductive because of all the associated factors known.

Changes derived from central sensitization such as hyperalgesia and allodynia have been demonstrated in vulvodynia not only in the perineal area but also in distant regions of the body [33]. Central sensitization involves abnormal long-term potentiation that can begin after physical precipitating events such as recurrent vulvovaginal candidiasis, lower urinary tract infections, or dermatologic pathology.

Then, we can conclude that vulvodynia is thus considered to be one of the nociplastic pain syndromes, characterized by nociceptive/inflammatory pain, neuropathic pain, and dysfunctional pain, in the absence of clinically evident pathology [34].

Regarding the therapeutic approach of vulvodynia, a stepwise method of pelvic floor dysfunction treatment, adequate psychological support, and sexual healthcare is recommended along with medical therapies [35]. Intermittent use of topical lidocaine cream may be useful for women with intense vestibular touch pain, prior to sexual intercourse [36].

Other pharmaceutical strategies are oral or topical NSAIDs, amitriptyline and other tricyclic antidepressants, hydrocortisone, vulvar interferon, anticonvulsants – such as gabapentin, botulinum neurotoxin injection, antifungal, or combined approach [37].

3.3 Painful bladder syndrome (PBS) and interstitial cystitis (IC)

In women, symptoms of interstitial cystitis are difficult to distinguish from those of painful bladder syndrome and they appear to overlap with those of urinary tract infection, chronic urethral syndrome, overactive bladder, vulvodynia, and endometriosis [38].

In terms of symptoms, the two conditions can be superimposable; the differential diagnosis with other pathologies such as endometriosis, vulvodynia, overactive bladder can be very complex, although identifying interstitial cystitis and painful bladder syndrome in women with more than one of these diseases may be difficult.

Interstitial cystitis is nowadays associated with painful bladder syndrome and not distinguished. It can be categorized into two major subtypes, mainly based on the bladder histological findings. The first type or "classical" interstitial cystitis presents itself with Hunner's lesions: mucosal lesions accompanied by abnormal capillary structures. The second type presents itself without Hunner's lesions, has no obvious bladder etiology, and is most frequently accompanied by common systemic comorbidities or chronic pelvic pain with symptoms that involve other pelvic structures [39].

The etiology and pathophysiology remain uncertain with many different hypotheses proposed over the years, including injury of the bladder epithelium and increased barrier permeability, neurogenic inflammation with mast cell infiltration without a bacterial infection, autoimmune involvement [40].

Painful bladder syndrome is a disease that affects the bladder and manifests itself with persistent pain and difficulty urinating. This syndrome can be counted among the causes of nociplastic pain in women.

Painful bladder syndrome was defined by the European Society for the Study of Bladder Pain Syndrome/Interstitial Cystitis (ESSIC) as a chronic (>6 months) pelvic pain, feeling of pressure or discomfort perceived to be related to the urinary bladder, with at least one other urinary symptom such as persistent voiding urgency or frequency [41].

The precise cause of painful bladder syndrome is still unknown, but it is believed to be the result of a combination of factors, such as inflammation of the bladder, increased nerve sensitivity, and immune system dysfunction.

Painful bladder syndrome urinary symptoms can vary from person to person, but the most common include the following:

- Pain in the pelvic area and bladder, which may be constant or intermittent;
- Urgency to urinate frequently, even when the bladder is not full;
- Pain when urinating;
- Feeling of burning or pressure in the bladder;
- Difficulty urinating or holding urine.

Diagnosing painful bladder syndrome can be difficult as symptoms can be similar to those of other urinary disorders.

Treatment of painful bladder syndrome can include a combination of therapies, such as pain medications, physical therapies, dietary modifications, and behavioral therapies.

The European Association of Urology (EAU) proposed a stepwise approach for treatment of interstitial cystitis/bladder painful syndrome which consists of [42]:

- First-line therapy: education, physiotherapy, behavioral modification (e.g., bladder training), psychological therapies for stress modulation;
- Second-line therapy: pharmacotherapy: pentosan polysulfate sodium, low-dose tricyclic antidepressants, antispasmodics;
- Third-line therapy: intravesical injections with local anesthetic, dimethyl sulfoxide or heparin, or intradetrusor botulinum toxin A injection;
- Fourth-line therapy: neuromodulation (e.g., percutaneous tibial nerve stimulation).

In some cases, surgery may be required only when all conservative treatments have failed [43].

3.4 Irritable bowel disease (IBD)

Irritable bowel disease is defined by Rome IV Criteria as pain on at least 1 day per week in the last 3 months associated with two or more of the following symptoms: abdominal pain; change in stool frequency; change in stool appearance; variations of defecation with predominant constipation (IBS-C) or with predominant diarrhea (IBS-D) or with mixed bowel habits (IBS-M if the patient refers >25% constipation and > 25% diarrhea; IBS-U if the patient refers <25% constipation and < 25% diarrhea). The onset of symptoms has to be at least 6 months before diagnosis. Diagnosis is clinical and based on these criteria [44].

In irritable bowel syndrome, motility disturbance is associated with sensory hypersensitivity, altered mucosa and gut microbiota, local and systemic immune system dysfunction, and impaired central nervous system processing (with central and viscero-visceral sensitization). Moreover, irritable bowel syndrome has been associated with high prevalence of psychological disorders and significantly higher anxiety and depression levels than the general population [45].

Initiation of treatment of IBS should start with identifying the severity and predominant symptoms of the disorder. According to NICE guidelines first-line treatment consists of dietary and lifestyle modification, even exercise can be beneficial. If lifestyle advice is not effective, pharmacological therapy can be practiced and based on severity. Psychological interventions are useful, moreover, if not responsive to pharmacological treatments after 12 months. NICE discourages use of acupuncture and reflexology [46].

4. Conclusions

The traditional conceptualization of chronic pain syndromes has been historically dualistic either as a result of organic-physical mechanisms or as psychological mechanisms. Despite the advances in the understanding of idiopathic pain and the recognition of neuroplastic changes as the cause of chronic and complex pain conditions, multiple pathophysiological mechanisms are still unclear. Nociplastic pain is an important substrate of many gynecological and nongynecological chronic pain syndromes. That is why a multidisciplinary approach is needed. Moreover, these conditions are due to somatic or visceral noxious agents interacting with psychosocial, epigenetic, and emotional factors. In order to manage these patients, our aims for the future is to better understand pathognomonic clinical findings or biomarkers of nociplastic pain syndromes, and to implement the multidisciplinary team work, not only with specialists from the various branches of medicine but also with a psychological support for our patients.

Author details

Lucia Merlino[1*], Alba Crognale[1], Maria Grazia Piccioni[1], Maria Grazia Porpora[1], Roberto Senatori[2], Luca Titi[3] and Carlo Della Rocca[4]

1 Department of Maternal Infantile and Urological Sciences, Sapienza University of Rome, Rome, Italy

2 Italian Society of Colposcopy and Cervicovaginal Pathology (SICPV), Rome, Italy

3 Department of Anesthesia and Intensive Care Medicine, Sapienza University of Rome, Rome, Italy

4 Department of Medical-Surgical Sciences and Biotechnologies, Sapienza University of Rome, Rome, Italy

*Address all correspondence to: luciamerlinostudio@gmail.com

References

[1] Kosek E, Cohen M, Baron R, Gebhart GF, Mico JA, Rice ASC, et al. Do we need a third mechanistic descriptor for chronic pain states? Pain. 2016;**157**(7):1382-1386. DOI: 10.1097/j.pain.0000000000000507

[2] Nicholas M, Vlaeyen JWS, Rief W, Barke A, Aziz Q, Benoliel R, et al. IASP taskforce for the classification of chronic pain. The IASP classification of chronic pain for ICD-11: Chronic primary pain. Pain. 2019;**160**(1):28-37. DOI: 10.1097/j.pain.0000000000001390

[3] Fitzcharles MA, Cohen SP, Clauw DJ, et al. Nociplastic pain: Towards an understanding of prevalent pain conditions. Lancet. 2021;**397**(10289):2098-2110. DOI: 10.1016/S0140-6736(21)00392-5

[4] Littlejohn G. Neuroinflammation in fibromyalgia and CRPS: Top-down or bottom-up? Nature Reviews Rheumatology. 2016;**12**(4):242. DOI: 10.1038/nrrheum.2016.26

[5] Kwon M, Altin M, Duenas H, Alev L. The role of descending inhibitory pathways on chronic pain modulation and clinical implications. Pain Practice. 2014;**14**(7):656-667. DOI: 10.1111/papr.12145. Epub 2013 Nov 20

[6] Geisser ME, Strader Donnell C, Petzke F, Gracely RH, Clauw DJ, Williams DA. Comorbid somatic symptoms and functional status in patients with fibromyalgia and chronic fatigue syndrome: Sensory amplification as a common mechanism. Psychosomatics. 2008;**49**(3):235-242. DOI: 10.1176/appi.psy.49.3.235

[7] Yam MF, Loh YC, Tan CS, Khadijah Adam S, Abdul Manan N, Basir R. General pathways of pain sensation and the major neurotransmitters involved in pain regulation. International Journal of Molecular Sciences. 2018;**19**(8):2164. DOI: 10.3390/ijms19082164

[8] Woolf CJ. Evidence for a central component of post-injury pain hypersensitivity. Nature. 1983;**306**(5944):686-688. DOI: 10.1038/306686a0

[9] Nijs J, Lahousse A, Kapreli E, Bilika P, Saraçoğlu İ, Malfliet A, et al. Nociplastic pain criteria or recognition of central sensitization? Pain phenotyping in the past, present and future. Journal of Clinical Medicine. 2021;**10**(15):3203. DOI: 10.3390/jcm10153203

[10] Sterling M, Jull G, Vicenzino B, Kenardy J. Sensory hypersensitivity occurs soon after whiplash injury and is associated with poor recovery. Pain. 2003;**104**(3):509-517. DOI: 10.1016/S0304-3959(03)00078-2

[11] Meeus M, Nijs J. Central sensitization: A biopsychosocial explanation for chronic widespread pain in patients with fibromyalgia and chronic fatigue syndrome. Clinical Rheumatology. 2007;**26**(4):465-473. Epub 2006 Nov 18. DOI: 10.1007/s10067-006-0433-9

[12] Dickenson AH, Sullivan AF. Evidence for a role of the NMDA receptor in the frequency dependent potentiation of deep rat dorsal horn nociceptive neurones following C fibre stimulation. Neuropharmacology. 1987;**26**(8):1235-1238. DOI: 10.1016/0028-3908(87)90275-9

[13] Eckert NR, Vierck CJ, Simon CB, Calderon S, Cruz-Almeida Y, Staud R,

et al. Methodological considerations for the temporal summation of second pain. The Journal of Pain. 2017;**18**(12):1488-1495. Epub 2017 Aug 9. DOI: 10.1016/j.jpain.2017.07.009

[14] Neziri AY, Haesler S, Petersen-Felix S, Müller M, Arendt-Nielsen L, Manresa JB, et al. Generalized expansion of nociceptive reflex receptive fields in chronic pain patients. Pain. 2010;**151**(3):798-805. DOI: 10.1016/j.pain.2010.09.017

[15] As-Sanie S, Harris RE, Napadow V, Kim J, Neshewat G, Kairys A, et al. Changes in regional gray matter volume in women with chronic pelvic pain: A voxel-based morphometry study. Pain. 2012;**153**(5):1006-1014. Epub 2012 Mar 2. DOI: 10.1016/j.pain.2012.01.032

[16] Maier SF, Watkins LR. Cytokines for psychologists: Implications of bidirectional immune-to-brain communication for understanding behavior, mood, and cognition. Psychological Review. 1998;**105**(1):83-107. DOI: 10.1037/0033-295x.105.1.83

[17] Ji RR, Nackley A, Huh Y, Terrando N, Maixner W. Neuroinflammation and central sensitization in chronic and widespread pain. Anesthesiology. 2018;**129**(2):343-366. DOI: 10.1097/ALN.0000000000002130

[18] Brumovsky PR, Gebhart GF. Visceral organ cross-sensitization - an integrated perspective. Autonomic Neuroscience. 2010;**153**(1-2):106-115. Epub 2009 Aug 12. DOI: 10.1016/j.autneu.2009.07.006

[19] Ansari R, Attari F, Razjouyan H, Etemadi A, Amjadi H, Merat S, et al. Ulcerative colitis and irritable bowel syndrome: Relationships with quality of life. European Journal of Gastroenterology & Hepatology. 2008;**20**(1):46-50. DOI: 10.1097/MEG.0b013e3282f16a62

[20] Matsuka Y, Afroz S, Dalanon JC, Iwasa T, Waskitho A, Oshima M. The role of chemical transmitters in neuron-glia interaction and pain in sensory ganglion. Neuroscience and Biobehavioral Reviews. 2020;**108**:393-399. Epub 2019 Nov 27. DOI: 10.1016/j.neubiorev.2019.11.019

[21] Yu X, Liu H, Hamel KA, Morvan MG, Yu S, Leff J, et al. Dorsal root ganglion macrophages contribute to both the initiation and persistence of neuropathic pain. Nature Communications. 2020;**11**(1):264. DOI: 10.1038/s41467-019-13839-2

[22] Chronic Pelvic Pain. ACOG practice bulletin, number 218. Obstetrics and Gynecology. 2020;**135**(3):e98-e109. DOI: 10.1097/AOG.0000000000003716

[23] Treede RD, Rief W, Barke A, Aziz Q, Bennett MI, Benoliel R, et al. Chronic pain as a symptom or a disease: The IASP classification of chronic pain for the international classification of diseases (ICD-11). Pain. 2019;**160**(1):19-27. DOI: 10.1097/j.pain.0000000000001384

[24] Malykhina AP. Neural mechanisms of pelvic organ cross-sensitization. Neuroscience. 2007;**149**(3):660-672. Epub 2007 Sep 8. DOI: 10.1016/j.neuroscience.2007.07.053

[25] Sutton KS, Pukall CF, Chamberlain S. Pain, psychosocial, sexual, and psychophysical characteristics of women with primary vs. secondary provoked vestibulodynia. The Journal of Sexual Medicine. 2009;**6**(1):205-214. DOI: 10.1111/j.1743-6109.2008.01038.x

[26] Stratton P, Khachikyan I, Sinaii N, Ortiz R, Shah J. Association of chronic pelvic pain and endometriosis with signs of sensitization and myofascial pain. Obstetrics and Gynecology.

2015;**125**(3):719-728. DOI: 10.1097/AOG.0000000000000663

[27] Wolfe F, Clauw DJ, Fitzcharles MA, Goldenberg DL, Katz RS, Mease P, et al. The American College of Rheumatology preliminary diagnostic criteria for fibromyalgia and measurement of symptom severity. Arthritis Care Res (Hoboken). 2010;**62**(5):600-610. DOI: 10.1002/acr.20140

[28] Arnold LM, Bennett RM, Crofford LJ, Dean LE, Clauw DJ, Goldenberg DL, et al. AAPT diagnostic criteria for fibromyalgia. The Journal of Pain. 2019;**20**(6):611-628. Epub 2018 Nov 16. DOI: 10.1016/j.jpain.2018.10.008

[29] Bergeron S, Reed BD, Wesselmann U, Bohm-Starke N. Vulvodynia. Nature Reviews. Disease Primers. 2020;**6**(1):36. DOI: 10.1038/s41572-020-0164-2

[30] Bornstein J, Goldstein AT, Stockdale CK, Bergeron S, Pukall C, Zolnoun D, et al. 2015 ISSVD, ISSWSH and IPPS consensus terminology and classification of persistent vulvar pain and vulvodynia. Obstetrics and Gynecology. 2016;**127**(4):745-751. DOI: 10.1097/AOG.0000000000001359

[31] Reed BD, Harlow SD, Sen A, Edwards RM, Chen D, Haefner HK. Relationship between vulvodynia and chronic comorbid pain conditions. Obstetrics and Gynecology. 2012;**120**(1):145-151. DOI: 10.1097/AOG.0b013e31825957cf

[32] Weström LV, Willén R. Vestibular nerve fiber proliferation in vulvar vestibulitis syndrome. Obstetrics and Gynecology. 1998;**91**(4):572-576

[33] Pukall CF, Binik YM, Khalifé S, Amsel R, Abbott FV. Vestibular tactile and pain thresholds in women with vulvar vestibulitis syndrome. Pain. 2002;**96**(1-2):163-175. DOI: 10.1016/s0304-3959(01)00442-0

[34] Torres-Cueco R, Nohales-Alfonso F. Vulvodynia-it is time to accept a new understanding from a neurobiological perspective. International Journal of Environmental Research and Public Health. 2021;**18**(12):6639. DOI: 10.3390/ijerph18126639

[35] Merlino L, Titi L, Pugliese F, D'Ovidio G, Senatori R, Rocca CD, et al. Vulvodynia: Pain management strategies. Pharmaceuticals (Basel). 2022;**15**(12):1514. DOI: 10.3390/ph15121514

[36] Foster DC, Kotok MB, Huang LS, Watts A, Oakes D, Howard FM, et al. Oral desipramine and topical lidocaine for vulvodynia: A randomized controlled trial. Obstetrics and Gynecology. 2010;**116**(3):583-593. DOI: 10.1097/AOG.0b013e3181e9e0ab

[37] Merlino L, Matys V, D'Ovidio G, et al. Chapter 6; other important pharmaceutical strategies are: A brief overview on vulvodynia: Pain. Pharmacological Management Approach. Current overview on pharmaceutical Science. 2023;**8**(6):59-66. DOI: 10.9734/bpi/cops/v8/4976E

[38] Bogart LM, Berry SH, Clemens JQ. Symptoms of interstitial cystitis, painful bladder syndrome and similar diseases in women: a systematic review. J Urol. 2007;**177**(2):450-456. Erratum in: J Urol. 2007 Jun;177(6):2402. DOI: 10.1016/j.juro.2006.09.032

[39] Kuret T, Peskar D, Erman A, Veranič P. A systematic review of therapeutic approaches used in experimental models of interstitial cystitis/bladder pain syndrome. Biomedicine. 2021;**9**(8):865. DOI: 10.3390/biomedicines9080865

[40] Birder LA. Pathophysiology of interstitial cystitis. International Journal of Urology. 2019;**26**(Suppl 1):12-15. DOI: 10.1111/iju.13985

[41] van de Merwe JP, Nordling J, Bouchelouche P, Bouchelouche K, Cervigni M, Daha LK, et al. Diagnostic criteria, classification, and nomenclature for painful bladder syndrome/ interstitial cystitis: An ESSIC proposal. European Urology. 2008;**53**(1):60-67. Epub 2007 Sep 20. DOI: 10.1016/j. eururo.2007.09.019

[42] Fall M, Baranowski AP, Elneil S, Engeler D, Hughes J, Messelink EJ, et al. de C Williams AC; European Association of Urology. EAU guidelines on chronic pelvic pain. European Urology. 2010;**57**(1):35-48. Epub 2009 Aug 31. DOI: 10.1016/j.eururo.2009.08.020

[43] Clemens JQ, Erickson DR, Varela NP, Lai HH. Diagnosis and treatment of interstitial cystitis/bladder pain syndrome. The Journal of Urology. 2022;**208**(1):34-42. Epub 2022 May 10. DOI: 10.1097/JU.0000000000002756

[44] Drossman DA, Hasler WL. Rome IV-functional GI disorders: Disorders of gut-brain interaction. Gastroenterology. 2016;**150**(6):1257-1261. DOI: 10.1053/j. gastro.2016.03.035

[45] Fond G, Loundou A, Hamdani N, Boukouaci W, Dargel A, Oliveira J, et al. Anxiety and depression comorbidities in irritable bowel syndrome (IBS): A systematic review and meta-analysis. European Archives of Psychiatry and Clinical Neuroscience. 2014;**264**(8):651-660. Epub 2014 Apr 6. DOI: 10.1007/ s00406-014-0502-z

[46] Irritable bowel syndrome in adults. Diagnosis and Management. London: National Institute for Health and Care Excellence (NICE); Apr 2017

Section 2

Pharmacology and Research

Chapter 12

Perspective Chapter: Aspirin – The Wonder Drug

Ahmed Adebayo Ishola

Abstract

"Aspirin: The Wonder Drug" is a chapter that explores the history, pharmacology, medical uses, risks and side effects, and impact of aspirin on society. The chapter provides a brief history of aspirin, tracing its roots back to ancient times, and discusses how it works as an anti-inflammatory, analgesic, and antiplatelet agent. Aspirin has been used for over a century to treat a variety of conditions, including pain, fever, inflammation, and cardiovascular disease. It works by inhibiting the production of prostaglandins, which are chemicals involved in inflammation and pain. Aspirin is a non-selective inhibitor of cyclooxygenase (COX), blocking both COX-1 and COX-2, which reduces the amount of prostaglandins in the body, leading to a reduction in pain, inflammation, and fever. In addition, aspirin has antiplatelet effects, preventing blood clots from forming by irreversibly inhibiting the production of thromboxane A2. Overall, aspirin's impact on medicine and society cannot be overstated, as it has been used to alleviate pain and suffering in millions of people worldwide, and has saved countless lives through its use in the prevention of heart attacks and strokes.

Keywords: aspirin, pain, inflammation, cyclooxygenase, impact

1. Introduction

In 1897, Felix Hoffman, a German chemist working for the Bayer company, was able to modify salicylic acid to create acetylsalicylic acid, which was named aspirin [1]. Hoffmann's innovation led to the widespread modern use of aspirin for pain relief. His acetylation of salicylic acid (a compound found in willow bark) also proved fortunate in another way, because the modification is important to aspirin's ability to prevent cardiovascular events [2].

Aspirin quickly gained popularity due to its effectiveness in relieving pain and reducing fever, and it soon became one of the most commonly used drugs in the world. Over time, researchers discovered that aspirin had many other medical benefits, including anti-inflammatory and antiplatelet effects. It has been used to treat conditions such as arthritis, menstrual cramps, and headaches, as well as to prevent heart attacks and strokes [3].

Aspirin's impact on medicine and society cannot be overstated. It has been used to alleviate pain and suffering in millions of people around the world and has saved countless lives through its use in the prevention of heart attacks and strokes. It has also been the subject of extensive research, leading to a better understanding of how it works in the body and the discovery of new uses for the drug. Today, aspirin is still widely used and continues to be the subject of research, as scientists uncover new uses and applications for this "wonder drug" [4].

In this chapter, we will explore the chemical composition of aspirin, how it works in the body, and its medical uses. We will also examine the risks and side effects associated with aspirin use, as well as the impact that aspirin has had on medicine and society.

2. How aspirin works

Aspirin's ability to relieve pain, reduce fever, and treat inflammation has been known for over a century. It wasn't until the 1970s, however, that researchers uncovered the specific mechanism by which aspirin exerts its effects on the body (**Table 1**).

Aspirin works by inhibiting the production of prostaglandins, which are chemicals produced in the body that play a role in inflammation and pain [5]. Prostaglandins are produced by an enzyme called cyclooxygenase (COX), which comes in two forms: COX-1 and COX-2. COX-1 is involved in the production of prostaglandins that are necessary for normal physiological processes, such as protecting the stomach lining and promoting blood clotting [5]. COX-2, on the other hand, is induced by inflammation and is responsible for producing prostaglandins that promote pain and inflammation [9].

Aspirin is a nonselective inhibitor of COX, meaning that it blocks both COX-1 and COX-2 [10]. By inhibiting COX, aspirin reduces the amount of prostaglandins in the body, leading to a reduction in pain, inflammation, and fever. This is why aspirin is often used to treat conditions such as arthritis, menstrual cramps, and headaches [11].

In addition to its effects on prostaglandins, aspirin also has antiplatelet effects, meaning that it can prevent blood clots from forming. Aspirin accomplishes this by irreversibly inhibiting the production of thromboxane A2, which is a chemical that promotes platelet aggregation [7]. By preventing platelets from clumping together, aspirin reduces the risk of blood clots forming, which can lead to heart attacks and strokes.

Mechanism	Description	Reference
Inhibition of COX-1 and COX-2	Aspirin irreversibly acetylates a serine residue in the active site of COX-1 and COX-2, resulting in the inhibition of prostaglandin synthesis	[5]
Anti-inflammatory effects	Reduction of prostaglandin synthesis leads to decreased inflammation and pain	[6]
Analgesic effects	Inhibition of prostaglandin synthesis in the central nervous system leads to decreased perception of pain	[6]
Antiplatelet effects	Aspirin irreversibly acetylates COX-1 in platelets, preventing the synthesis of thromboxane A2, which is necessary for platelet aggregation	[7]
Cancer prevention	Aspirin's inhibition of COX-2 may play a role in reducing the risk of certain types of cancer	[8]

Table 1.
Mechanisms of action of aspirin.

The mechanisms by which aspirin works in the body have been extensively studied, and researchers continue to uncover new information about how this drug exerts its effects. For example, recent research has suggested that aspirin may also have anti-inflammatory effects that are independent of its effects on COX-1 and COX-2.

3. Chemical properties of aspirin

Aspirin is a widely used medication that has been in use for over a century. It is a white crystalline solid with a molecular formula of $C_9H_8O_4$ and a molecular weight of 180.16 g/mol [12]. The chemical name for aspirin is acetylsalicylic acid, and it is classified as a nonsteroidal anti-inflammatory drug (NSAID) [13]. Aspirin is an organic acid and is therefore slightly acidic in nature. The pKa of aspirin is 3.5, which means that it is a weak acid and can ionize in solution. Aspirin is soluble in organic solvents such as ethanol, chloroform, and ether, but it is relatively insoluble in water. Aspirin is synthesized through the acetylation of salicylic acid, a natural compound found in willow bark. The acetylation process involves the reaction of salicylic acid with acetic anhydride, which results in the formation of acetylsalicylic acid and acetic acid.

4. Medical uses of aspirin

4.1 Pain relief

Aspirin is one of the most commonly used pain relievers in the world. Its ability to block the production of prostaglandins makes it effective in treating mild to moderate pain, such as headaches, toothaches, and menstrual cramps [6]. Aspirin is often used in place of nonsteroidal anti-inflammatory drugs (NSAIDs) for pain relief, particularly in people who cannot take NSAIDs due to gastrointestinal or renal problems. According to a review of studies published in the journal Pain and Therapy [14], aspirin has been shown to be effective in reducing pain intensity and improving overall pain relief compared to placebo in several conditions, including headache, dental pain, and menstrual pain. However, the review also noted that aspirin may be less effective than other NSAIDs in some cases, such as for pain caused by osteoarthritis [14].

4.2 Anti-inflammatory

Aspirin is also an effective anti-inflammatory drug. Its ability to inhibit the production of prostaglandins makes it useful in treating conditions such as arthritis, gout, and other inflammatory disorders [6]. The anti-inflammatory effect of aspirin has been studied extensively. One of the key ways aspirin exerts its anti-inflammatory effect is by inhibiting the cyclooxygenase (COX) enzyme. COX plays a crucial role in the production of prostaglandins, which are involved in inflammation, pain, and fever. By inhibiting COX, aspirin reduces the production of prostaglandins, leading to a decrease in inflammation and pain [11]. Aspirin has been shown to be effective in reducing inflammation in a variety of conditions, including rheumatoid arthritis, osteoarthritis, and inflammatory bowel disease (IBD). In addition, aspirin has been shown to have antiplatelet effects, which can reduce the risk of cardiovascular events such as heart attack and stroke [15].

4.3 Antiplatelet effects

Aspirin is particularly useful in people who have had a heart attack or stroke in the past, as it can help prevent future events [3]. The antiplatelet effect of aspirin has been extensively studied and is well-established. Aspirin is commonly used for the prevention of cardiovascular events, including heart attack and stroke, in individuals with a high risk of these events. In addition, aspirin is used to prevent the formation of blood clots in individuals with certain medical conditions, such as atrial fibrillation and deep vein thrombosis [16].

4.4 Cardiovascular disease

In addition to its antiplatelet effects, aspirin may also have a protective effect against cardiovascular disease. Some studies have suggested that regular aspirin use can reduce the risk of heart attacks and strokes by up to 30% [6]. Aspirin is commonly used to prevent cardiovascular disease, such as heart attacks and strokes. The mechanism of action of aspirin in cardiovascular disease prevention is related to its ability to inhibit the enzyme cyclooxygenase (COX), which is involved in the production of prostaglandins and thromboxane A2 (TxA2) [3]. TxA2 is a potent platelet activator and vasoconstrictor that promotes thrombosis and contributes to the pathogenesis of cardiovascular disease [3]. By inhibiting COX, aspirin reduces the production of TxA2 and thus inhibits platelet activation and aggregation, which are important steps in the formation of blood clots that can cause heart attacks and strokes [3]. Aspirin also has anti-inflammatory effects that may contribute to its cardiovascular disease prevention benefits. Chronic inflammation is a key component of atherosclerosis, the underlying cause of most cardiovascular disease [17]. By reducing inflammation, aspirin may slow the progression of atherosclerosis and prevent cardiovascular events [17]. However, the use of aspirin for primary prevention of cardiovascular disease is controversial and should be carefully considered on a case-by-case basis.

4.5 Cancer prevention

Epidemiological studies have suggested that regular use of aspirin may be associated with a reduced risk of developing certain types of cancer, including colorectal, esophageal, gastric, and breast cancer [8, 18]. The exact mechanisms by which aspirin exerts its anticancer effects are not fully understood. However, one of the proposed mechanisms is through its inhibition of COX. COX is overexpressed in many types of cancer, leading to increased production of prostaglandins, which promote inflammation and cell proliferation. By inhibiting COX, aspirin reduces the production of prostaglandins and may prevent the growth and spread of cancer cells [8]. In addition to its COX inhibition, aspirin has also been shown to have other anticancer effects, including the induction of apoptosis (programmed cell death) in cancer cells, the inhibition of angiogenesis (the growth of new blood vessels that supply tumors), and the enhancement of immune system function [15].

4.6 Alzheimer's disease

Aspirin has also been studied for its potential to prevent or delay the onset of Alzheimer's disease. Some studies have reported that long-term low-dose acetylsalicylic use shows protective potential for the development of both vascular dementia and Alzheimer's disease in patients with coronary heart disease [19]. Also through its anti-inflammatory property, ASA could potentially prevent or delay the onset of Alzheimer's disease (AD) [20–23].

One of the proposed mechanisms by which aspirin may protect against Alzheimer's disease is through its anti-inflammatory effects. Chronic inflammation is believed to play a role in the development of Alzheimer's disease, and aspirin's ability to inhibit COX and reduce inflammation may help prevent or slow down the progression of the disease. However, other studies have not found a significant association between aspirin use and the risk of Alzheimer's disease. A meta-analysis of 12 observational studies found no significant association between aspirin use and the risk of Alzheimer's disease [24]. Furthermore, aspirin may have potential side effects, including gastrointestinal bleeding and increased risk of stroke, which may outweigh the potential benefits for some individuals. As such, the use of aspirin for the prevention or treatment of Alzheimer's disease is not recommended, and more research is needed to determine its potential efficacy and safety [25].

5. Risks and side effects of aspirin

5.1 Aspirin toxicity

Aspirin is generally safe when taken as directed, but it can cause toxicity when taken in excessive amounts. Overdose of aspirin can lead to serious adverse effects, such as respiratory and metabolic acidosis, dehydration, electrolyte imbalances, and even death [26].

The toxicity of aspirin is related to its ability to inhibit the enzyme cyclooxygenase (COX), which is involved in the production of prostaglandins. Prostaglandins are important mediators of inflammation, pain, and fever, and their inhibition can lead to the adverse effects associated with aspirin toxicity [27]. Aspirin toxicity can also be exacerbated by certain factors, such as age, liver or kidney disease, alcohol consumption, and concomitant use of other medications [26]. Therefore, it is important to use aspirin with caution and under the guidance of a healthcare provider, particularly in individuals with underlying medical conditions or taking other medications. Aspirin toxicity can occur when taken in excessive amounts, and it can result in serious adverse effects. The risk of aspirin toxicity can be reduced by using aspirin as directed and under the guidance of a healthcare provider.

While aspirin can be highly effective in treating pain, inflammation, and preventing blood clots, there are also several potential risks and side effects associated with its use. Here are some of the most important risks and side effects of aspirin:

5.1.1 Gastrointestinal bleeding

One of the most significant risks of aspirin use is gastrointestinal bleeding. This can occur when the lining of the stomach or small intestine is damaged by the drug, which can lead to ulcers and bleeding [28]. People who have a history of ulcers, gastrointestinal bleeding, or other gastrointestinal problems are at a higher risk of developing these side effects.

5.1.2 Allergic reactions

Some people may be allergic to aspirin or other nonsteroidal anti-inflammatory drugs (NSAIDs). This can cause symptoms such as hives, swelling, and difficulty breathing. People who have a history of asthma, nasal polyps, or other allergies are at a higher risk of developing these side effects [6].

5.1.3 Increased bleeding risk

Aspirin's antiplatelet effects mean that it can increase the risk of bleeding, particularly in people who are taking other blood-thinning medications [3]. People who have a history of bleeding disorders, recent surgery, or other bleeding problems are at a higher risk of developing these side effects.

5.1.4 Reye's syndrome

Reye's syndrome is a rare but serious condition that primarily affects children and adolescents, and is characterized by acute encephalopathy and liver damage. It has been linked to the use of aspirin during certain viral infections, particularly influenza and chickenpox [29].

The exact mechanism by which aspirin triggers Reye's syndrome is not fully understood, but it is believed to be related to the ability of aspirin to interfere with mitochondrial function and fatty acid metabolism, leading to liver and brain damage [30]. As a result of these potential risks, the use of aspirin for the treatment of viral infections in children and adolescents is not recommended. Instead, alternative treatments, such as acetaminophen, are recommended for pain and fever relief. While aspirin is generally safe for use in adults, it should be used with caution in children and adolescents, particularly during viral infections. The potential risk of Reye's syndrome should be carefully considered, and alternative treatments should be used when possible.

5.1.5 Interactions with other medications

Aspirin is a widely used medication, and it is important to be aware of potential interactions with other drugs. Aspirin can interact with a variety of medications, including other pain relievers, blood thinners, and some prescription medications. One of the most significant drug interactions with aspirin is with other blood thinning medications, such as warfarin and clopidogrel. These medications are commonly used to prevent blood clots, but when taken with aspirin, the risk of bleeding may be increased [31]. Aspirin can also interact with some prescription medications, including some diabetes medications, methotrexate, and some antidepressants. It is important to talk to a healthcare provider before taking aspirin with any prescription medication, to ensure there are no potential interactions or adverse effects. Additionally, aspirin can interact with other over-the-counter medications, such as ibuprofen and naproxen. These medications belong to the same class of drugs as aspirin, and taking them together can increase the risk of side effects, such as stomach bleeding [31]. Aspirin can interact with a variety of medications, and it is important to be aware of potential interactions and to consult a healthcare provider before taking aspirin with other medications.

6. Potential future uses of aspirin

Aspirin's potential benefits extend beyond its current uses in pain relief and fever reduction. In addition to its potential for cancer prevention and treatment and its possible role in preventing and treating Alzheimer's disease, aspirin is also being investigated for its potential to prevent and treat a range of other conditions. One area of research is in aspirin's potential to prevent blood clots in people with conditions such as deep vein thrombosis and pulmonary embolism. Studies have shown that aspirin may be as effective as other blood-thinning medications in preventing blood clots, and it may also have fewer side effects [32]. Aspirin is also being investigated as a potential treatment for a range of autoimmune diseases, including rheumatoid arthritis and lupus. Studies have shown that aspirin may be able to reduce inflammation in the body, which is thought to play a role in the development of these conditions. However, more research is needed to determine the optimal dose and duration of aspirin therapy for these purposes.

Schizophrenia is a chronic and severe mental disorder that affects a person's thinking, behavior, and emotions. While the exact causes of schizophrenia are unknown, studies have suggested that inflammation may play a role in the development and progression of the disease [33, 34]. Aspirin, a widely used anti-inflammatory drug, has been investigated as a potential treatment for schizophrenia. One study found that aspirin, when used in combination with antipsychotic medication, led to a significant improvement in symptoms compared to antipsychotic medication alone [34]. Another study found that aspirin may be effective in reducing inflammation in individuals with schizophrenia, which could improve their cognitive function and quality of life [35]. However, more research is needed to confirm these findings and determine the optimal dosages and treatment regimens for aspirin in schizophrenia.

7. Aspirin and society

Aspirin has had a profound impact on society since its discovery, particularly in the fields of medicine and healthcare. Here are some of the key ways that aspirin has influenced society:

7.1 Pain relief

Aspirin's effectiveness as a pain reliever has made it one of the most widely used medications in the world. It has been used for over a century to treat a wide range of painful conditions, including headaches, menstrual cramps, and toothaches [36]. As a result, aspirin has helped countless individuals manage their pain and improve their quality of life.

7.2 Cardiovascular disease prevention

Aspirin's antiplatelet effects mean that it can help prevent blood clots from forming, which can reduce the risk of heart attacks and strokes [36]. This has made aspirin a vital tool in the prevention and management of cardiovascular disease, which is a leading cause of death worldwide. In fact, studies have shown that regular aspirin use can reduce the risk of heart attack and stroke in individuals with a history of cardiovascular disease [16].

7.3 Inflammatory disease treatment

Aspirin's anti-inflammatory effects have also made it an important treatment option for inflammatory conditions such as rheumatoid arthritis, osteoarthritis, and inflammatory bowel disease [36]. These conditions can cause chronic pain and disability, and aspirin has helped improve the quality of life for millions of individuals who suffer from them.

7.4 Pharmaceutical industry influence

Aspirin was one of the first medications to be mass-produced and marketed, and its success paved the way for the development of many other drugs. Today, the pharmaceutical industry is a multi-billion dollar industry that has had a significant impact on the global economy and has helped improve the health and wellbeing of individuals all over the world [37].

7.5 Cultural significance

Aspirin has become a cultural icon, with many individuals associating it with pain relief and medical care. It has been referenced in literature, music, and movies, and has become a symbol of modern medicine and healthcare. As a result, aspirin has become an integral part of modern culture, and its impact on society extends beyond the realm of medicine and healthcare [38]. Despite its many benefits, aspirin is not without risks and side effects. As we discussed earlier, aspirin use can increase the risk of gastrointestinal bleeding, allergic reactions, and other complications [39]. For this reason, it is important for individuals to discuss the potential risks and benefits of aspirin use with their healthcare provider before starting or stopping the medication.

In summary, aspirin has had a significant impact on society, particularly in the fields of medicine and healthcare. Its widespread use as a pain reliever, cardiovascular disease prevention tool, and treatment option for inflammatory conditions has helped improve the health and wellbeing of countless individuals worldwide. Its influence on the pharmaceutical industry and cultural significance further cement its importance in modern society.

8. Conclusion

In conclusion, aspirin is a wonder drug that has made a significant impact on society since its discovery over a century ago. Its effectiveness as a pain reliever, cardiovascular disease prevention tool, and treatment option for inflammatory conditions has helped improve the quality of life for millions of individuals worldwide. Its widespread use and cultural significance have also made it an important symbol of modern medicine and healthcare. However, as with any medication, aspirin is not without risks and potential side effects. It is important for individuals to discuss the potential benefits and risks of aspirin use with their healthcare provider before starting or stopping the medication. Overall, the discovery and widespread use of aspirin is a testament to the power of scientific research and innovation in improving the health and wellbeing of individuals and society as a whole.

Author details

Ahmed Adebayo Ishola
Molecular Biochemistry Department, Central Research Laboratory, Ilorin, Nigeria

*Address all correspondence to: djmedite@yahoo.com; djmedite@gmail.com

References

[1] Miner J, Hoffhines A. The discovery of aspirin's antithrombotic effects. Texas Heart Institute Journal. 2007;**34**:179

[2] Weiss HJ. The discovery of the antiplatelet effect of aspirin: A personal reminiscence. Journal of Thrombosis and Haemostasis. 2003;**1**:1869-1875

[3] Patrono C, Rocca B. Aspirin: Promise and resistance in the new millennium. Arteriosclerosis, Thrombosis, and Vascular Biology. 2008;**28**:s25-s32

[4] Fuster V, Sweeny JM. Aspirin: A historical and contemporary therapeutic overview. Circulation. 2011;**123**:768-778

[5] Vane JR, Botting RM. The mechanism of action of aspirin. Thrombosis Research. 2003;**110**:255-258

[6] Grosser T, Theken KN, FitzGerald GA. Cyclooxygenase inhibition: Pain, inflammation, and the cardiovascular system. Clinical Pharmacology and Therapeutics. 2017;**102**:611-622

[7] Warner TD, Nylander S, Whatling C. Anti-platelet therapy: Cyclo-oxygenase inhibition and the use of aspirin with particular regard to dual anti-platelet therapy. British Journal of Clinical Pharmacology. 2011;**72**:619-633

[8] Rothwell PM, Wilson M, Elwin C-E, Norrving B, Algra A, Warlow CP, et al. Long-term effect of aspirin on colorectal cancer incidence and mortality: 20-year follow-up of five randomised trials. Lancet. 2010;**376**:1741-1750

[9] Zarghi A, Arfaei S. Selective COX-2 inhibitors: A review of their structure-activity relationships. The Iranian Journal of Pharmaceutical Research (IJPR). 2011;**10**:655

[10] Sharma S, Sharma SC. An update on eicosanoids and inhibitors of cyclooxygenase enzyme systems. Indian Journal of Experimental Biology. 1997;**35**:1025-1031

[11] FitzGerald GA, Patrono C. The coxibs, selective inhibitors of cyclooxygenase-2. The New England Journal of Medicine. 2001;**345**: 433-442

[12] Mose T, Knudsen LE, Hedegaard M, Mortensen GK. Transplacental transfer of monomethyl phthalate and mono (2-ethylhexyl) phthalate in a human placenta perfusion system. International Journal of Toxicology. 2007;**26**:221-229

[13] Kowalski ML, Stevenson DD. Classification of reactions to nonsteroidal antiinflammatory drugs. Immunology and Allergy Clinics of North America. 2013;**33**:135-145

[14] Moore RA, Wiffen PJ, Derry S, Maguire T, Roy YM, Tyrrell L. Non-prescription (OTC) oral analgesics for acute pain-an overview of Cochrane reviews. Cochrane Database of Systematic Reviews. 2015;**11**:CD010794

[15] Patrono C. Aspirin: New cardiovascular uses for an old drug. The American Journal of Medicine. 2001;**110**:S62-S65

[16] Antithrombotic-Trialists. Collaborative meta-analysis of randomised trials of antiplatelet therapy for prevention of death, myocardial infarction, and stroke in high risk patients. BMJ. 2002;**324**:71-86

[17] Ridker PM, Everett BM, Thuren T, MacFadyen JG, Chang WH, Ballantyne C, et al. Antiinflammatory

therapy with canakinumab for atherosclerotic disease. The New England Journal of Medicine. 2017;**377**:1119-1131

[18] Cuzick J, Otto F, Baron JA, Brown PH, Burn J, Greenwald P, et al. Aspirin and non-steroidal anti-inflammatory drugs for cancer prevention: An international consensus statement. The Lancet Oncology. 2009;**10**:501-507

[19] Nguyen TNM, Chen L-J, Trares K, Stocker H, Holleczek B, Beyreuther K, et al. Long-term low-dose acetylsalicylic use shows protective potential for the development of both vascular dementia and Alzheimer's disease in patients with coronary heart disease but not in other individuals from the general population: Results from two large cohort studies. Alzheimer's Research & Therapy. 2022;**14**:75

[20] Bernardo A, Minghetti L. PPAR-γ agonists as regulators of microglial activation and brain inflammation. Current Pharmaceutical Design. 2006;**12**:93-109

[21] Choi S-H, Bosetti F. Cyclooxygenase-1 null mice show reduced neuroinflammation in response to β-amyloid. Aging (Albany NY). 2009;**1**:234

[22] Sastre M, Dewachter I, Landreth GE, Willson TM, Klockgether T, van Leuven F, et al. Nonsteroidal anti-inflammatory drugs and peroxisome proliferator-activated receptor-γ agonists modulate immunostimulated processing of amyloid precursor protein through regulation of β-secretase. The Journal of Neuroscience. 2003;**23**:9796-9804

[23] Woodling NS, Andreasson KI. Untangling the web: Toxic and protective effects of neuroinflammation and PGE2 signaling in Alzheimer's disease. ACS Chemical Neuroscience. 2016;**7**:454-463

[24] Etminan M, Gill S, Samii A. Effect of non-steroidal anti-inflammatory drugs on risk of Alzheimer's disease: Systematic review and meta-analysis of observational studies. BMJ. 2003;**327**:128

[25] Jaturapatporn D, Isaac MGEKN, McCleery J, Tabet N. Aspirin, steroidal and non-steroidal anti-inflammatory drugs for the treatment of Alzheimer's disease. Cochrane Database of Systematic Reviews. 2012;**2**:CD006378

[26] Lugassy DM. Salicylates. In: Nelson LS, Howland MA, Lewin NA, Smith SW, Goldfrank LR, Hoffman RS, editors. Goldfrank's Toxicol. Emergencies. 11th ed. New York, NY: McGraw-Hill Education; 2019. Available from: http://accessemergencymedicine.mhmedical.com/content.aspx?aid=1163010580

[27] Gum PA, Kottke-Marchant K, Poggio ED, Gurm H, Welsh PA, Brooks L, et al. Profile and prevalence of aspirin resistance in patients with cardiovascular disease. The American Journal of Cardiology. 2001;**88**:230-235

[28] Lanas A, Scheiman J. Low-dose aspirin and upper gastrointestinal damage: Epidemiology, prevention and treatment. Current Medical Research and Opinion. 2007;**23**:163-173

[29] Belay ED, Bresee JS, Holman RC, Khan AS, Shahriari A, Schonberger LB. Reye's syndrome in the United States from 1981 through 1997. The New England Journal of Medicine. 1999;**340**:1377-1382

[30] Starko KM, Ray CG, Dominguez LB, Stromberg WL, Woodall DF. Reye's syndrome and salicylate use. Pediatrics. 1980;**66**:859-864

[31] NIH. Aspirin. Natl. Institutes Heal.; 2023. Available from: https://doi.org/https://medlineplus.gov/druginfo/meds/a682878.html

[32] Brighton TA, Eikelboom JW, Mann K, Mister R, Gallus A, Ockelford P, et al. Low-dose aspirin for preventing recurrent venous thromboembolism. The New England Journal of Medicine. 2012;**367**:1979-1987

[33] Müller N. Inflammation in schizophrenia: Pathogenetic aspects and therapeutic considerations. Schizophrenia Bulletin. 2018;**44**:973-982

[34] Schmidt L, Phelps E, Friedel J, Shokraneh F. Acetylsalicylic acid (aspirin) for schizophrenia. Cochrane Database of Systematic Reviews. 2019;**8**:CD012116

[35] Sommer IE, van Westrhenen R, Begemann MJH, de Witte LD, Leucht S, Kahn RS. Efficacy of anti-inflammatory agents to improve symptoms in patients with schizophrenia: An update. Schizophrenia Bulletin. 2014;**40**:181-191

[36] Derry S, Wiffen PJ, Moore RA. Aspirin for acute treatment of episodic tension-type headache in adults. Cochrane Database of Systematic Reviews. 2017;**1**:CD011888

[37] González Peña OI, López Zavala MÁ, Cabral Ruelas H. Pharmaceuticals market, consumption trends and disease incidence are not driving the pharmaceutical research on water and wastewater. International Journal of Environmental Research and Public Health. 2021;**18**:2532

[38] Montinari MR, Minelli S, De Caterina R. The first 3500 years of aspirin history from its roots—A concise summary. Vascular Pharmacology. 2019;**113**:1-8

[39] Huang ES, Strate LL, Ho WW, Lee SS, Chan AT. A prospective study of aspirin use and the risk of gastrointestinal bleeding in men. PLoS ONE. 2010;**5**:e15721

Chapter

Therapeutic Uses of Aspirin

Maria I. Trapali

Abstract

Aspirin, also known as acetylsalicylic acid (ASA), is a nonsteroidal anti-inflammatory drug (NSAID) used to reduce pain, fever, and/or inflammation and as an antithrombotic agent. The specific inflammatory conditions under which aspirin is used for treatment include many different diseases. Lower doses of aspirin have also been indicated to decrease the risk of loss of life from a heart strike or the risk of stroke in people who are at high risk or who have cardiovascular illness but not in elderly people who are healthy. Recent research suggests that aspirin may help prevent the development of cancerous tumors, such as those of the stomach, intestines, or even the breast. However, although aspirin is considered a "good" medicine for the prevention and treatment of many diseases, doctors recommend that no one should take aspirin without a doctor's approval because taking it is not only unsafe for all people but can also interact with other medicines and cause harm. The most useful therapeutic properties of aspirin depend on its ability to inhibit prostaglandin formation. Along with interfering with thromboxane production, aspirin inhibits the synthesis of prostaglandins. In a normal environment, thromboxane and prostacyclin are in homeostatic equilibrium, with incompatible effects on platelet aggregation and vascular action. In this chapter, the therapeutic uses of aspirin are presented.

Keywords: aspirin, inflammation, cancer, prostaglandins, platelets, cyclooxygenase

1. Introduction

Aspirin is one of the most widely used medicines [1], with some disputes about its real birth date, and it has celebrated its 120th birthday. Chemically, aspirin is called acetylsalicylic acid and is widely used as an analgesic, antipyretic, and anti-inflammatory agent, as well as for treating headache and muscle and joint pain [2].

It is also used long-term in people at high risk for ischemic disease. It is considered to be one of the major drugs that has been discovered [3], and no drug is currently as widely used as aspirin. It is a nonsteroidal anti-inflammatory drug (NSAID) that suppresses normal platelet function. It is used as an analgesic, antipyretic, and anti-inflammatory agent. At low doses, it is also taken as a platelet anticoagulant (antithrombotic). It should not be taken by people who are deficient in the G6PD enzyme or by people under 16 years of age because of the risk of Reye's syndrome (high fever, headache, sudden death) and with caution by people taking anticoagulation agents. Many people take aspirin to reduce the risk of heart attack. Aspirin helps to prevent

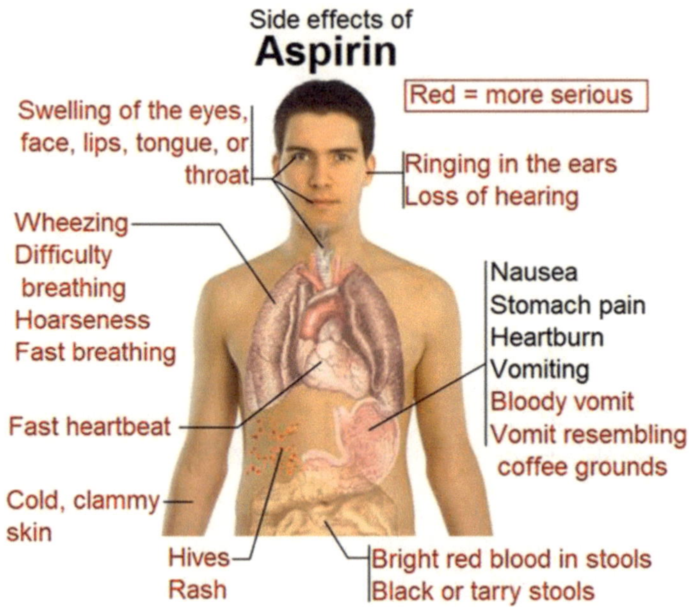

Figure 1.
Main side effects of aspirin [4].

thrombosis in the heart or even in the brain; thus, strokes can be avoided. This discovery was made by Dr. Lawrence Craven in approximately 1950 when he noticed unusual bleeding in children who were taking aspirin to treat pain after tonsil surgery. Recent research suggests that aspirin may help prevent the development of cancerous tumors, such as those of the stomach, intestines, or even the breast. However, although aspirin is considered a "good" medicine for the prevention and treatment of many diseases, doctors recommend that no one should take aspirin without a doctor's approval because taking it is not only unsafe for all people but can also interact with other medicines and cause harm. Women who are pregnant should avoid taking aspirin. Despite these problems, aspirin is still one of the oldest and most widely used drugs in the world [3]. The side effects of aspirin are presented in **Figure 1**.

2. Effects and uses of aspirin

2.1 Antiplatelet effect of aspirin

The most useful therapeutic properties of aspirin depend on its ability to inhibit prostaglandin formation. Prostaglandins are a large group of biologically active, unsaturated fatty acids with 20 carbon atoms produced during the metabolism of arachidonic acid and through the cyclooxygenase pathway. They are local hormones that are rapidly formed, act on adjacent regions and are subsequently broken down and destroyed by enzymes. The prostaglandins PGD2, PGE2, PGF2a, PGI1, PGI2, prostacyclin, and thromboxane (TXA2) are important mediators of inflammation. Nonsteroidal anti-inflammatory drugs inhibit the production of prostaglandins. Prostaglandins affect a wide number of biological processes, including vasodilation, vascular permeability, bronchospasm, platelet aggregation, dysmenorrhea, inhibition of gastric secretion, and stimulation of nerve receptors of algae during tissue destruction, inhibition of sleep, and maintenance of an open arterial duct. Exogenous administration of PGE2 in the form of a gel is used to soften the cervix before the onset of labor.

The normal endothelium is a stable, strong antithrombotic (thromboresistant) blood flow surface. It exhibits anticoagulant, fibrinolytic, and antiplatelet properties. Prothrombotic and antithrombotic properties. However, whenever the endothelium is activated or disrupted, it rapidly transforms into a prothrombotic surface, which effectively promotes coagulation, inhibits fibrinolysis, and activates platelets. Hemostatic transformation of the vessel wall is caused by mechanical damage or by disruption and activation of vascular cells by factors such as cytokines, cytokine bacterial endotoxins, hypoxia, and various hemodynamic forces. Prostaglandin I2 (PGI2, prostacyclin) is an important endothelial oxygenation product that is synthesized through cyclooxygenase (COX) and prostacyclin synthase from arachidonic acid [5]. Prostacyclin, like nitric oxide (NO), is both a vasodilator and an inhibitor of platelet aggregation (but not platelet adhesion). These actions are achieved through the activation of adenylate cyclase, thereby increasing the levels of cyclin adenosine monophosphate (cAMP) in target cells, which are vascular smooth muscle cells and platelets. The hyperpolarizing endothelial proliferative factor (EDHF) and carbon monoxide, a byproduct of the metabolism of hemoglobin to chlorpromazine by haem oxygenase [6], are also direct factors in vasodilators, which are used by endothelial cells. Endothelial adenosine diphosphate (ADPase) or CD39 [7] is a membrane inhibitor of platelets that may indirectly promote vasodilation by producing adenosine. These properties of the endothelium are compensated by endothelial vasoconstrictor factors, including platelet-activating factor, platelet-activating factor endothelin-1, and thromboxane A2 (TXA2).

2.1.1 Biological inflammation mediators

2.1.1.1 Derived from plasma

- Quinines (bradykinin)
- Complement factors (C3a, C3b, C5a, C5, C6, and C7)
- Fibrin degradation products
- Hageman factor
- Protease inhibitors (α2 macroglobulin and α1 antitrypsin)
- CRP

2.1.1.2 Produced locally in tissues

- Arachidonic acid products (PGE2, PGI2, TxB2, and LTB4)
- Vasodilator amines (histamines)
- Cytokines (interleukins 1 (IL-1) and 2 (IL-2))

- Oxygen and nitric oxide free radicals
- Platelet-activating factor

Cyclooxygenase and lipoxygenase act on arachidonic acid and release prostaglandins (PGE), prostacyclin (PGI2), thromboxane (TxB2), and leukotrienes (LT). These biological products exert a variety of actions, both inflammatory and anti-inflammatory, while some eicosanoids cause severe pain. Thromboxanes are physiologically active compounds found in many organs of the body. They are formed *in vivo* from prostaglandin endo-peroxides and cause platelet aggregation, arterial constriction, and other biological effects. Thromboxanes are important mediators of the actions of polyunsaturated fatty acids transformed by cyclooxygenase. They are produced by platelets, which cause blood to clot and blood vessels to constrict. It also encourages the accumulation of platelets. Thromboxane A2 (TXA2) is active but is very unstable and has a half-life of only 30 seconds before it undergoes hydrolysis to form thromboxane B2 (TXB2), which is inactive [8].

COX-1 is an enzyme that occurs in a wide range of cells throughout the whole organism. It maintains the formation of PGs involved in the performance of essential functions (e.g., control of blood flow through individual organs). COX-2 (**Figure 2**) is synthesized from the beginning (de novo) in anti-inflammatory cells [10], such as neutrophils and mast cells, after exposure to bacterial endotoxins and/or cytokines (e.g., tumor necrosis factor (TNF) and interleukin 1b). The production of PGs at sites of inflammation and/or tissue can cause damage. COX-2 is released in large quantities locally in the area of inflammation or systemically after infection. Originally, it was thought that this was a result of an increase in arachidonic acid. In 1990, however, it was shown that this increase in the formation of prostaglandins was due to an increase in the expression of the enzyme cyclooxygenase [11]. We now know that increased cyclooxygenase is not cyclooxygenase-1 but rather an isomer of cyclooxygenase-2. In the sequence of reactions that produce prostaglandins from arachidonic acid, aspirin inhibits the essential enzyme cyclo-oxygenase.

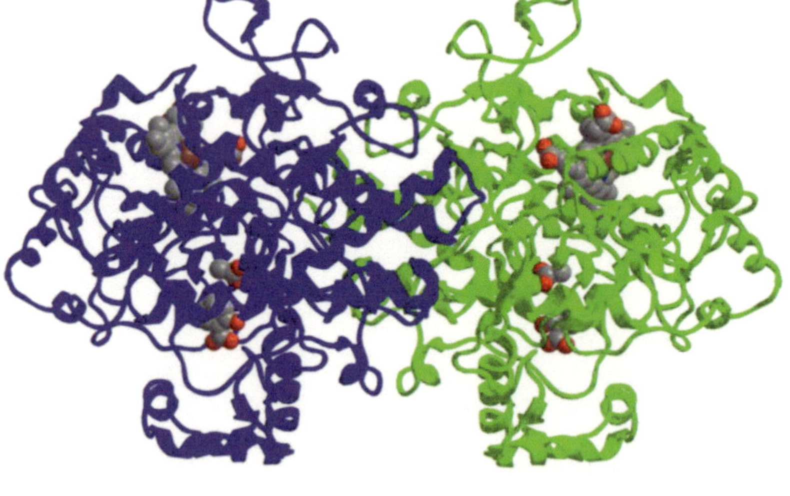

Figure 2.
The "Cox-2 crystal structure" of cox-2 inhibited by aspirin [9].

The antiplatelet effect of aspirin results from the elimination of COX-1 and COX-2. It causes permanent acetylation of serine at position 530 in COX-1 and at site 516 in COX-2, regulating the connection of arachidonic acid to the catalytic active site of the enzyme. Aspirin has a greater effect on COX-1 than on COX-2, as it is approximately 170 times more effective at inhibiting COX-1 [12]. Additionally, along with interfering with thromboxane production, aspirin also inhibits the synthesis of prostaglandins, most importantly, prostacyclin. In a normal environment, thromboxane and prostacyclin are in homeostatic equilibrium, with incompatible effects on platelet aggregation and vascular action (thromboxane is synthesized within platelets, but prostacyclin is synthesized within endothelial cells) [13].

2.2 Anti-inflammatory uses of aspirin

One of the properties of the immune system is the ability to communicate, coordinate, and move cells to achieve protection against foreign invaders. Communication between immune cells is achieved by means of small protein molecules produced by different types of cells called cytokines. The class of cytokines includes a wide variety of regulatory factors produced by many different types of cells. They are usually secreted by immune cells when they encounter a pathogen, activating other immune cells and thus increasing the immune response. T cells and macrophages are important sources of cytokine production. Cytokines are divided into chemokines, interleukins, and lymphokines based on their function and the cells that secrete them or the target cells on which they act. Examples of inflammatory cytokines are interferon (IFN)-a, tumor necrosis factor (TNF)-a, interleukin (IL)-1b, IL-6, and IL-8 (**Figure 3**).

Aspirin affects the inflammatory pathway by irreversibly inhibiting cyclooxygenase (COX)-1, altering the enzyme activity of COX-2, and decreasing the production of prostaglandins and thromboxane. The above mechanisms are effective in increasing the risk of atherosclerosis and heart disease [15]. Aspirin can lower oxidative stress

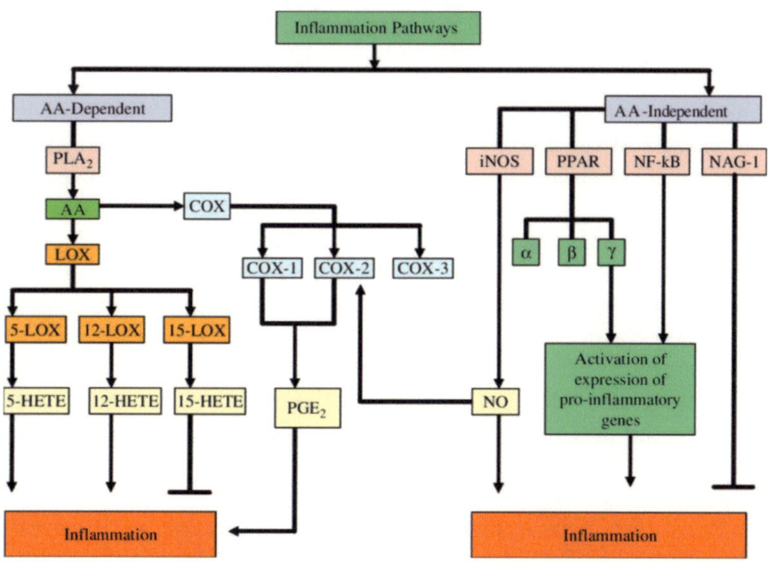

Figure 3.
Pathways of inflammation [14].

and defend against oxidative damage. There are useful effects of aspirin in preclinical and clinical studies of mood disorders and schizophrenia. Epidemiological data suggest that high-dose aspirin is associated with a decreased risk of Alzheimer's disease. COX-2 inhibitors may cause neuroinflammatory reactions, reduce antioxidant resistance, and promote neuronal progression. COX-2 inhibition may also interfere with inflammation decreases the production of prostaglandin E2 (PGE2). Therefore, to understand the clinical efficacy of aspirin in patients with neuropsychiatric disorders such as depression and schizophrenia, it is important to consider how its inhibition of COX-1 affects these patients [15].

2.3 Aspirin in preeclampsia prevention

Preeclampsia (PE) is defined as hypertension during pregnancy (systolic blood pressure >140 mmHg and diastolic >90 mmHg), together with albuminuria (>300 mg of albumin in a 24-hour urine collection or >30 mg/mmol in a random urine sample or more than one cross in a urine stick), with or without abnormal edema. A severe form of preeclampsia can threaten the life of both mothers and children. Approximately 1 in 200 women (0.5%) develop severe preeclampsia during pregnancy. Symptoms tend to become apparent in the latter stages of pregnancy but may appear for the first time even after delivery.

Symptoms of a severe form of preeclampsia include the following:

- Severe headaches that do not subside with simple painkillers
- Vision problems, such as blurred vision or flashes in front of the eyes
- Severe pain just below the ribs
- Burning in the chest that does not go away with antacids
- Rapidly increasing swelling in the face, hands, or feet
- A very strong feeling of sickness.

Preeclampsia affects the development of the placenta, which can prevent normal fetal development. There may also be less fluid around the fetus in the uterine environment. If the placenta is severely damaged, then the fetus will be in a very difficult situation. In some cases, this can even lead to the death of the fetus in the womb. Medical monitoring aims to identify and rescue the most at-risk fetuses and deliver them since the delivery of the fetus, especially the placenta, is the treatment for preeclampsia.

In PE, the creation of thromboxane A2 and prostaglandin I2 is modified by the excessive accumulation of TXA2 metabolites in the maternal systemic circulation. This leads to increased actuation and aggregation of platelets and vasoconstriction, resulting in decreased placental perfusion and oxidative stress. Aspirin acetylates the platelet enzyme COX, altering the synthesis of different prostaglandins, and behaves as an analgesic and anti-inflammatory agent. Aspirin permanently suppresses COX-1 and reversibly suppresses COX-2 to a minor extent. The consequent reticence of the COX-dependent creation of thromboxane A2 prevents platelet aggregation. This result is maintained for the entire platelet lifespan of 8–9 days [16]. Low-dose aspirin decreases fatality and despair in pregnant women at high risk of PE. The FDA has assigned this drug as pregnancy category C, and treatment is relatively safe. Although aspirin can cross the placenta, it is safe at low doses [16, 17].

2.4 Antitumor effect of aspirin

Many studies have established that aspirin can minimize the morbidity and mortality of tumors, including bladder cancer, breast cancer, esophageal cancer, gastric cancer, colorectal cancer, liver cancer, lung cancer, and prostate cancer.

Angiogenesis is a crucial process in the course of tumorigenesis. Cancer cells have the ability to exploit preexisting vessels (coadoption) to initiate the creation of a well-vascularized tumor. The defensive response of the initial vessels to this process is the regression of the vessels, resulting in the formation of an unvascularized tumor. The tumors that will succeed in growing are those that have overcome the process of vascular regression, inducing angiogenesis again. The main factor that induces angiogenesis is hypoxia. Von-Hippel Lindau protein (VHL) plays an important role in regulating HIF-1a gene expression and is increased in hypoxic cancer cells (hypoxia inducible factor), leading to the transcriptional overexpression of several genes, the products of which induce angiogenesis. The most important are vascular endothelial growth factor A (VEGF-A) and platelet-derived growth factor (PDGF). VEGF binds to the receptors VEGFR-1/flt-1 and VEGFR-2/KDR/flk-1, which are located on the surface of existing endothelial cells and promote proliferation, migration, differentiation, and survival. This process is mediated through changes in the expression of integrins (a family of receptors for endothelial cell adhesion to the surrounding layer). Eventually, these immature vessels need to mature, a process through which the action of PDGF on its receptors in pericytes leads to the coating of neoplastic vessels by pericytes [18, 19].

The mode of action of aspirin in cancer prevention has not been established. The anticancer effects of aspirin are proposed to occur through acetylation-mediated inactivation of COX, as COX-2 is upregulated in 80–90% of colorectal cancers [20]. Another study in human intestinal mucosal cells revealed that low-dose aspirin produced acetylation of COX-1 and strongly inhibited PGE2 synthesis to reduce the levels of S6 kinase, which is involved in the blockage of early colorectal carcinogenesis [21].

Salicylic acid, the hydrolyzed outcome of aspirin, is also involved in the chemopreventive effects of aspirin. Salicylic acid was shown to bind to many cellular proteins (salicylic acid binding proteins or SABPs), such as IκB kinase (IKK), a constituent of the NF-κB complex AMP-activated protein kinase, glyceraldehyde-3-phosphate dehydrogenase (GAPDH), and CDK2, affecting their levels and/or functional activity [22]. Aspirin may also inhibit mammalian target of rapamycin (mTOR), HIF-1α, and VEGF-A signaling related to antiangiogenesis and the development of autophagy at the protein level in murine hepatocarcinomatous and sarcoma models. mTOR is a 282 kPa intracellular serine/threonine kinase that acts as a central regulator of cell proliferation and the cell cycle. When the mTOR biochemical pathway is activated, the risk of cancer may increase [23].

3. Conclusions

Aspirin, or acetylsalicylic acid, is one of the most widely known analgesic and anti-inflammatory drugs. Depending on the dosage used, it can reduce pain, as well as fever, and may also be beneficial in preventing cerebral thrombosis and stroke. Aspirin was launched in 1899, and to date, it is a benchmark analgesic drug with sales exceeding 400,000 tons worldwide. High doses of aspirin are used for its anti-inflammatory effect, while low doses of aspirin are usually used for its antiplatelet effect. The most common side effect of the drug (**Figure 3**) is the induction of digestive erosion and ulcers. The most serious complication is bleeding from these lesions, especially for bleeding from aspirin-treated patients.

Aspirin exerts both therapeutic and toxic effects on the body's actions mainly through the inhibition of COX, a key enzyme for the metabolism of arachidonic acid to produce prostaglandins. There are two main forms of COX: (a) COX-1 or basic COX-1, which is continuously produced (such as prostaglandin E2 in the kidneys, prostaglandin E2 in the mouth and kidneys, prostaglandin I2 or prostacyclin in blood vessels, and thromboxane in platelets), and (b) COX-2 or inducible COX-2, the production of which is induced during the inflammatory phase reaction and may induce the production of COX-1-like prostaglandins depending on the inflammatory organ.

The antiplatelet effect of aspirin results in the elimination of COX-1 and COX-2. It causes permanent acetylation of a serine at position 530 in COX-1 and at position 516 in COX-2, regulating the connection of arachidonic acid to the catalytic active site of the enzyme. Aspirin can also lower oxidative stress and protect against oxidative damage. There are advantageous outcomes of aspirin in preclinical and clinical studies on mood derangement and schizophrenia, and epidemiological data suggest that high-dose aspirin is related to a decreased risk of AD. COX-2 inhibitors may cause neuroinflammatory reactions, reduce antioxidant resistance, and provoke neuroprogression. COX-2 inhibition may also interfere with inflammation, decreasing the production of PGE2. Aspirin may also inhibit mTOR, HIF-1α, and VEGF-A signaling related to antiangiogenesis and the development of autophagy at the protein level in murine hepatocarcinomatous and sarcoma models. mTOR is a 282 kPa intracellular serine/threonine kinase that acts as a central regulator of cell proliferation and the cell cycle. When the mTOR biochemical pathway is activated, the risk of cancer may increase [24–26].

Future prospects related to aspirin could include further research on the possible treatment of new diseases and the study of genetic polymorphisms possibly involved in the drug's mechanism of action.

Author details

Maria I. Trapali
Department of Biomedical Sciences, School of Health and Care Sciences, University of West Attica, Athens, Greece

*Address all correspondence to: ymaria@uniwa.gr

References

[1] Montinari M, Minelli S, De Caterina R. The first 3500 years of aspirin history from its roots—A concise summary. Vascular Pharmacology. 2019;**113**:1-8

[2] The Editors of Encyclopaedia Britannica. Aspirin. Available from: https://www.britannica.com/science// aspirin

[3] Sneader W. The discovery of aspirin: A reappraisal. British Medical Journal. 2000;**321**(7276):1591-1594. Available from: https://www.ncbi.nlm.nih.gov// pmc/articles/PMC1119266/

[4] Side Effects of Aspirin. Available from: https://upload.wikimedia.org/ wikipedia/commons/thumb/c/ce/ Side_effects_of_aspirin.png/640pxSide_ effects_of_aspirin.png

[5] Davidge S. Prostaglandin H synthase and vascular function. Circulation Research. 2001;**89**:650

[6] Durante W, Schafer A. Carbon monoxide and vascular cell function. International Journal of Molecular Medicine. 1998;**2**:55

[7] Marcus A, Brookman M, Drosopoulos J. Metabolic control of excessive extracellular nucleotide accumulation by CD39/ ectonucleotidase-1: Implications for ischemic vascular diseases. The Journal of Pharmacology and Experimental Therapeutics. 2003;**305**(1):9-16

[8] Ylikorkala O, Mäkilä U. Prostacyclin and thromboxane in gynecology and obstetrics. American Journal of Obstetrics and Gynecology. 1985;**152**(3):318-329

[9] Available from: https://upload. wikimedia.org/wikipedia/commons/ thumb/4/42/COX-2_inhibited_by_ Aspirin.png/640pxCOX-2_inhibited_by_ Aspirin.png

[10] Hawkey C. COX-2 inhibitors. Lancet. 1999;**353**:307-314

[11] Warner T, Mitchell J. Cyclooxygenases: New forms, new inhibitors, and lessons from the clinic. The FASEB Journal. 2004;**18**:790-804

[12] Vane JR, Bakhle YS, Botting RM. Cyclooxygenases 1 and 2. Annual Review of Pharmacology and Toxicology. 1998;**38**:97-120

[13] Hybiaka J et al. Aspirin and its pleiotropic application. European Journal of Pharmacology. 2020;**866**:172762

[14] Issa AY, Volate SR, Wargovich MJ. The role of phytochemicals in inhibition of cancer and inflammation: New directions and perspectives. Journal of Food Composition and Analysis. 2006;**19**:405-419. Available from: https://www.researchgate.net/profile/ Ala-Issa/publication/248580172/figure/ fig1/AS:393253955358724@1470770 457398/Pathways-of-inflammation-Inflammatory-cell-signaling-pathwayscan-be-mechanistically_W640. jpg

[15] Berk M et al. Aspirin: A review of its neurobiological properties and therapeutic potential for mental illness. BMC Medicine. 2013;**11**:74

[16] Dutta S, Kumar S, Hyett J, Salomon C. Molecular targets of aspirin and prevention of preeclampsia and their potential association with circulating extracellular vesicles during

pregnancy. International Journal of Molecular Sciences. 2019;**20**(18):4370. DOI: 10.3390//ijms20184370

[17] Yurdakok M. Fetal and neonatal effects of anticoagulants used in pregnancy: A review. Turkish Journal of Pediatrics. 2012;**54**:207-215

[18] Carmeliet P. Mechanisms of angiogenesis and arteriogenesis. Nature Medicine. 2000;**6**(4):389-395

[19] Jain R. Tumor angiogenesis and accessibility: Role of vascular endothelial growth factor. Seminars in Oncology. 2002;**29**(6 Suppl. 16):3-9

[20] Sostres C, Gargall C, Lanas A. Aspirin, cyclooxygenase inhibition and colorectal cancer. World Journal of Gastrointestinal Pharmacology and Therapeutics. 2014;**5**:40-49

[21] Patrignani P et al. Low-dose aspirin acetylates cyclooxygenase-1 in human colorectal mucosa: Implications for the chemoprevention of colorectal cancer. Clinical Pharmacology and Therapeutics. 2017;**102**:52-61

[22] Dachineni R et al. Salicylic acid metabolites and derivatives inhibit CDK activity: Novel insights into aspirin's chemo preventive effects against colorectal cancer. International Journal of Oncology. 2017;**51**(6):1661-1673

[23] Zhao Q et al. Aspirin may inhibit angiogenesis and induce autophagy by inhibiting mTOR signaling pathway in murine hepatocarcinomatous and sarcoma models. Oncology Letters. 2016;**12**(4):2804-2810

[24] Villa PM. Aspirin in the prevention of pre-eclampsia in high-risk women: A randomised placebo-controlled PREDO trial and a meta-analysis of randomised trials. BJOG : An International Journal of Obstetrics and Gynaecology. 2013;**120**:64-74

[25] Henderson JT, Whitlock EP, O'Connor E. Low-dose aspirin for prevention of morbidity and mortality from preeclampsia. Annals of Internal Medicine. 2014;**160**:695-703

[26] Ricoult SJ, Yecies JL, Ben-Sahra I, Manning BD. Oncogenic PI3K and K-Ras stimulate de novo lipid synthesis through mTORC1 and SREBP. Oncogene. 2016;**35**(10):1250-1260

Chapter 14

Genetics of CPSP

Stephen Sciberras

Abstract

Various polymorphisms in several genes appear to be involved in the development of chronic post-surgical pain (CPSP). These genes are involved in the transduction, transmission and modulation of a nociceptive impulse. Understanding the influence of such polymorphisms would lead to a better awareness of the underlying processing in CPSP, with the possibility of stratifying the risk of CPSP for individual patients. It may also identify new treatment options by targeting specific points in this pathway. We look into six genes—*SCN9A*, *KCNS1*, *GCH1*, *COMT*, *OPRM1*, *OPRK1*—that are involved in nociception, and look at current literature to support their involvement in the development of CPSP. We also describe the potential use of such information in clinical practice.

Keywords: CPSP, SCN9A, KCNS1, GCH1, COMT, OPRM1, OPRK1

1. Introduction

Nociception involves various receptors encoded by different DNA sequences. Hence, changes in these genes could play a significant role in nociception by altering the function of receptors and other proteins involved in nociception [1].

Mutations in a gene may involve three main different mechanisms: base substitution, insertion or deletion [2]. It is more frequent to have single nucleotide changes, or polymorphisms (SNPs) than changes that involve a series of bases.

We shall be focusing on three main pathways that could be affected by different genotypes:

- Ionic channels involved in the initialization and transmission of nociceptive impulse
- Modulation of pain pathway involving catecholamines
- Pharmacogenetic response to analgesics.

2. Genetic variations in ionic channels

We shall concentrate on two ionic channels: the sodium voltage-gated channel and the potassium voltage-gated channel.

2.1 SCN9A

Voltage-gated sodium channels (VGSC) are important in the generation and transmission of an action potential. The nine different VGSC alpha subunits are encoded for by nine genes spread over four chromosomes [3]. In particular, one type of VGSC alpha subunit, Nav 1.7 is implicated in channelopathy-associated insensitivity to pain and is encoded by *SCN9A*. Nav1.7 is involved in the initiation of an action potential and hence it is important in setting the sensitivity for nociceptive signals to be transmitted [4]. In fact, a number of Nav1.7 inhibitors have been looked into as possible analgesics [5].

The *SCN9A* gene is found on chromosome 2 (2q24.3), and is 113.5-kbases long. There are 29 exons in the gene, as characterised by Raymond et al. This work also showed how *SCN9A*, like other genes responsible for voltage-gated sodium channels, exhibit alternative splicing of some of these exons. This mechanism allows for even more variability in the resulting protein structure. Indeed, exon 5A of *SCN9A* is preferentially expressed in the peripheral nerves and central nervous system, whereas exon 5A was transcripted only in dorsal root ganglion neurones [6].

SCN9A polymorphism is responsible for structural differences in Nav1.7, which may lead to differences in channel activity. Reimann et al. [7] investigated the functional effects of rs6746030, which is a mutation in exon 18 involving a substitution of an amino acid at position 1150. Although peak currents and time of activation or fast inactivation were not different, slow inactivation was shorter in subjects with the minor allele A of rs6746030. Slow inactivation regulates the firing frequency of neurons, so this could explain how this mutation predisposes to a greater sensitivity to pain.

Polymorphisms in this gene are implicated in erythromelalgia and similar neuropathic pain syndromes [8], congenital insensitivity to pain [9] and possibly epilepsy [10–12], schizophrenia [13]. *SCN9A* is also associated with Paroxysmal Extreme Pain Disorder, which is characterised by skin flushing and episodes of severe pain [14]. Zhong et al. [15] also related propofol sensitivity to rs6746030, with carriers of the minor allele requiring lower propofol plasma concentrations for the same effect.

Estacion et al. [16] demonstrated that the single nucleotide change from the G allele to the A allele at rs6746030 results in a structurally different Nav1.7 that is more excitable. Indeed, rs6746030 has been implicated in higher pain scores in patients with lumbar disc herniation [17]. In a study of 27 different SNP's of the *SCN9A* gene, rs6746030 was the most influential in over 1200 patients investigated, including in postoperative pain [7]. Specifically in a postoperative setting, Duan et al. investigated the role of rs6746030 in the prediction of post-operative pain following gynaecological laparoscopic surgery. The presence of the minor allele of the SNP resulted in a higher Numerical Rating Score [18].

Other SNP's investigated have been less researched. rs11898284 has been shown to be associated with increased heat pain sensitivity [19]. Patients who carry the minor allele of rs11898284 appear to have worse outcomes after total knee arthroplasty [20].

One issue with research in SCN9A is the low frequency of some of the mutations investigated. This would mean that a large number of patients would need to be enrolled in a study to see any difference, especially in homozygous carriers of these mutations.

2.2 KCNS1

Potassium voltage-gated channels do not participate directly in signal transduction but are important in modulating the resting membrane potential. In this way, these channels either facilitate or inhibit an action potential from being generated [21].

Kcns1 is a Kv9.1 channel subunit, which is electrically silent on its own, but modulates channel properties when combined with other potassium channels [22, 23]. This is coded for by the *KCNS1* gene, a small gene with around 11,000 base pairs found on chromosome 20 (20q13.12).

Experimental data shows that mice that lack *KCNS1* suffer from a slight increase in acute pain under normal circumstances but show an exaggerated response after nerve injury [24]. Costigan et al. [22] also explored neighbouring genes and found that nearly 80% of these were involved in membrane signalling, with nearly half of these associated with nociception. They conclude that *KCNS1* is central to many pathways that are integral to pain perception.

The most common polymorphism in *KCNS1* studied so far is rs734784, which is found in exon 5. This missense SNP is common in the general population (around 40–45%) and leads to one isoleucine amino acid being changed to a valine residue. rs734784 has been associated with increased pain in volunteers and in patients with sciatica [22].

Costigan et al. [22] looked into the pain of 151 patients a year after lumbar discectomy and found an association of greater pain with rs734784. The mutation accounted for around 5% of the variance in pain scores in these patients. The same authors also demonstrated that rs734784 was more frequent in patients who had suffered from chronic phantom pain after an amputation.

In a study of 345 women who underwent an elective hysterectomy, Hoofwijk et al. [25] found no correlation between polymorphisms of *KCNS1*, including rs734784, and CPSP at 3 and at 12 months. Similarly, in 300 patients post-mastectomy, Langford et al. [26] did not find a difference in patients with or without this SNP. Costigan et al. [22] also did not find an association between pain at 12 months following surgery and rs734783.

On the other hand, Sciberras et al. found that patients homozygous for the C allele of rs734784 had significantly less WOMAC® scores throughout the study period [20]. Clinically, this translated to a WOMAC® score of nearly 4 points less, with a similar trend in pain scores.

Such contradictory findings are common in genetic studies. Differences in methodology, such as the use of a recessive or additive model may make a difference—Sciberras et al. used a recessive model, whereas Costigan et al. employed an additive model only.

3. Modulation of pain pathways involving catecholamines

Catecholamines are integral to the modulation of nociception. Levels of noradrenaline, adrenaline and dopamine modulate the transmission of nociceptive impulses through the spinal cord [27], and affect the perception of pain in the brain [28]. For instance, in normal healthy tissue, norepinephrine has little effect. However, after injury, levels of norepinephrine may correlate with either hyperalgesia or analgesia, depending on an interplay of different receptors and neuronal pathways.

Furthermore, noradrenergic neurotransmitters such as dopamine also affect the brain itself. For instance, dopamine D-1 receptors are pronociceptive, whereas stimulation of D-2 receptors appears to be effective against tonic pain [29].

3.1 GCH1

Synthesis of catecholamines starts by uptake of tyrosine [30]. This is converted to dopamine by tyrosine hydroxylase, a process that requires tetrahydrobiopterin (BH4). This cofactor is produced by GTP cyclohydrolase 1, encoded by the *GCH1* gene which is found on chromosome 14 and measuring around 60,800 base pairs.

In rats, BH4 levels have been associated with pain, specifically neuropathic pain. Tegeder et al. [31] demonstrated how axonal injury increased the upregulation of *GCH1* and consequently levels of BH4 in primary sensory neurons. Inhibiting the increase in BH4 levels alleviated pain, whereas administering BH4 intrathecally exacerbated the pain.

In human volunteers, subjects who carried polymorphisms of *GCH1* had less pain when a topical high concentration of capsaicin was applied to their skin [32]. In this small study, *GCH1* was shown to be responsible for 35% of the inter-individual response to pain.

Tegeder et al. [31] were the first to describe a pain-protective haplotype made up of 15 polymorphisms in the *GCH1* gene. In a study of 523 patients attending a tertiary care outpatient pain centre, homozygous carriers of this haplotype spent less time on specialised pain therapy [33], although the effect was small. This might be due to the small number of patients who had this haplotype of 15 specific SNPs: only around 14% of patients carried this haplotype, with only 10 subjects being homozygous carriers. Lötsch et al. [34] later reduced this haplotype to three main polymorphisms, including rs3783641. Their work showed that two SNPs predicted the pain-protective haplotype with nearly 100% sensitivity. These SNPs were rs8007267 and rs3783641. We also note that the presence of rs3783641 without rs8007267 occurs infrequently (1.4%), as shown in **Table 1**.

Tegeder et al. [31] also showed an effect of a pain-protective haplotype on pain scores 12 months after a lumbar discectomy. 162 patients were enrolled, with successful follow-up in 147 subjects. An additive effect of the haplotype was found: patients with no copy of the haplotype fared worse, patients homozygous for the haplotype were all better, and the heterozygous patients had an intermediate response. The authors themselves note that rs3783641 and rs8007267 would have contributed most to this effect.

Kim et al. [35] also showed a protective effect of rs998259 and the above-mentioned haplotype in 69 patients after surgical treatment of lumbar disc degeneration. These patients were followed up for 12 months. Functional scores improved more in patients with the minor allele of rs998259.

Contrary to these finding, the presence of rs3783641 actually increased the odds of CPSP at 3 and at 12 months, although this was not statistically significant, in patients after elective hysterectomy [25] and in patients after a total knee arthroplasty [20].

Multiple studies were either inconclusive or showed no effect of GCH1 on CPSP [36–38]. A meta-analysis of studies involving rs3783641 concludes that any associations demonstrated so far are probably spurious [39].

SNP	Change	Haplotypes				
rs8007267*	G > A	G	G	A	G	G
rs2878172	T > C	T	T	C	C	C
rs2183080	G > C	G	G	G	C	G
rs3783641*	A > T	A	A	T	A	A
rs7147286	C > T	C	C	T	T	C
rs998259	G > A	G	A	G	G	G
rs8004445	C > A	C	C	C	A	C
rs12147422	A > G	A	A	A	G	A
rs7492600	C > A	C	C	C	A	C
rs9671371	G > A	G	G	A	G	A
rs8007201	T > C	T	T	C	T	C
rs4411417	A > G	A	A	G	A	A
rs752688	G > A	G	G	A	G	G
rs7142517	G > T	G	T	G	T	G
rs10483639*	C > G	C	C	G	C	C
		31.5%	19.8%	14.6%	9.7%	7.6%

Dark grey shading: pain-protective haplotype.
**SNPs investigated by Lötsch et al.*

Table 1.
Pain-protective haplotype of GCH1, as per Tegeder et al. [31].

3.2 COMT

The *COMT* gene on chromosome 22 codes for the enzyme Catechol-O-MethylTransferase (COMT). This enzyme metabolises catecholamine neurotransmitters (dopamine, epinephrine and norepinephrine), by adding a methyl group [40]. COMT itself has been extensively studied as a possible therapeutic target, most notably in Parkinsonism.

The human *COMT* gene was first described by Tenhunen et al. [41]. It contains six exons, spanning over around 27,000 base pairs. Two promoters control the transcription of the gene into two different mRNA: MB-COMT and S-COMT. The former is found predominantly in brain neurones, whereas the latter is found more in other tissues such as the liver, kidney and blood.

Over 8000 single point mutations in the *COMT* gene are currently known. The fours most commonly studied in CPSP are rs4680, rs4633, rs4818 and rs6929.

The rs4680 mutation, also known as the Val 158 Met polymorphism has been extensively studied. rs4680 causes a structural change in the COMT enzyme, which lowers enzymatic activity. Hence, patients with the A variant will be able to metabolise catecholamines at a slower rate. The two variants are co-dominant, so heterozygous individuals will have an intermediate activity level [42]. It has been implicated in more severe low back pain [43], in patients with multiple sclerosis [44], and also in predicting the opioid consumption after surgery [45]. In the case of total knee replacements, Thomazeau et al. [46] found that the rs4680 mutation was more frequent (83%) in patients reporting chronic postsurgical pain, compared with 64% in the other patients. This conferred an odds risk ratio of 3.42 upon multivariate analysis.

Similar to rs4680, rs4633 affects COMT enzyme activity, although polymorphism at this site is not associated with structural changes of the enzyme itself. The T allele is associated with lower COMT activity, and the C allele with the higher COMT activity.

rs4818 is not associated with any structural changes, but polymorphism at this allele is associated with even more variation of the COMT enzyme when compared to rs4680. Patients who are homozygous for the G variant will have increased enzymatic activity. Heterozygous individuals will have intermediate activity, and homozygous individuals with the C variant will have the least enzymatic activity [47].

With regards to CPSP, the evidence for *COMT* is still somewhat inconclusive. Wang et al. [48] did not find a relationship between CPSP and the genotype of women who had undergone a caesarean section, but the number of patients with CPSP was admittedly small. On the other hand, in patients after TKA, Thomazeau et al. [46] found a borderline significance between the rs4680 A allele and chronic pain, with an odds ratio of 3.2, but the authors comment that the study was most likely underpowered to find significant differences. Rut et al. [49] demonstrated a protective association of the minor allele of rs4633 (T) in patients one year after a lumbar discectomy. However, the same study showed that the G allele of rs4680 was associated with a better outcome, not the minor A allele as in other studies. It is could be that COMT variations may have a different effect on different types of surgeries.

COMT polymorphisms are increasingly being researched as a haplotype, using rs6269, rs4633, rs4818 and rs4680 respectively as a haploblock: a region on a gene that has tends to be inherited as a whole. Diatchenko et al. [50] were the first to observe that these four polymorphisms produced seven haplotypes that had a frequency of more than 0.5%, as shown in **Table 2**. The most common three haplotypes account for over 95% of all haplotypes: these are the GCGG, ATCA and ACCG haplotypes. Patients with the GCGG haplotype possess the rs4818 mutation only, and these patients would have the highest COMT activity. Hence GCGG is classically defined as the Low Pain Sensitivity (LPS) haplotype. Conversely, ACCG is associated with the lowest COMT activity and is defined as the High Pain Sensitivity (HPS) haplotype. Finally, the ATCA haplotype confers intermediate COMT activity and is defined as the Average Pain Sensitivity (SPS) haplotype [52].

For instance, Zhang et al. showed that patients with the haplotype ACCG had a higher fentanyl consumption than in patients with the haplotypes GCGG or ATCA [52]. This effect was not seen when individual SNP's were analysed.

rs6269	rs4633	rs4818	rs4680	COMT activity	Pain	Frequency (%)
G	C	G	G	High	Least pain	36.8
A	T	C	A	Intermediate	Intermediate	54.6
G	C	C	G	Low	Most pain	7.0
A	C	C	A	Unknown	Unknown	1.7

Adapted from [51].

Table 2.
Various haplotypes of the COMT gene, with relative COMT activity.

Contrary to the observations by Diatchenko [50], Sciberras et al. found that the TCA haplotype was linked to lower pain scores [20]. This was a different cohort of patients, and indeed in a similar group of patients, Rut et al. [49] found that rs4633 showed a protective effect. Another study of 69 patients after lumbar spinal surgery, this time by Dai et al. [53], also found that patients with the T allele for rs4633 had better functional outcomes after twelve months. Furthermore, the ATCA haplotype was associated with better outcomes. On the other hand, Machoy-Mokryńska et al. [54] observed higher levels of pain with the TCA haplotype.

One limitation of most studies is the lack of correlation between genetic polymorphism and enzymatic activity. This has been done by Dharaniprasad et al. [55], in 216 patients after cardiac surgery. rs4680 was associated with a 14-fold lower activity in COMT activity. Indeed, patients with this polymorphism all developed CPSP.

4. Pharmacogenetic response to analgesics

Genetics also play a role in the individual response to analgesics, through changes in receptors involved in nociception, or through changes in enzymes involved in the metabolism of these analgesics.

4.1 OPRM1

The MOP receptor, previously known as the μ-opioid receptor, is a G-coupled protein receptor that binds to endomorphins and endorphins [56]. Activation of the receptor leads to reduced cAMP intracellularly which causes a hyperpolarisation of the cell membrane [57]. The MOP receptor is mainly present in the central nervous system, especially in the periaqueductal grey zone. This is involved in descending inhibitory pathways that act on second-order neurons in the spinal cord to reduce nociception and hence induce analgesia.

The *OPRM1* gene resides on the long arm of chromosome 6, and it is about 230,000 base pairs long over 18 exons [58]. Given the large size of the gene, it is not surprising that there are 3324 documented polymorphisms of the *OPRM1* gene. Only 1395 of these variants have a minor allele frequency greater than 1% [59, 60].

The most commonly investigated variant is rs1799971, a mutation in exon 1 of *OPRM1*. The change of residue 40 from asparagine to aspartic acid creates a novel CpG-methylation site that prevents the upregulation of *OPRM1* [56]. This change results in a three-fold increase in the binding of β-endorphin compared to the wild-type receptor [61]. One would expect that this would mean that subjects with rs1799971 would have an augmented response to opioids, but in fact, the opposite seems to be true. Lötsch et al. [62] demonstrated that the pupils constricted less in patients with the G allele and that this response was related to the number of G alleles.

rs1799971, also known as the A118G mutation, is frequently found in Asian populations (40–60%), less so in European populations (around 15%) and very infrequently in populations of African American descent (4%) [63]. It has been linked to a poor response to opiates in several studies, both in cancer pain and postoperatively. It has also been linked to alcoholism.

Other polymorphisms also show a strong association with pain sensitivity, although more work needs to be done to confirm such findings. Shabalina et al. [58] investigated 30 candidate SNPs over *OPRM1*, focussing on polymorphisms in exons and promoter genes. With nearly 200 Caucasian subjects, the authors showed that rs563649 and the rs2075572- rs533586 haplotype were associated with pain sensitivity. Furthermore, they showed that morphine produced less analgesia in subjects with at least one copy of rs563649, although statistical significance was not reached.

4.2 OPRK1 gene

The KOP receptor mediates analgesia without causing respiratory depression [64]. Indeed, although all opioids act on MOP receptors, some opioids such as morphine and oxycodone exhibit some activity also on KOP receptors.

The primary ligand to KOP is dynorphin, which induces analgesia. The KOP receptor is widely distributed in the central nervous system, including in the spinal cord and brainstem [65]. Dynorphin is emerging as an important factor in the development of chronic pain [66]. The pain appears to induce an increase in dynorphin levels in the spinal cord, as shown by Wagner et al. [67] in a neuropathic pain model in rats. This increase in dynorphin occurred 21 days after injury and was observed bilaterally in the spinal cord. It is not clear if such a consequence further augments chronic pain, or if this is protective [68]. Dynorphin injected intrathecally induces analgesia, but it has only been tested in animal models—unfortunately, it is associated with paralysis of the hind limbs when used in this manner. Caudle et al. postulate that dynorphin may act to reduce pain in the initial phases of injury: this effect has also been seen in knockout mice who had the KOP receptors deleted [69]. Such mice exhibited increased hyperalgesia after injury.

The gene that encodes for the KOP receptor is the *OPRK1*, which is present on 8q11.23. The human gene has been characterised only in 2004, and it is the gene responsible for the KOP opioid receptor [70]. It is 26,000 base pairs long on chromosome 8, spread over 4 exons.

Literature on *OPRK1* polymorphisms and pain development is still scarce. One possible candidate polymorphism would be rs6985606, but most of such literature reflects research on opioid dependence [71] and on the analgesic response to opioids. rs6985606 has been shown to be a risk factor for pre-operative pain in a study of women with breast cancer who underwent breast surgery [72].

For instance, Kringel et al. [73] explored the use of a number of biomarkers that could be used to identify patients requiring high doses of opioids. Nine potential SNP's in the *OPRK1* gene were flagged for future research. However, Sciberras et al. [20] could not find any association between rs6985606 and CPSP in a cohort of orthopaedic patients.

5. Potential use in clinical practice

So far, there is little evidence of the use of genomic testing for CPSP in clinical practice. However, this has been done for other conditions, including pharmacogenetic-guided treatment of pain post-operatively (PGx). Senagore et al. reviewed the use of PGx in a series of patients, and found better pain scores and lower use of opioids in patients who had received pharmacogenetic testing prior to surgery [74].

Given that conclusive polymorphisms that predict CPSP with confidence are still to be determined, it might be difficult to recommend a specific panel of assays for pre-operative evaluation. However, the techniques in genotyping are continuously being refined, and automated batch-testing is possible. Furthermore, the costs of such testing is becoming more commercially-viable, so it may be possible in the near future to test individual patients for a number of polymorphisms and calculate a predicted risk of CPSP.

The clinical impact of such information is still debatable. CPSP is difficult to treat, and may resolve spontaneously with time. However, if a patient is identified as having a high risk of developing CPSP, one may refer such cases to a dedicated chronic pain clinic for follow-up and treatment.

6. Conclusion

Genetic factors appear to be important in predicting the individual progression from acute to chronic post-surgical pain. However, the exact impact and the interplay between different combinations of polymorphisms are still to be determined.

Author details

Stephen Sciberras
University of Malta, Msida, Malta

*Address all correspondence to: stephen.sciberras@um.edu.mt

References

[1] James S. Human pain and genetics: Some basics. British Journal of Pain. 2013;7:171-178. DOI: 10.1177/2049463713506408

[2] Durland J, Ahmadian-Moghadam H. Genetics. Mutagenesis. In: StatPearls [Internet]. Treasure Island, Florida: StatPearls Publishing; 2023. Available from: https://www.ncbi.nlm.nih.gov/books/NBK560519/

[3] Catterall WA, Goldin AL, Waxman SG. International Union of Pharmacology. XLVII. Nomenclature and structure-function relationships of voltage-gated sodium channels. Pharmacological Reviews. 2005;**57**:397-409. DOI: 10.1124/pr.57.4.4

[4] Cummins TR, Howe JR, Waxman SG. Slow closed-state inactivation: A novel mechanism underlying ramp currents in cells expressing the hNE/PN1 sodium channel. The Journal of Neuroscience. 1998;**18**:9607-9619

[5] McKerrall SJ, Sutherlin DP. Nav1.7 inhibitors for the treatment of chronic pain. Bioorganic & Medicinal Chemistry Letters. 2018;**28**:3141-3149. DOI: 10.1016/j.bmcl.2018.08.007

[6] Raymond CK, Castle J, Garrett-Engele P, Armour CD, Kan Z, Tsinoremas N, et al. Expression of alternatively spliced sodium channel alpha-subunit genes. Unique splicing patterns are observed in dorsal root ganglia. Journal of Biological Chemistry. 2004;**279**:46234-46241. DOI: 10.1074/jbc.M406387200

[7] Reimann F, Cox JJ, Belfer I, Diatchenko L, Zaykin DV, McHale DP, et al. Pain perception is altered by a nucleotide polymorphism in SCN9A. Proceedings of the National Academy of Sciences of the United States of America. 2010;**107**:5148-5153. DOI: 10.1073/pnas.0913181107

[8] Hisama FM, Dib-Hajj SD, Waxman SG. SCN9A neuropathic pain syndromes. In: GeneReviews®. Seattle, Washington: University of Washington; 1993. PMID: 20301342

[9] Drissi I, Woods WA, Woods CG. Understanding the genetic basis of congenital insensitivity to pain. British Medical Bulletin. 2020;**133**:65-78. DOI: 10.1093/bmb/ldaa003

[10] Wallace RH, Wang DW, Singh R, Scheffer IE, George AL Jr, Phillips HA, et al. Febrile seizures and generalized epilepsy associated with a mutation in the Na^+–channel beta1 subunit gene SCN1B. Nature Genetics. 1998;**19**(4):366-370. DOI: 10.1038/1252. PMID: 9697698

[11] Lossin C, Wang DW, Rhodes TH, Vanoye CG, George AL Jr. Molecular basis of an inherited epilepsy. Neuron. 2002;**34**(6):877-884. DOI: 10.1016/S0896-6273(02)00714-6. PMID: 12086636

[12] Zhang T, Chen M, Zhu A, Zhang X, Fang T. Novel mutation of SCN9A gene causing generalized epilepsy with febrile seizures plus in a Chinese family. Neurological Sciences. 2020;**41**:1913-1917. DOI: 10.1007/s10072-020-04284-x

[13] Chen C-H, Huang Y-S, Fang T-H. Involvement of rare mutations of SCN9A, DPP4, ABCA13, and SYT14 in schizophrenia and bipolar disorder. International Journal of Molecular Sciences. 2021;**22**(24):13189. DOI: 10.3390/ijms222413189. PMID: 34947986. PMCID: PMC8709054

[14] Fertleman CR, Baker MD, Parker KA, Moffatt S, Elmslie FV, Abrahamsen B,

et al. SCN9A mutations in paroxysmal extreme pain disorder: Allelic variants underlie distinct channel defects and phenotypes. Neuron. 2006;**52**:767-774. DOI: 10.1016/j.neuron.2006.10.006

[15] Zhong Q, Chen X, Zhao Y, Liu R, Yao S. Association of Polymorphisms in pharmacogenetic candidate genes with propofol susceptibility. Scientific Reports. 2017;7:3343. DOI: 10.1038/s41598-017-03229-3

[16] Estacion M, Harty TP, Choi J-SS, Tyrrell L, Dib-Hajj SD, Waxman SG. A sodium channel gene SCN9A polymorphism that increases nociceptor excitability. Annals of Neurology. 2009;**66**:862-866. DOI: 10.1002/ana.21895

[17] Kurzawski M, Rut M, Dziedziejko V, Safranow K, Machoy-Mokrzynska A, Drozdzik M, et al. Common missense variant of SCN9A gene is associated with pain intensity in patients with chronic pain from disc herniation. Pain Medicine. 2018;**19**:1010-1014. DOI: 10.1093/pm/pnx261

[18] Duan G, Xiang G, Guo S, Zhang Y, Ying Y, Huang P, et al. Genotypic analysis of SCN9A for prediction of postoperative pain in female patients undergoing gynecological laparoscopic surgery. Pain Physician. 2016;**19**:E151-E162

[19] Duan G, Guo S, Zhang Y, Ying Y, Huang P, Wang Q, et al. The effect of SCN9A variation on basal pain sensitivity in the general population: An experimental study in young women. The Journal of Pain: Official Journal of the American Pain Society. 2015;**16**:971-980. DOI: 10.1016/j.jpain.2015.06.011

[20] Sciberras S. The effect of regional anaesthesia and genetic factors on the development of chronic pain following total knee arthroplasty [Doctoral thesis]. Hosted on Open Access Repository, University of Malta; 2022. Available from: https://www.um.edu.mt/library/oar/handle/123456789/106920

[21] Tsantoulas C, McMahon SB. Opening paths to novel analgesics: The role of potassium channels in chronic pain. Trends in Neurosciences. 2014;**37**:146-158. DOI: 10.1016/j.tins.2013.12.002

[22] Costigan M, Belfer I, Griffin RS, Dai F, Barrett LB, Coppola G, et al. Multiple chronic pain states are associated with a common amino acid-changing allele in KCNS1. Brain. 2010;**133**:2519-2527. DOI: 10.1093/brain/awq195

[23] Bocksteins E. Kv5, Kv6, Kv8, and Kv9 subunits: No simple silent bystanders. The Journal of General Physiology. 2016;**147**:105-125. DOI: 10.1085/jgp.201511507

[24] Tsantoulas C, Denk F, Signore M, Nassar MA, Futai K, McMahon SB. Mice lacking Kcns1 in peripheral neurons show increased basal and neuropathic pain sensitivity. Pain. 2018;**159**:1641-1651. DOI: 10.1097/j.pain.0000000000001255

[25] Hoofwijk DMN, Reij RRI, Rutten BPF, Kenis G, Theunissen M, Joosten EA, et al. Genetic polymorphisms and prediction of chronic post-surgical pain after hysterectomy—A subgroup analysis of a multicenter cohort study. Acta Anaesthesiologica Scandinavica. 2019;**63**:1063-1073. DOI: 10.1111/aas.13413

[26] Langford DJ, Paul SM, West CM, Dunn LB, Levine JD, Kober KM, et al. Variations in potassium channel genes are associated with distinct trajectories of persistent breast pain after breast cancer surgery. Pain. 2015;**156**:371-380. DOI: 10.1097/01.j.pain.0000460319.87643.11

[27] Takano Y, Yaksh TL. Characterization of the pharmacology of intrathecally administered alpha-2 agonists and antagonists in rats. The Journal of Pharmacology and Experimental Therapeutics. 1992;**261**:764-772

[28] Jarcho JM, Mayer EA, Jiang ZK, Feier NA, London ED. Pain, affective symptoms, and cognitive deficits in patients with cerebral dopamine dysfunction. Pain. 2012;**153**:744-754. DOI: 10.1016/j.pain.2012.01.002

[29] Wood PB. Role of central dopamine in pain and analgesia. Expert Review of Neurotherapeutics. 2008;**8**:781-797. DOI: 10.1586/14737175.8.5.781

[30] Fernstrom JD, Fernstrom MH. Tyrosine, phenylalanine, and catecholamine synthesis and function in the brain. Journal of Nutrition. 2007;**137**:1539S-1547S; discussion 1548S. DOI: 10.1093/jn/137.6.1539S

[31] Tegeder I, Costigan M, Griffin RS, Abele A, Belfer I, Schmidt H, et al. GTP cyclohydrolase and tetrahydrobiopterin regulate pain sensitivity and persistence. Nature Medicine. 2006;**12**:1269-1277. DOI: 10.1038/nm1490

[32] Campbell CM, Edwards RR, Carmona C, Uhart M, Wand G, Carteret A, et al. Polymorphisms in the GTP cyclohydrolase gene (GCH1) are associated with ratings of capsaicin pain. Pain. 2009;**141**:114-118. DOI: 10.1016/j.pain.2008.10.023

[33] Doehring A, Freynhagen R, Griessinger N, Zimmermann M, Sittl R, von Hentig N, et al. Cross-sectional assessment of the consequences of a GTP Cyclohydrolase 1 haplotype for specialized tertiary outpatient pain care. The Clinical Journal of Pain. 2009;**25**:781-785. DOI: 10.1097/AJP.0b013e3181b43e12

[34] Lötsch J, Belfer I, Kirchhof A, Mishra BK, Max MB, Doehring A, et al. Reliable screening for a pain-protective haplotype in the GTP Cyclohydrolase 1 gene (GCH1) through the use of 3 or fewer single nucleotide polymorphisms. Clinical Chemistry. 2007;**53**:1010-1015. DOI: 10.1373/clinchem.2006.082883

[35] Kim DH, Dai F, Belfer I, Banco RJ, Martha JF, Tighiouart H, et al. Polymorphic variation of the guanosine triphosphate Cyclohydrolase 1 gene predicts outcome in patients undergoing surgical treatment for lumbar degenerative disc disease. Spine (Phila Pa 1976). 2010;(35):1909-1914. DOI: 10.1097/Brs.0b013e3181eea007

[36] Hickey OT, Nugent NF, Burke SM, Hafeez P, Mudrakouski AL, Shorten GD. Persistent pain after mastectomy with reconstruction. Journal of Clinical Anesthesia. 2011;**23**:482-488. DOI: 10.1016/j.jclinane.2011.01.009

[37] Belfer I, Dai F, Kehlet H, Finelli P, Qin L, Bittner R, et al. Association of functional variations in COMT and GCH1 genes with postherniotomy pain and related impairment. Pain. 2015;**156**:273-279. DOI: 10.1097/01.j.pain.0000460307.48701.b0

[38] Montes A, Roca G, Sabate S, Lao JI, Navarro A, Cantillo J, et al. Genetic and clinical factors associated with chronic postsurgical pain after hernia repair, hysterectomy, and thoracotomy. Anesthesiology. 2015;**122**:1123-1141. DOI: 10.1097/ALN.0000000000000611

[39] Chidambaran V, Gang Y, Pilipenko V, Ashton M, Ding L. Systematic review and meta-analysis of genetic risk of developing chronic postsurgical pain. The Journal of Pain. 2020;**21**:2-24. DOI: 10.1016/j.jpain.2019.05.008

[40] Boussetta S, Cherni L, Pakstis AJ, Ben Salem N, Elkamel S,

Khodjet-El-Khil H, et al. Usefulness of COMT gene polymorphisms in north African populations. Gene. 2019;**696**:186-196. DOI: 10.1016/j.gene.2019.02.021

[41] Tenhunen J, Salminen M, Lundström K, Kiviluoto T, Savolainen R, Ulmanen I. Genomic organization of the human catechol O-methyltransferase gene and its expression from two distinct promoters. European Journal of Biochemistry. 1994;**223**:1049-1059. DOI: 10.1111/j.1432-1033.1994.tb19083.x

[42] Lachman HM, Papolos DF, Saito T, Yu YM, Szumlanski CL, Weinshilboum RM. Human catechol-O-methyltransferase pharmacogenetics: Description of a functional polymorphism and its potential application to neuropsychiatric disorders. Pharmacogenetics. 1996;**6**:243-250. DOI: 10.1097/00008571-199606000-00007

[43] Jacobsen LM, Schistad EI, Storesund A, Pedersen LM, Rygh LJ, Røe C, et al. The COMT rs4680 met allele contributes to long-lasting low back pain, sciatica and disability after lumbar disc herniation. European Journal of Pain. 2012;**16**:1064-1069. DOI: 10.1002/j.1532-2149.2011.00102.x

[44] Fernández-de-las-Peñas C, Ambite-Quesada S, Ortíz-Gutiérrez R, Ortega-Santiago R, Gil-Crujera A, Caminero AB. Catechol-O-methyltransferase Val158Met polymorphism (rs4680) is associated with pain in multiple sclerosis. The Journal of Pain: Official Journal of the American Pain Society. 2013;**14**:1719-1723. DOI: 10.1016/j.jpain.2013.09.007

[45] Candiotti KA, Yang Z, Buric D, Arheart K, Zhang Y, Rodriguez Y, et al. Catechol-o-methyltransferase polymorphisms predict opioid consumption in postoperative pain. Anesthesia and Analgesia. 2014;**119**:1194-1200. DOI: 10.1213/ANE.0000000000000411

[46] Thomazeau J, Rouquette A, Martinez V, Rabuel C, Prince N, Laplanche J-L, et al. Predictive factors of chronic post-surgical pain at 6 months following knee replacement: Influence of postoperative pain trajectory and genetics. Pain Physician. 2016;**19**:E729-E741

[47] Barbosa FR, Matsuda JB, Mazucato M, de Castro FS, Zingaretti SM, da Silva LM, et al. Influence of catechol-O-methyltransferase (COMT) gene polymorphisms in pain sensibility of Brazilian fibromialgia patients. Rheumatology International. 2012;**32**:427-430. DOI: 10.1007/s00296-010-1659-z

[48] Wang LZ, Wei CN, Xiao F, Chang XY, Zhang YF. Incidence and risk factors for chronic pain after elective caesarean delivery under spinal anaesthesia in a Chinese cohort: A prospective study. International Journal of Obstetric Anesthesia. 2018;**34**:21-27. DOI: 10.1016/j.ijoa.2018.01.009

[49] Rut M, Machoy-Mokrzyńska A, Ręcławowicz D, Słoniewski P, Kurzawski M, Droździk M, et al. Influence of variation in the catechol-O-methyltransferase gene on the clinical outcome after lumbar spine surgery for one-level symptomatic disc disease: A report on 176 cases. Acta Neurochirurgica. 2014;**156**:245-252. DOI: 10.1007/s00701-013-1895-6

[50] Diatchenko L, Slade GD, Nackley AG, Bhalang K, Sigurdsson A, Belfer I, et al. Genetic basis for individual variations in pain perception and the development of a chronic pain condition. Human Molecular Genetics. 2005;**14**:135-143. DOI: 10.1093/hmg/ddi013

[51] Roten LT, Fenstad MH, Forsmo S, Johnson MP, Moses EK, Austgulen R, et al. A low COMT activity haplotype is associated with recurrent preeclampsia in a Norwegian population cohort (HUNT2). Molecular Human Reproduction. 2011;**17**:439-446. DOI: 10.1093/molehr/gar014

[52] Zhang F, Tong J, Hu J, Zhang H, Ouyang W, Huang D, et al. COMT gene haplotypes are closely associated with postoperative fentanyl dose in patients. Anesthesia and Analgesia. 2015;**120**:933-940. DOI: 10.1213/ANE.0000000000000563

[53] Dai F, Belfer I, Schwartz CE, Banco R, Martha JF, Tighioughart H, et al. Association of catechol-O-methyltransferase genetic variants with outcome in patients undergoing surgical treatment for lumbar degenerative disc disease. Spine Journal. 2010;**10**:949-957. DOI: 10.1016/j.spinee.2010.07.387

[54] Machoy-Mokrzyńska A, Starzyńska-Sadura Z, Dziedziejko V, Safranow K, Kurzawski M, Leźnicka K, et al. Association of COMT gene variability with pain intensity in patients after total hip replacement. Scandinavian Journal of Clinical and Laboratory Investigation. 2019;**79**:202-207. DOI: 10.1080/00365513.2019.1576920

[55] Dharaniprasad G, Samantaray A, Srikanth L, Hanumantha Rao M, Chandra A, Sarma PVGK. Chronic persistent surgical pain is strongly associated with COMT alleles in patients undergoing cardiac surgery with median sternotomy. General Thoracic and Cardiovascular Surgery. 2020;**68**:1101-1112. DOI: 10.1007/s11748-020-01321-6

[56] Crist RC, Berrettini WH. Pharmacogenetics of OPRM1. Pharmacology, Biochemistry, and Behavior. 2014;**123**:25-33. DOI: 10.1016/j.pbb.2013.10.018

[57] McDonald J, Lambert D. Opioid receptors. Continuing Education in Anaesthesia Critical Care & Pain. 2005;**5**:22-25. DOI: 10.1093/bjaceaccp/mki004

[58] Shabalina SA, Zaykin DV, Gris P, Ogurtsov AY, Gauthier J, Shibata K, et al. Expansion of the human mu-opioid receptor gene architecture: Novel functional variants. Human Molecular Genetics. 2009;**18**:1037-1051. DOI: 10.1093/hmg/ddn439

[59] The 1000 genomes project consortium. A global reference for human genetic variation. Nature. 2015;**526**:68-74. DOI: 10.1038/nature15393

[60] Spampinato SM. Overview of genetic analysis of human opioid receptors. Methods in Molecular Biology. 2015;**1230**:3-12. DOI: 10.1007/978-1-4939-1708-2_1

[61] Bond C, LaForge KS, Tian M, Melia D, Zhang S, Borg L, et al. Single-nucleotide polymorphism in the human mu opioid receptor gene alters beta-endorphin binding and activity: Possible implications for opiate addiction. Proceedings of the National Academy of Sciences of the United States of America. 1998;**95**:9608-9613. DOI: 10.1073/pnas.95.16.9608

[62] Lötsch J, Skarke C, Grösch S, Darimont J, Schmidt H, Geisslinger G. The polymorphism A118G of the human mu-opioid receptor gene decreases the pupil constrictory effect of morphine-6-glucuronide but not that of morphine. Pharmacogenetics. 2002;**12**:3-9. DOI: 10.1097/00008571-200201000-00002

[63] Levran O, Kreek MJ. Population-specific genetic background for the

OPRM1 variant rs1799971 (118A>G): Implications for genomic medicine and functional analysis. Molecular Psychiatry. 2021;**26**:3169-3177. DOI: 10.1038/s41380-020-00902-4

[64] Pathan H, Williams J. Basic opioid pharmacology: An update. British Journal of Pain. 2012;**6**:11-16. DOI: 10.1177/2049463712438493

[65] Cahill CM, Taylor AM, Cook C, Ong E, Morón JA, Evans CJ. Does the kappa opioid receptor system contribute to pain aversion? Frontiers in Pharmacology. 2014;**5**:253. DOI: 10.3389/fphar.2014.00253. PMID: 25452729. PMCID: PMC4233910

[66] Podvin S, Yaksh T, Hook V. The emerging role of spinal dynorphin in chronic pain: A therapeutic perspective. Annual Review of Pharmacology and Toxicology. 2016;**56**:511-533. DOI: 10.1146/annurev-pharmtox-010715-103042

[67] Wagner R, DeLeo JA, Coombs DW, Willenbring S, Fromm C. Spinal dynorphin immunoreactivity increases bilaterally in a neuropathic pain model. Brain Research. 1993;**629**:323-326. DOI: 10.1016/0006-8993(93)91339-t

[68] Caudle RM, Mannes AJ. Dynorphin: Friend or foe? Pain. 2000;**87**:235-239. DOI: 10.1016/S0304-3959(00)00360-2

[69] Schepers RJ, Mahoney JL, Gehrke BJ, Shippenberg TS. Endogenous kappa-opioid receptor systems inhibit hyperalgesia associated with localized peripheral inflammation. Pain. 2008;**138**:423-439. DOI: 10.1016/j.pain.2008.01.023

[70] Yuferov V, Fussell D, LaForge KS, Nielsen DA, Gordon D, Ho A, et al. Redefinition of the human kappa opioid receptor gene (OPRK1) structure and association of haplotypes with opiate addiction. Pharmacogenetics. 2004;**14**:793-804. DOI: 10.1097/00008571-200412000-00002

[71] Crist RC, Clarke T-K, Berrettini WH. Pharmacogenetics of opioid use disorder treatment. CNS Drugs. 2018;**32**:305-320. DOI: 10.1007/s40263-018-0513-9

[72] Aouizerat B, Kober K, Levine J, Paul S, Cooper B, Schmidt B, et al. (269) variations in opioid receptor genes are associated with breast pain in women prior to and with mild and severe persistent breast pain after breast cancer surgery. The Journal of Pain. 2015;**16**:S43. DOI: 10.1016/j.jpain.2015.01.186

[73] Kringel D, Ultsch A, Zimmermann M, Jansen J-P, Ilias W, Freynhagen R, et al. Emergent biomarker derived from next-generation sequencing to identify pain patients requiring uncommonly high opioid doses. The Pharmacogenomics Journal. 2017;**17**:419-426. DOI: 10.1038/tpj.2016.28

[74] Senagore AJ, Champagne BJ, Dosokey E, Brady J, Steele SR, Reynolds HL, et al. Pharmacogenetics-guided analgesics in major abdominal surgery: Further benefits within an enhanced recovery protocol. The American Journal of Surgery. 2017;**213**:467-472. DOI: 10.1016/j.amjsurg.2016.11.008

Chapter 15

Recent Advances in Electroanalysis Techniques Used for Morphine in Managing Postoperative Pain

Mamta Latwal and Ganesh Panday

Abstract

Determination of a particular drug in pharmaceutical preparations and biological fluids is critically important in pharmaceutical and medical sciences to avoid its overdose. Effective analysis requires sensitivities at ppb level or even less in the biological fluids with high selectivity. Morphine is a potent analgesic drug that is used to relieve severe pains like postoperative pain, labor pain, and cardiac pain. It is a μ-opioid agonist which acts directly on the central nervous system to relieve pain. It is very important to monitor the doses of morphine in the patient's body under examination since the overdose may cause disruption to the central nervous system. As the applications of analytical instruments are progressing, modern electrochemical methods are attracting interest for the analysis of therapeutic agents or their metabolites in medical samples since these methods are economic and can detect extremely low concentrations approximately 10 ng/ml. A review of the principles and application of modern electroanalytical techniques, namely, cyclic voltammetry, differential pulse voltammetry, square wave voltammetry, and amperometry, is presented. The use and advantages of these techniques at different electrodes for the detection of morphine have been discussed. The analytical applications of these techniques to pharmaceutical compounds in dosage forms and biological media are also discussed.

Keywords: morphine, drug, electroanalysis, electrocatalytic oxidation, sensor

1. Introduction

Morphine is a narcotic analgesic drug mainly used for the relief of postoperative pain, cardiac pain, pain of childbirth, and terminal cancers. It is one among the 50 different alkaloids present in opium and poppy derivatives. It is the active metabolite derived from heroin (3,6-diacetylmorphine). Morphine is a μ-opioid agonist which acts directly on the central nervous system to relieve pain [1]. Consequently, it can cause disruption to the central nervous system if not used properly. The minimum lethal dose is 200 mg but in case of hypersensitivity 60 mg can bring sudden death. In the case of drug addiction, 2–3 g/day can be tolerated [2]. Therefore, the determination of concentration of morphine in the patient's body is a very important issue.

Morphine is a benzylisoquinoline alkaloid with two additional ring closures. It has a rigid pentacyclic structure consisting of a benzene ring, two partially unsaturated cyclohexane rings, a piperidine ring and a tetrahydrofuran ring. The structure of morphine is given in **Figure 1**. The first three rings make the phenanthrene ring system which has little conformational flexibility. There are two hydroxyl functional groups (a phenolic –OH and an allylic –OH), an ether linkage, a basic 3o-amine function, and 5 centers of chirality with morphine exhibiting a high degree of stereoselectivity of analgesic action.

Morphine is metabolized into morphine-3-glucuronide (M3G) and morphine-6-glucuronide (M6G). The metabolism of morphine occurs not only in the liver but may also take place in the brain and the kidneys. The glucuronides are mainly eliminated via bile and urine. A highly polar metabolite that is unable to pass the blood-brain barrier is glucuronides. Although morphine glucuronidation in human brain tissue has been shown, the capability is much lower than in the liver. This shows that morphine glucuronides, despite their high polarity, can enter the brain and that the M3G and M6G concentrations detected in the cerebrospinal fluid (CSF) following systemic injection represent hepatic metabolism of morphine [3].

Moreover, it has been found that there has been a significant increase in morphine-related crimes in recent years. More and more people have started taking this drug including youngsters. Drug-related crime has been a serious worldwide problem. Therefore, there is an urgent demand to develop a rapid and sensitive analytical method for prohibiting the overuse of morphine as well as its determination in pharmaceutical and clinical samples. Traditional analytical methods like gas chromatography (GC), high-performance liquid chromatography (HPLC), mass spectrometry (MS), etc. have been developed for the determination of morphine. This concentration of drug can be detected by HPLC [4–6] as well as GC-MS in urine samples [7]. However, these methods need expensive equipment and professional operators, which may not satisfy the needs of modern drug prohibition programs. The development of simple, convenient, highly sensitive, versatile, fast, and economic techniques is very necessary to control the overuses of this drug causing many side effects. Recently, electroanalytical methods have been widely used for the analysis of

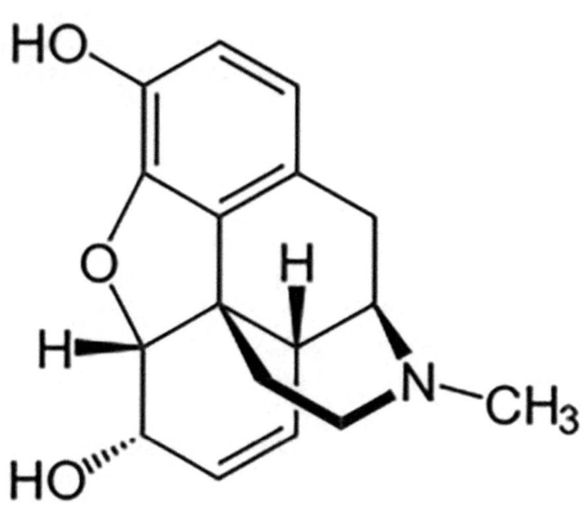

Figure 1.
Structure of morphine.

morphine. Different methods in electroanalytical techniques have been discussed in this chapter for the detection of morphine in clinical samples.

2. Postoperative pain relievers

The effective relief of pain to a patient undergoing surgery is of extreme importance as it has substantial physiological benefits. Reducing pain with a minimum amount of side effects is the main goal of postoperative pain relievers. Various agents (opioid vs. nonopioid), routes (oral, intravenous, neuraxial, regional), and modes (patient controlled vs. "as needed") are available for the treatment of postoperative pain. Despite years of advances in pain management, the mainstay of postoperative pain therapy in many settings is still opioids. Opioids bind to receptors in the central nervous system and peripheral tissues and modulate the effect of the nociceptors [8].

Moderate to severe pain, either acute or chronic, is among the conditions for which morphine sulfate is FDA approved. Morphine, which is most frequently used in pain management, significantly reduces pain in individuals [9]. The management of palliative/end-of-life care, ongoing cancer treatment, and vaso-occlusive pain during sickle cell crises are clinical scenarios that benefit greatly from morphine medication [10]. The off-label use of morphine is common for practically any painful disease. When patients in the emergency room do not respond to first- and second-line medications for musculoskeletal pain, stomach discomfort, chest pain, arthritis, and even migraines, morphine is administered [11].

In a certain case study, 280 individuals undergoing various types of surgery, including thoracic, upper, and lower abdominal, perineal, obstetric, and orthopedic procedures, were evaluated for postoperative pain alleviation. Through an indwelling epidural catheter, morphine (2/4 mg) was administered following the procedure. Only 3.5% of patients reported being unsatisfied, compared to 87% who had excellent analgesia. In 30% of cases, a single injection provided total pain relief for the whole postoperative time. The remaining patients had a mean analgesic duration of 10.7 hours (SD ± 4.3). Although the immediate effect after 4-mg doses may well involve systemic reactions due to rapid vascular uptake of morphine from the spinal fluid, plasma morphine concentrations obtained after 2-mg doses suggest a localized spinal action as the basis for the lengthy duration of analgesia [12].

3. Electroanalysis of morphine

Few electroanalytical methods have been identified by researchers for the determination of morphine. The mechanism of electrochemical oxidation of morphine has been shown in **Figure 2**. The electrochemical oxidative comportment of morphine in aqueous solution was very helpful to predict the oxidation peaks of this drug. The anodic peaks obtained in the voltammogram are due to the oxidation of phenolic and tertiary amine groups present. It has also been verified that a weak peak obtained is due to the formation of a dimer in phenolic group oxidation but not due to further oxidation of pseudomorphine [13].

The electroanalytical methods include amperometry, differential pulse voltammetry (DPV), square wave voltammetry, and cyclic voltammetry (CV). These methods have been critically reviewed in this chapter.

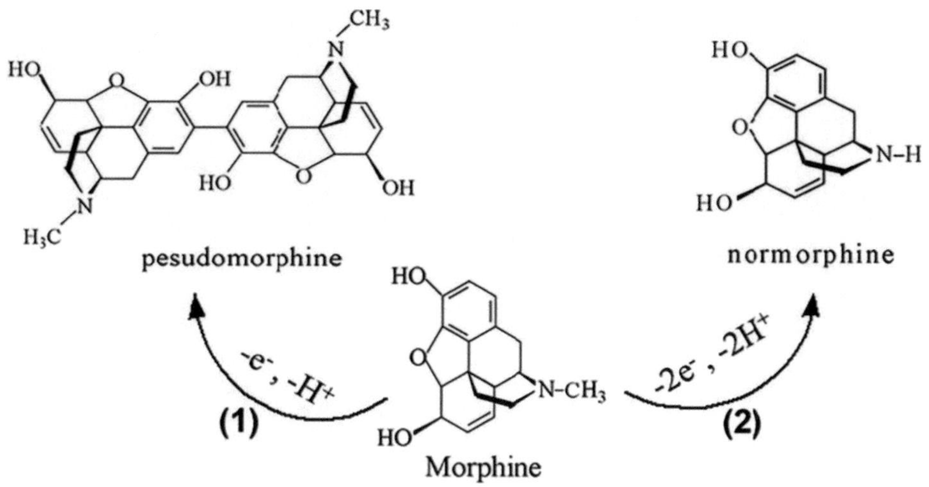

Figure 2.
Electrochemical oxidation of morphine.

3.1 Amperometry

In this electroanalytical technique, an indicator (working electrode) is subjected to a constant reducing or oxidizing potential, and the resulting steady-state current is recorded. This method can be used to detect electroactive chemicals in the solution because the measured current's amplitude frequently varies on the concentration of the reduced or oxidized component. A small number of researchers have used it to find morphine in biological samples that were spiked or real.

A relatively stable and highly sensitive cobalt hexacyanoferrate-modified electrode was employed for the first time to study the pharmacokinetics of morphine in rat brain after an intravenous administration of morphine (25 mg/kg). The peak current was linearly related to the morphine concentration in the range of 1.0×10^{-6} M–5.0×10^{-4} M at +0.60 V (vs. Ag/AgCl) with a detection limit of 5.0×10^{-7} M [14]. Another highly sensitive and durable sensor for amperometric determination of morphine has been reported using CNT [15]. A glassy carbon electrode (preheated at 50°C for 5 min) was modified with multiwalled carbon nanotubes (MWCNTs) by simply rubbing electrode surface on filter paper powdered with CNT. This modified electrode showed its potential as a selective and sensitive electrocatalyst for the determination of morphine with a detection limit of 0.2 μM in concentration range 0.5–150 μM and sensitivity of 10 nA/μM. The amperometric response of the modified electrode was found to be incredibly stable over a continuous operation of 30 min. This proves the electrocatalytic potential of CNT-modified GC electrode for sensing morphine.

Molecularly imprinted polymers (MIP) have also been employed for morphine detection [16, 17]. For synthesizing molecular imprinted polymer, monomer with specific functional group is made to interact with a template and then polymerized with thermally/UV stimulated initiators. An electrode modified with MIP particles within the conducting poly(3,4-ethylenedioxythiophene) polymer, PEDOT (MIP/PEDOT-modified electrode), which immobilizes particles onto an indium tin oxide (ITO) glass has been prepared as presented in **Figure 3**. This modified electrode showed good capability for amperometric detection of morphine in terms of sensitivity, operating potential, and reproducibility of the MIP/PEDOT-modified

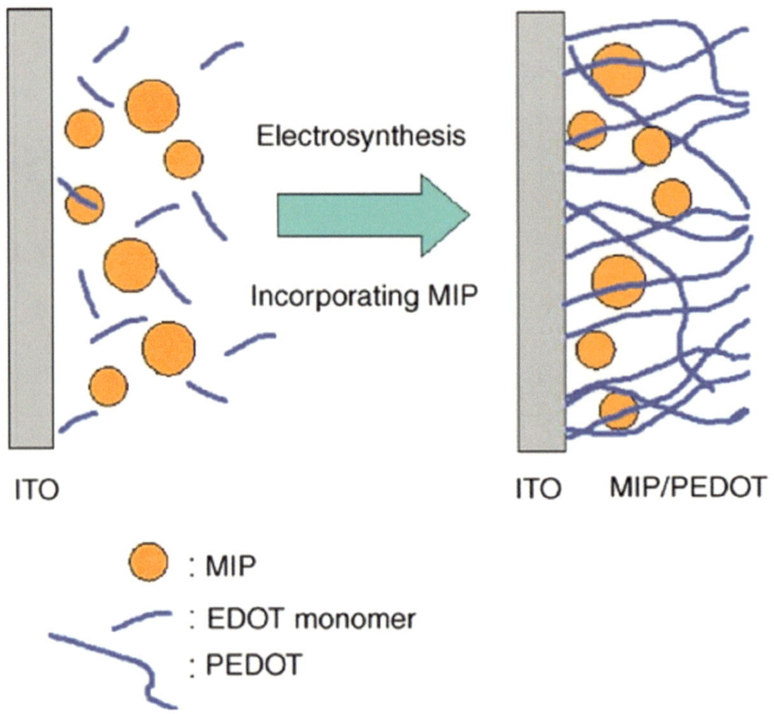

Figure 3.
Schematic for the preparation of the MIP/PEDOT-modified electrode [16].

electrode [16]. On the other hand, PEDOT has been applied as electroactive film onto the surface of electrode and the intended amperometric sensor showed a sensitivity of 91.86 μA/cm^2 per mM with a detection limit of 0.2 mM for morphine detection [17].

In another unique method, the electrooxidation pathway for morphine was first investigated in neutral medium (pH = 6), then hydrodynamic amperometry was used for the determination of morphine using Prussian blue film-modified palladized aluminum electrode. Result showed that the detection limit of this method was about 0.8 μM with a linear concentration range 2–50 μM which was less efficient than the above reported one [18].

3.2 Differential pulse voltammetry

In DPV, short pulses with limited amplitude are superimposed upon a staircase waveform. This method can provide improved selectivity for observing different redox processes than other voltammetric methods. Various results have shown good sensitivity for the detection of morphine when the DPV method was used for electroanalysis [19, 20]. In few cases, typical electrochemical cells can be replaced with contracted screen-printed electrochemical strips for sensors that have proven to be of great potential in application areas like pharmaceutical, environmental, and food analysis applications. These screen-printed electrodes provide a simple, inexpensive, and user-friendly path of electrochemical measurements. However, for the electroanalysis of drug residuals in biological fluids, particularly in the case of drug abuse, low concentration of drug residuals, interferences of other electroactive biological species, fouling the electrode's surface, and sample amount limitations are the major difficulties. These challenges can be overcome by using electromembrane extraction (EME) before electroanalysis on screen printed strips. This method has been developed for morphine to quantify its concentration in urine samples. DPV peak current at 0.18 V was selected as the signal and the calibration curve which was plotted by the variation of DPV currents as a function of morphine concentration was linear within the range of 0.005–2.0 μg/mL. The limit of detection and the limit of quantification were 0.0015 (S/N = 3) and 0.005 μg/mL, respectively [21]. Another type of screen-printed electrode containing metal sulfide nanosheets modified graphite has been found able to determine morphine simply and effectively at concentration levels encountered in toxicology and doping. Results indicated linear response in a concentration range between 0.05 and 600.0 μM of morphine with 0.03 μM limit of detection [22].

A screen-printed electrode modified by electrochemically exfoliated graphene oxide has shown good potential for detecting morphine in real samples [23]. Synthetic and real urine samples with a maintained pH of 6.6 and 7.0, respectively, were taken with added concentration of morphine. The modified electrode exhibited a high-performance sensing ability with sensitivity of 2.61 nA/μM and a detection limit of 2.5 μM. The voltammetric response of modified electrode with different concentrations of morphine has been shown in **Figure 4**.

Real sample analysis has been performed for measuring the potential of synthesized material for the detection of morphine [24]. Urine samples of drug-addicted patients were taken for this study where the sample was collected after 5 h from the last abuse. This sample was firstly centrifuged and then the supernatant was filtered and

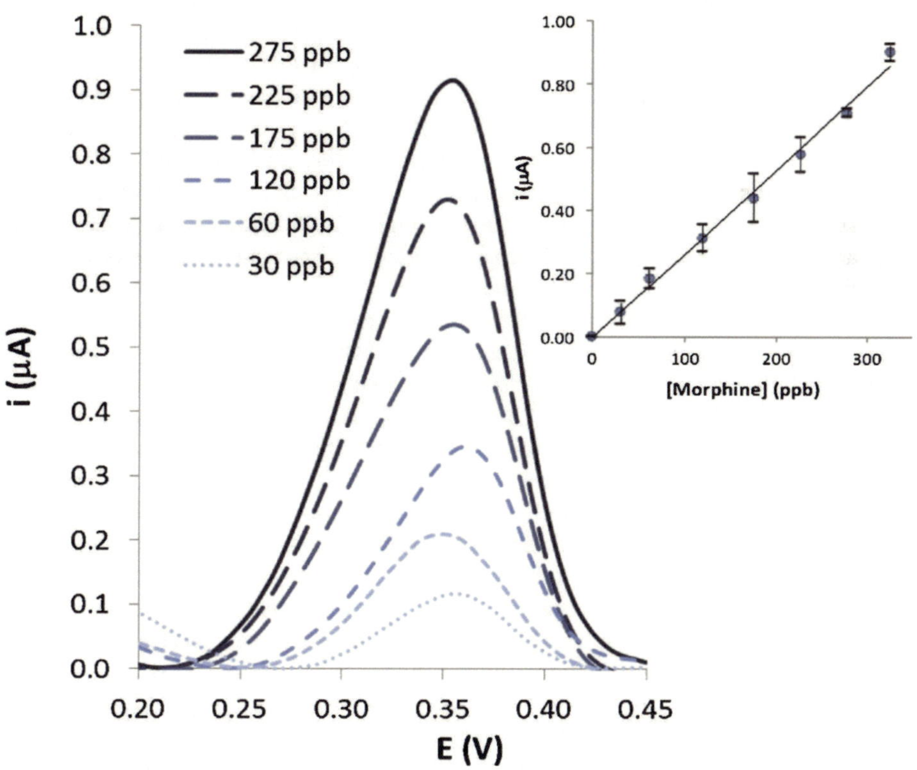

Figure 4.
Differential pulse voltammogram for different morphine concentrations [23].

hydrolyzed before electrochemical analysis. Currently, urine samples are frequently used to assess drug usage. Diacetylmorphine, which is heroin, is converted to morphine in urine samples. Heroin quickly deacetylates to 6-monoacetylmorphine (6-MAM), which has a potency of about six times that of morphine. More deacetylation of 6-MAM results in the formation of morphine. Concentration of morphine to codeine in urine of heroin abusers is therefore analyzed. MWCNTs/SnO_2–Zn_2SnO_4 modified carbon paste electrodes have shown promising potential for detection of morphine and codeine in urine samples. Under optimum conditions, the fabricated electrode showed wide linear ranges from 0.1 to 310.0 μM for morphine oxidation and from 0.1 to 600.0 μM for codeine oxidation. The electrochemical performance was better with a detection limit of 0.009 μM in real samples than other working electrodes with satisfactory recoveries [24].

Under optimized conditions, a sensitive and selective voltammetric sensor has been developed for the detection of morphine. This method used MWCNTs and polydopamine to modify the GC electrode. Electrocatalytic efficiency was evaluated using DPV that showed the potential of modified electrode for the determination of morphine in human plasma and urine samples with a liner dynamic range of 0.075–75.0 μM and detection limit of 0.06 μM [25]. A portable device containing such a sensible and disposable sensor needs to be developed to control drug abuse by persons at work and during driving.

3.3 Square wave voltammetry

Square wave voltammetry is a form of linear potential sweep voltammetry that uses a combined square wave and staircase potential applied to a stationary electrode. Studies on electroanalytical methods for detection of morphine have also been carried out using square wave voltammetry. Many materials, individually and as composites, have been investigated by researchers that can be used for sensing morphine concentration. In a particular study, MWCNTs, MIP, and gold nanoparticles have been employed for modification of pencil graphite electrodes. Under optimized conditions of several effective parameters, the calibration curve by square wave voltammetry was linear in two linear domains, over the range of 0.008–5 μM vs. Ag/AgCl, and the detection limit was 2.9 nM [26]. The aforesaid electrochemical sensor was successfully applied for MO determination in real samples such as human urine and plasma.

As discussed in the previous subsection 2.2, screen-printed electrodes have shown great potential as sensors. An immunosensor based on graphene screen-printed electrode modified with gold nanoparticles has been reported for morphine detection [27]. After modification of electrode with gold nanoparticles, cysteamine was also self-assembled on electrode surface via thiol interaction to introduce terminal amino groups to the electrode surface. The electrodes were then used to fabricate the immunosensor by covalent immobilization of antibodies against morphine. This sensor worked because of a competition between morphine and the morphine-bovine serum albumin conjugate for the immobilized antibodies on the sensor surface and the resulting change in the square wave voltammetry reduction current using the hexacyanoferrate system as an electrochemical probe. A sensitive and selective detection of morphine in the concentration range 0.1–100 ng/mL with a detection limit of 90 pg/mL was obtained. This method was also applied for the determination of morphine in spiked saliva samples and showed high recoveries. Such a sensitive determination method for morphine is of great interest for public health.

Recently, iron tungstate ($FeWO_4$) has been used for developing an electrochemical sensor for sub micromolar detection of morphine [28]. The effect of iron-tungsten

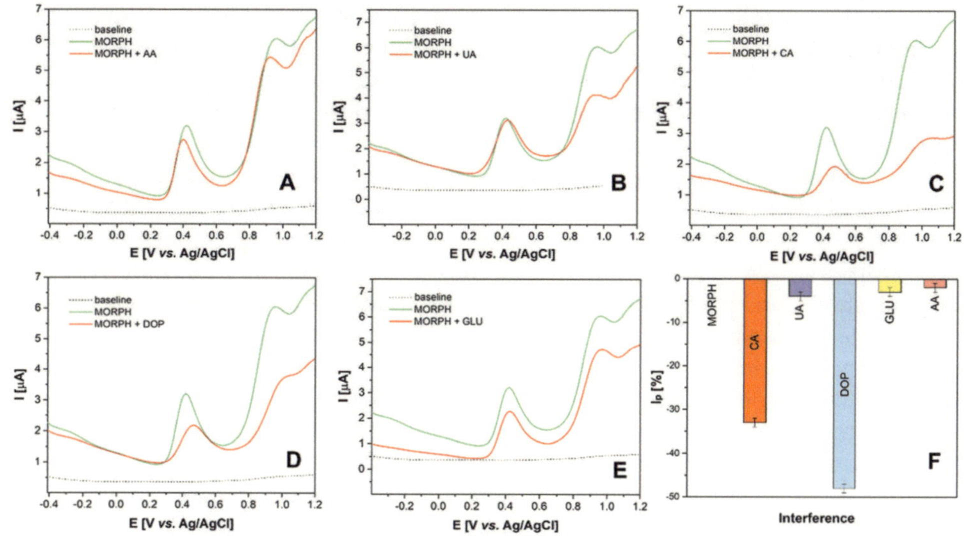

Figure 5.
Square wave voltammograms of morphine at Fe1W3@CPE in absence (green line) and presence (red line) of (A) ascorbic acid (AA); (B) uric acid (UA); (C) citric acid (CA); (D) dopamine (DOP); (E) glucose (GLU); and (F) peak current signal (%) before and after addition of interferents [28].

ratio has been extensively studied for achieving the best possible characteristics and Fe_1W_3 with 7.5% of modifier in carbon paste electrode showed the best results. The limit of detection of this modified electrode was 0.58 μM and limit of quantification was 1.94 μM. The linear operating range was between 5 and 85 μM of morphine in the Britton-Robinson buffer solution at pH 8. The developed electrode resulted in good selectivity and excellent repeatability when applied in real biological samples like human urine. Selectivity of the method is a crucial parameter for the application in real-word sample analysis. To investigate this, the possibility for the detection of 50 μM of morphine was investigated in the presence of ascorbic acid, uric acid, citric acid, dopamine, and glucose under optimized conditions. The results of square wave voltammetric studies in the presence and absence of the above-mentioned interferents have been shown in **Figure 5**. The oxidation potential of morphine and other alkaloids, that can be present in urine samples were obtained at different potentials. As found in the literature, morphine and alkaloids are simultaneously determined. The developed electrochemical sensor has appeared to be a suitable competitor for efficient, precise, and accurate monitoring of morphine in biological fluids [28]. There are studies that show the detection of morphine with codeine by the researchers [29, 30].

3.4 Cyclic voltammetry

To get both qualitative and quantitative data regarding electrochemical reactions, CV, a potentiodynamic electrochemical technique, is frequently used. During a CV measurement, the working electrode's potential in relation to the reference electrode is determined in the system under investigation, and the potential is scanned back and forth between predetermined higher and lower limits. The current flowing between the working electrode and the counter electrode is monitored concurrently. CV has been used by several researchers for determination of morphine using modified electrodes [31–34].

Due to their excellent redox mediator properties, some metal hexacyanoferrates have been used for the development of electroanalytical methods for detection of morphine [14, 16]. In the above cases, the cyclic voltammograms of the modified electrode showed the presence of well-defined redox peaks. We have also studied the electrocatalytic potential of synthesized cadmium hexacyanoferrate-CNT nanocomposite for oxidation of morphine [35]. The synthesized material can be drop cast over the surface of glassy carbon electrode which remains stable with no significant loss in electrocatalytic activity up to 10 days. This voltammetric sensor worked well in spiked urine samples with a detection limit of 0.21 μM that confirms that this modified electrode will show good performance for the determination of morphine in human urine fluid samples. Few electrochemical sensors have also been developed that can measure the concentration of morphine in urine samples but due to high detection limit they will show less sensitivity than others [36]. A ZnO/CNT nanocomposite modified carbon paste electrode showed linear range for morphine determination from 0.1 to 700 μmol/L and the detection limit was calculated as 0.06 μmol/L [37].

A simple and sensitive voltammetric sensor has been reported for simultaneous determination of Morphine (Mp) and Buprenorphine (Bp) [38]. The complete method has been described graphically in **Figure 6**. It involved embedment of rhodium nanoparticles in a carbon matrix followed by its carbonization. Then after the composite was cast over the surface of GCE for its voltammetric characterization. The modified glassy carbon electrode with rhodium nanoparticles-mesoporous carbon composite showed high potential for simultaneous determination of Morphine (Mp) and Buprenorphine (Bp), with a linear range and limit of detection of 0.1–20 μM and

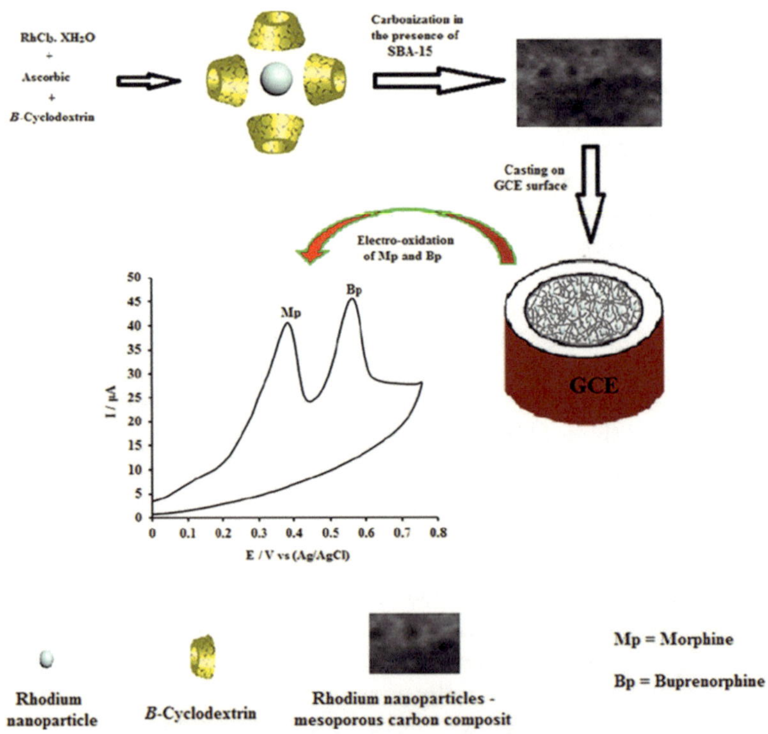

Figure 6.
Cyclic voltammetric determination of morphine (Mp) and buprenorphine (Bp) [38].

40 nM, respectively for morphine, and these data were obtained about 0.1–14 μM and 45 nM, respectively, for buprenorphine. This method involved easy and fast preparation with high efficiency as a sensor [38].

4. Conclusion

Diversity of electrochemical sensors developed for the detection of morphine is presented in this chapter. Efforts are being made by researchers to develop a simple, sensitive, economical, and accurate electroanalytical method for the determination of morphine which can be used for pharmaceutical and clinical applications. One of the major challenges is the selection of electrode material that is responsible for limit of detection and sensitivity. For designing a potential sensor, molecular-level understanding of the correlation between the surface structure and reactivity is very important factor which governs the selectivity and sensitivity. Future studies in this area should be more focused on understanding interfacial reaction kinetics to design novel sensors suitable for use in all practical applications.

Acknowledgements

The University of Petroleum and Energy Studies, Dehradun is gratefully acknowledged for supporting the present work. This research did not receive any specific grant from funding agencies in the public, commercial, or not-for-profit sectors.

Conflict of interest

The authors declare no conflict of interest.

Author details

Mamta Latwal[1*] and Ganesh Panday[2]

1 Department of Chemistry, University of Petroleum and Energy Studies, Dehradun, Uttarakhand, India

2 School of Agriculture, Dev Bhoomi Uttarakhand University, Dehradun, Uttarakhand, India

*Address all correspondence to: mamta.latwal@gmail.com

References

[1] Stjernswärd J. WHO cancer pain relief programme. Cancer Surveys. 1988;**7**:195-208

[2] Macchiarelli L, Arbarello P, Bondi GC, di Luca NM, Feola T. Medicina Legale (compendio). II ed. Turin, Italy: Minerva Medica Publications; 2002

[3] Christrup LL. Morphine metabolites. Acta Anaesthesiologica Scandinavica. 1997;**41**(1-2):116-122. DOI: 10.1111/j.1399-6576.1997.tb04625.x PMID: 9061094

[4] Todd RD, Muldoon SM, Watson RL. Determination of morphine in cerebrospinal fluid and plasma by high-performance liquid chromatography with electrochemical detection. Journal of Chromatography. B, Biomedical Sciences and Applications. 1982;**232**:101-110

[5] Rashid BA, Aherne GW, Katmeh MF, Kwasowski P, Stevenson D. Determination of morphine in urine by solid-phase immunoextraction and high-performance liquid chromatography with electrochemical detection. Journal of Chromatography. A. 1998;**797**:245-250

[6] Baciu T, Borrull F, Aguilar C, Calull M. Recent trends in analytical methods and separation techniques for drugs of abuse in hair. Analytica Chimica Acta. 2015;**856**:1-26. DOI: 10.1016/j.aca.2014.06.051

[7] Meatherall R. GC-MS confirmation of codeine, morphine, 6-acetylmorphine, hydrocodone, hydromorphone, oxycodone, and oxymorphone in urine. Journal of Analytical Toxicology. 1999;**23**:177-186

[8] Garimella V, Cellini C. Postoperative pain control. Clinics in Colon and Rectal Surgery. 2013;**26**(3):191-196. DOI: 10.1055/s-0033-1351138

[9] Hosseininejad SM, Mohammadian AM, Bozorgi F, Montazar SH, Firouzian A, Moosazadeh M, et al. Does co-treatment with ultra-low-dose naloxone and morphine provide better analgesia in renal colic patients? The American Journal of Emergency Medicine. 2019;**37**(6):1025-1032

[10] Murphy PB, Bechmann S, Barrett MJ. Morphine. In: StatPearls [Internet]. Treasure Island, FL: StatPearls Publishing; 2022. Available from: https://www.ncbi.nlm.nih.gov/books/NBK526115/

[11] Barut GA, Tunç M, Şahin Ş, Ulus F, Sazak H. Effects of epidural morphine and levobupivacaine combination before incision and after incision and in the postoperative period on thoracotomy pain and stress response. Turkish Journal of Medical Sciences. 2018;**48**(4):716-723

[12] Rawal N, Sjöstrand U, Dahlström B. Postoperative pain relief by epidural morphine. Anesthesia and Analgesia. 1981;**60**(10):726-731

[13] Garrido JMPJ, Delerue-Matos C, Borges F, Macedo TRA, Oliveira-Brett AM. Voltammetric oxidation of drugs of abuse I. Morphine and Metabolites. Electroanalysis. 2004;**16**:1419-1426. DOI: 10.1002/elan.200302966

[14] Xu F, Gao M, Wang L, Zhou T, Jin L, Jin J. Amperometric determination of morphine on cobalt hexacyanoferrate modified electrode in rat brain microdialysates. Talanta. 2002;**58**(3):427-432. DOI: 10.1016/S0039-9140(02)00312-0

[15] Salimi A, Hallaj R, Khayatian GR. Amperometric detection of morphine at preheated glassy carbon electrode modified with multiwall carbon nanotubes. Electroanalysis. 2005;**17**:873-879. DOI: 10.1002/elan.200403166

[16] Ho KC, Chen CY, Hsu HC, Chen LC, Shiesh SC, Lin XZ. Amperometric detection of morphine at a Prussian blue-modified indium tin oxide electrode. Biosensors & Bioelectronics. 2004;**20**(1):3-8. DOI: 10.1016/j.bios.2003.11.027

[17] Yeh W, Ho KC. Amperometric morphine sensing using a molecularly imprinted polymer-modified electrode. Analytica Chimica Acta. 2005;**542**(1):76-82. DOI: 10.1016/j.aca.2005.01.071

[18] Pournaghi-Azar MH, Saadatirad A. Simultaneous voltammetric and amperometric determination of morphine and codeine using a chemically modified-palladized aluminum electrode. Journal of Electroanalytical Chemistry. 2008;**624**(1-2):293-298. DOI: 10.1016/j.jelechem.2008.09.016

[19] Niazi A, Ghasemi J, Zendehdel M. Simultaneous voltammetric determination of morphine and noscapine by adsorptive differential pulse stripping method and least-squares support vector machines. Talanta. 2007;**74**:247-254

[20] Alipour E, Gasemlou S. Easy modification of pencil graphite electrode for discrimination and determination of morphine in biological and street samples. Analytical Methods. 2012;**4**:2962-2969

[21] Ahmar H, Tabani H, Koruni MH, Davarani SSH, Fakhari AR. A new platform for sensing urinary morphine based on carrier assisted electromembrane extraction followed by adsorptive stripping voltammetric detection on screen-printed electrode. Biosensors & Bioelectronics. 2014;**54**:189-194. DOI: 10.1016/j.bios.2013.10.035

[22] Baezzat MR, Tavakkoli N, Zamani H. Construction of a new electrochemical sensor based on MoS2 nanosheets modified graphite screen printed electrode for simultaneous determination of diclofenac and morphine. Analytical and Bioanalytical Chemistry Research. 2022;**9**(2):153-162

[23] Maccaferri G, Terzi F, Xia Z, Vulcano F, Liscio A, Palermo V, et al. Highly sensitive amperometric sensor for morphine detection based on electrochemically exfoliated graphene oxide. Application in screening tests of urine samples. Sensors and Actuators B: Chemical. 2019;**281**:739-745. DOI: 10.1016/j.snb.2018.10.163

[24] Taei M, Hasanpour F, Hajhashemi V, Movahedi M, Baghlani H. Simultaneous detection of morphine and codeine in urine samples of heroin addicts using multi-walled carbon nanotubes modified SnO2–Zn2SnO4 nanocomposites paste electrode. Applied Surface Science. 2016;**363**:490-498. DOI: 10.1016/j.apsusc.2015.12.074

[25] Sabeti M, Ensafi AA, Rezaei B. Polydopamine-modified MWCNTs-glassy carbon electrode, a selective electrochemical morphine sensor. Electroanalysis. 2021;**33**:2286

[26] Rezaei B, Foroughi-Dehnavi S, Ensafi AA. Fabrication of electrochemical sensor based on molecularly imprinted polymer and nanoparticles for determination trace amounts of morphine. Ionics. 2015;**21**:2969-2980. DOI: 10.1007/s11581-015-1458-3

[27] Eissa S, Zourob M. Competitive voltammetric morphine immunosensor using a gold nanoparticle decorated graphene electrode. Microchimica Acta. 2017;**184**:2281-2289. DOI: 10.1007/s00604-017-2261-9

[28] Ognjanović M, Nikolić K, Bošković M, Pastor F, Popov N, Marciuš M, et al. Electrochemical determination of morphine in urine samples by tailoring FeWO4/CPE sensor. Biosensors. 2022;**12**:932. DOI: 10.3390/bios12110932

[29] Wester N, Mynttinen E, Etula J, Lilius T, Kalso E, Kauppinen EI, et al. Simultaneous detection of morphine and codeine in the presence of ascorbic acid and uric acid and in human plasma at nafion single-walled carbon nanotube thin-film electrode. ACS Omega. 2019;**4**:17726-17734

[30] Bagheri H, Khoshsafar H, Afkhami A, Amidi S. Sensitive and simple simultaneous determination of morphine and codeine using a Zn2SnO4 nanoparticle/graphene composite modified electrochemical sensor. New Journal of Chemistry. 2016;**40**:7102-7112

[31] Jahani PM, Mohammadi SZ, Khodabakhshzadeh A, Cha JH, Asl MS, Shokouhimehr M, et al. Simultaneous detection of morphine and diclofenac using graphene nanoribbon modified screen-printed electrode. International Journal of Electrochemical Science. 2020;**15**(9):9037-9048

[32] Norouzi P, Ganjali RM, Moosavi-movahedi AA, Larijani B. Fast Fourier transformation with continuous cyclic voltammetry at an Au microelectrode for the determination of morphine in a flow injection system. Talanta. 2007;**73**:54-61

[33] Li F, Song J, Gao D, Zhang Q, Han D, Niu L. Simple and rapid voltammetric determination of morphine at electrochemically pretreated glassy carbon electrodes. Talanta. 2009;**79**(3):845-850. DOI: 10.1016/j.talanta.2009.05.011

[34] Li F, Song J, Shan C, Gao D, Xu X, Niu L. Electrochemical determination of morphine at ordered mesoporous carbon modified glassy carbon electrode. Biosensors & Bioelectronics. 2010;**25**:1408-1413

[35] Ali SR, Chandra P, Latwal M, Jain SK, Bansal VK. Growth of cadmium hexacyanidoferrate(III) nanocubes and its application in voltammetric determination of morphine. Bulletin of the Chemical Society of Japan. 2011;**84**(12):1355-1361

[36] Aliabadi A, Rounaghi GH. A novel electrochemical sensor for determination of morphine in a sub-microliter of human urine sample. Journal of Electroanalytical Chemistry. 2019;**832**:204-208. DOI: 10.1016/j.jelechem.2018.10.052

[37] Afsharmanesh E, Karimi-Maleh H, Pahlavan A, Vahedi J. Electrochemical behavior of morphine at ZnO/CNT nanocomposite room temperature ionic liquid modified carbon paste electrode and its determination in real samples. Journal of Molecular Liquids 2013;181:8-13. https://doi.org/10.1016/j.molliq.2013.02.002

[38] Jahanbakhshi M. In situ synthesis of rhodium nanoparticles - Mesoporous carbon hybrid via a novel and facile nanocasting method for simultaneous determination of morphine and buprenorphine. Materials Science and Engineering: C. 2019;**97**:479-485. DOI: 10.1016/j.msec.2018.12.019

Chapter 16

Integrating the Numerical Pain Rating Scale (NPRS) with an Eye Tracker: Feasibility and Initial Validation

Yoram Braw, Motti Ratmansky and Itay Goor-Aryeh

Abstract

This chapter details the integration of a Numerical Rating Scale ($NPRS_{ETI}$) with a portable eye tracker, enabling the assessment of pain in conditions in which verbal communication and use of hands are limited (e.g., advanced Amyotrophic lateral sclerosis, ALS). After detailing the construction of the $NPRS_{ETI}$, we describe its validation in an outpatient pain clinic. More specifically, thirty chronic pain patients performed the $NPRS_{ETI}$ and filled a conventional NPRS (order was pseudo-randomized). Eye movements, including gaze direction and additional eye movement measures (e.g., saccade rate), were recorded, while participants rated their pain using the $NPRS_{ETI}$. The study's findings indicated no significant differences in pain severity ratings of the $NPRS_{ETI}$ and conventional NPRS. Notably, ratings using the two scales were highly correlated (r = 0.99). $NPRS_{ETI}$'s ratings were also strongly associated with participants' currently experienced pain rating using the Brief Pain Inventory (BPI). The findings provide initial proof of concept for integrating conventional pain rating scales with an eye tracker and validate the $NPRS_{ETI}$ compared with the well-validated and commonly used NPRS. Enhanced usability and decreasing costs of eye trackers will ease the additional research mandated to validate these preliminary findings and hopefully advance their integration into clinical practice.

Keywords: pain, evaluation, numerical pain rating scale, eye movements, validation

1. Introduction

An accurate assessment of pain is the basis for the treatment of pain in a systematic manner [1]. However, pain is a subjective experience that is challenging to evaluate in a clinical setting [2, 3]. Unidimensional pain scales were developed as a quick and efficient method to assess a vital aspect of the subjective experience of pain, its intensity [4]. They are well-established and extensively used in the clinical care of wide-ranging patient populations [5–7] and ages [8, 9]. As noted in a recent review, they are quick to administer and do not encroach on the time required for usual care [7]. Unidimensional pain scales, however, have several limitations. In addition to

IntechOpen

requiring intact comprehension, they necessitate a graphomotor response or speech production for the patient to input their response. While some physical limitations may be overcome (e.g., using nurse-administered pain scales [10]), others present a more formidable challenge. For example, pain was not consistently evaluated in Amyotrophic Lateral Sclerosis (ALS) studies despite its prevalence [11], partially due to using instruments that were not adapted to ALS-related impairment [12]. Other conditions, such as mechanically ventilated patients [13], also necessitate adapted pain assessment methods.

Eye tracking technology allows us to capture and record an individual's gaze and other key eye movement measures [14]. It was implemented in studying cognitive functioning and process in diverse academic fields such as industrial engineering, marketing, and psychology [15]. More recently, eye movement analysis was also used to enhance clinical practice and effort that coincides with the growing exploration of biomarkers in various neuropsychiatric disorders [16, 17]. Eye movements offer two advantages for assessing pain. First, eye movement-directed pain scales may allow patients to provide pain ratings without a motor activity (i.e., use of the patient's hands) or verbal response. In other words, an eye tracker may be used to input their ratings; individuals use their gaze as they would use a computer mouse or other means of responding (e.g., marking with a pencil or providing a verbal response). Challenging medical patients may particularly benefit from such human-computer interactive systems. For example, Ull, Weckwerth [18] assessed the technology's utility for treating mechanically ventilated patients in an intensive care unit (ICU). These patients were able to learn eye movement-directed responding to indicate their basic needs, respond to rating scales, as well as respond to quality of life and self-esteem questionnaires [18]. Similarly, eye tracking was used to control household electric appliances by ALS patients [19]. Second, eye movements indicate what the examinee is paying attention to while engaging with a task and offering a glimpse into both cognitive and processes [20, 21]. The latter are sensitive to aspects of cognitive processing (e.g., experienced cognitive load), as well as affective states such as anxiety [22]. Eye movement analysis, therefore, offers to advance clinical practice by enhancing clinicians' ability to diagnose medical conditions, especially those impacting brain functioning. For example, Tomer, Lupu [23] indicated the utility of integrating an eye tracker with the Word Memory Test (WMT), a well-established test for assessing feigning during cognitive assessments [24]. In addition to enhancing the detection of feigning when combined with conventional accuracy measures, Tomer, Lupu [23] suggested a three-stage cognitive process involved in feigning cognitive impairment. Similarly, we integrated an eye tracker with the MOXO-dCPT, an established continuous performance test (CPT) and found support for the utility of combining conventional and eye movement measures to enhance the diagnosis of ADHD and detection of feigned ADHD-associated cognitive impairment [25–27]. Overall, eye trackers-integrated medical appliances and similar novel technologies offer to provide objective psychophysiological data that may aid clinical practice, a prospect we hoped to capitalize on in the current project [28–30].

The current research project aimed to assess the utility and validity of an eye tracker-integrated Numerical Pain Rating Scale ($NPRS_{ETI}$). The conventional NPRS utilizes a paper-and-pencil format with numerals that reflect a range of pain intensities. As thoroughly reviewed earlier, it is one of the most commonly used unidimensional pain intensity scales in clinical settings, a fact that is related to its ease of administration and scoring [2, 4]. It also has higher compliance rates—particularly among older adults—than the Verbal Analog Scale (VAS), a unidimensional pain scale in which patients mark their experienced pain on a straight line with anchors at each edge. Its measurement properties are robust and well established across multiple patient populations, and it has slightly superior measurement properties—i.e., reliability, validity, and responsiveness—compared to other scales. Key figures in the field and relevant guidelines (e.g., Initiative on Methods, Measurement, and Pain Assessment in Clinical Trials; IMMPACT) recommended its use [2, 4]. Importantly, NPRS allows the patient to verbally report their pain rating without using their hands, making it amendable for integration with an eye tracker. These advantages led us to choose the NPRS for integration with an eye tracker.

The following sections will detail the construction of the $NPRS_{ETI}$ and its initial validation in an outpatient pain clinic. We compared patients' ratings using the $NPRS_{ETI}$ to those using a conventional paper-and-pencil NPRS. Ratings using the $NPRS_{ETI}$ were also compared to an NPRS embedded in the Brief Pain Inventory (BPI), correlated with key demographic and clinical variables, and qualitatively analyzed using a relative gaze duration heatmap and general eye movement measures (i.e., saccade rate and pupil size).

2. Methods

2.1 Participants

Participants were recruited from the outpatient pain unit of Tel-Hashomer Rehabilitation Hospital (N = 30). Inclusion criteria were: (a) Adult age (18 to 65). (b) Pain persisting > 3 months, based on the definition by the International Association for the Study of Pain (IASP; [31]). (c) Normal or corrected vision (candidates with a severe visual impairment such as nystagmus and hemianopsia were excluded). Exclusion criteria were: (a) Significant developmental, neuro-psychiatric disorders, or other medical conditions deemed to impair cognitive functioning and thereby impact their ability to provide pain ratings or comply with the experimental procedures (e.g., major neurocognitive disorder), according to the treating physician or electronic medical records. (b) Drug or alcohol dependence. (c) Poor comprehension of Hebrew.

The study was approved by the Tel-Hashomer Rehabilitation Hospital's Institutional Review Board (IRB) committee, with all participants signing a written informed consent form before participating in the study.

2.2 Tools

2.2.1 Construction of the numerical rating scale eye tracker-integrated ($NPRS_{ETI}$)

The $NPRS_{ETI}$ was constructed to maintain the critical characteristics of the conventional NPRS corresponded to those NPRS versions presented in the literature (e.g., [32]) with pain ratings that ranged from 0 ("no pain at all") and 10 ("unbearable pain"). The first version of the $NPRS_{ETI}$ included five stages: (a) A welcome screen requesting participant code and date of birth to minimize later errors in participant identification. (b) A screen presenting the $NPRS_{ETI}$ and the method of responding to it (i.e., gazing at the number corresponding to the pain rating will select the rating). This screen also included an illustration of the $NPRS_{ETI}$ so participants could conceptualize the scale and raise any questions regarding its use. (c) A blank screen with a black circle appearing in its center was presented. The circle followed the gaze of the participant, and the participant was instructed to experiment with moving it around the screen using their gaze. Verbal instruction was: "The marker, a black circle, indicates where you are gazing on the screen. The pain scale we presented before will soon appear again. When it appears, gaze for a few seconds at the number that best fits the pain you are currently experiencing." (d) Once the participant felt confident using the gaze-directed marker and understood the $NPRS_{ETI}$ instructions, a blank screen with a fixation cross at its center appeared. The participant was then instructed to gaze at the fixation point. (e) The actual $NPRS_{ETI}$ appeared at the center of the screen, with instructions for its use appearing in its upper section. The participant then provided their response by fixating for 250 ms on a number corresponding to their currently experienced pain intensity. The color of the box surrounding the selected rating then changed to red, indicating response selection. Next, the question "Are you confident with this choice?" and two response boxes ("Yes, I'm sure" and "No, I want to change my response") appeared at the bottom of the screen. If the participant was satisfied with their choice, a thank you screen appeared (i.e., "Thank you for participating in this study"). Otherwise, the pain rating procedure was repeated until the participant approved of their response. This initial $NPRS_{ETI}$ version was tested on six healthy participants leading us to modify the $NPRS_{ETI}$ since the program combined the eye movement data of the separate trials when participants altered their response (e.g., the $NPRS_{ETI}$ was performed twice). Five other healthy participants were assessed using this newer $NPRS_{ETI}$ version. This pretest indicated that participants tended to erroneously select a pain rating, usually "5" because the fixation point was located in the center of the screen (i.e., the location in which the $NPRS_{ETI}$ later presents the "5" pain rating). We, therefore, constructed a third and final $NPRS_{ETI}$ version in which the minimal fixation duration required for responding was set to 500 ms, thereby eliminating further errors in pain rating selection. See **Figure 1** for a diagram portraying the pain measurement process by $NPRS_{ETI}$.

2.2.2 Eye-tracking apparatus and eye movement measures

Binocular eye movements were recorded at a sampling rate of 250 Hz using the Portable Duo eye-tracking system (SR Research Ltd., Mississauga, Canada). The eye-tracking apparatus has an accuracy of approximately 0.5° and includes a host PC and display PC; the first tracks and computes participants' gaze position, and the latter displays the stimuli (i.e., the $NPRS_{ETI}$). Eye movements were analyzed using SR research event detection algorithm, widely used in academic research [33, 34] and by our research team in earlier studies [23, 25–27]. Stimuli were presented on an Alienware OptX AW2310, 23″ display screen (1920 x 1080 resolution) with a 120 Hz refresh rate. Eye-to-screen viewing distance was approximately 65 cm with the participants' eyes recorded in remote monocular mode using a designated sticker. **Figure 2** presents the experimental setup.

The participants' field of view (FoV) was divided into three areas of interest (AOIs) to assess the extent that their visual attention was directed toward the pain scale and other relevant stimuli (i.e., instructions for rating pain and anchors) vs. task-irrelevant regions: (a) *$NPRS_{ETI}$ AOI*: The AOI included the screen region in which the pain scale appeared. It was located at the center of the screen (length = 1540 pixels). Each of its squares was 140*140 pixels. (b) *Anchors AOI*: The AOI includes two regions in which the anchors of the pain scale were located ("no pain at all" and "unbearable pain"). (c) *Instructions AOI*: The region in which the $NPRS_{ETI}$

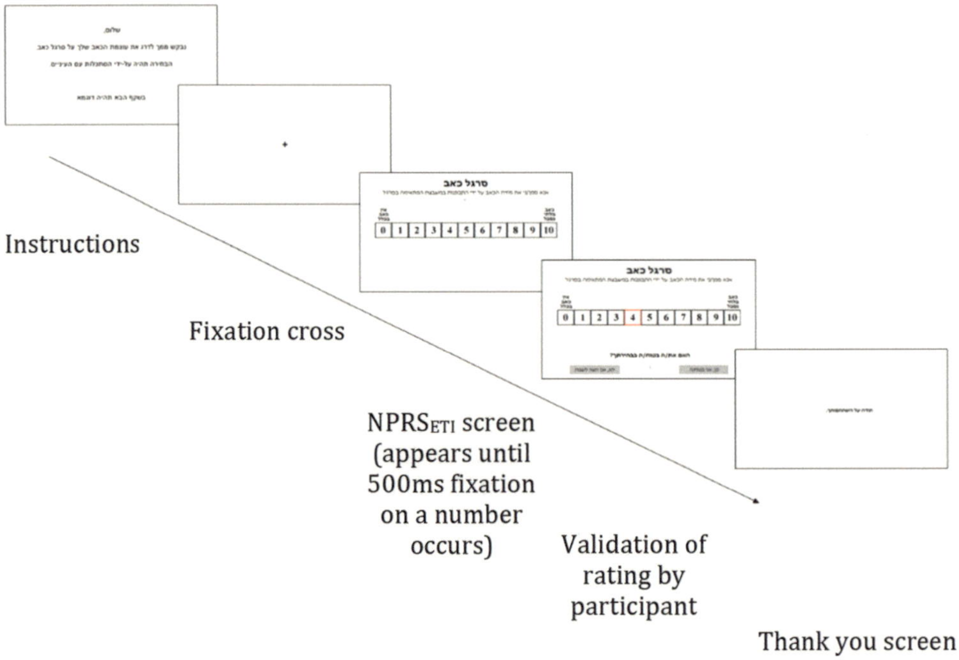

Figure 1.
$NPRS_{ETI}$ design. Notes: Eye tracker-integrated Numerical Pain Rating Scale = $NPRS_{ETI}$.

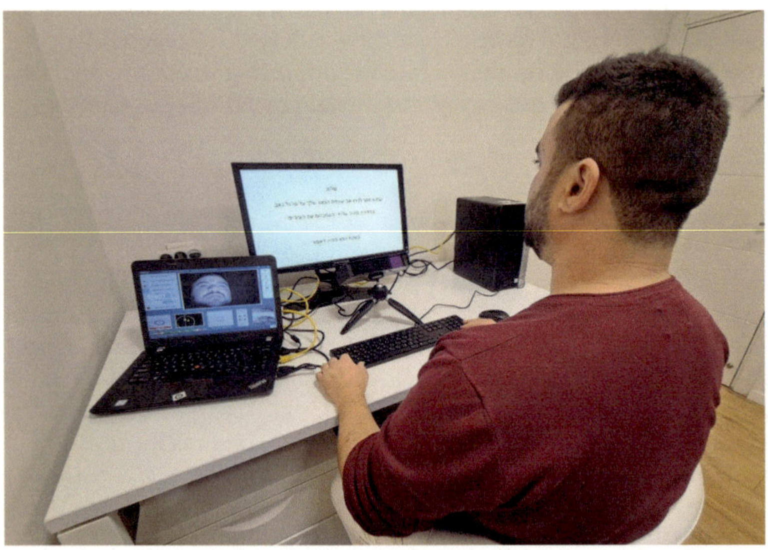

Figure 2.
The experimental setting. Notes: The actual experiment was performed with the computer located behind the participant and out of their field of view. The photographed person was part of the research team and not an actual participant in the experiment. Eye tracker-integrated Numerical Pain Rating Scale = $NPRS_{ETI}$.

instructions were presented. See **Figure 3** for the $NPRS_{ETI}$'s AOIs. Based on these AOIs, $NPRS_{ETI}$ dwell time (%), anchors dwell time (%), and instructions dwell time (%) were calculated. These measures reflected the percent time spent gazing at each

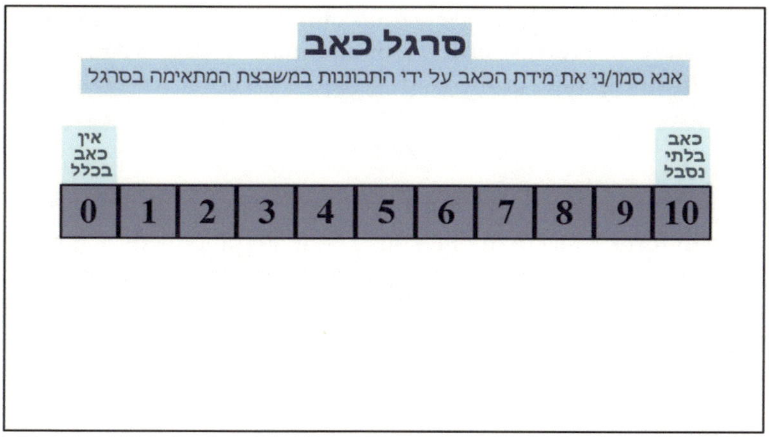

Figure 3.
AOIs of the $NPRS_{ETI}$. Notes: Blue regions delineate AOI in the participants' FoV as described in the Methods section (dark shade = $NPRS_{ETI}$ AOI, medium intensity shade = instructions AOI, light shade = anchors AOI,) areas of interest = AOI; Eye-integrated Numerical Pain Rating Scale = $NPRS_{ETI}$; field of view = FoV.

AOI out of the total task duration (i.e., time from the appearance of the scale to the selection of pain rating using the participant's gaze). Two additional general eye movement measures were calculated: (b) *Saccade rate (no.)*: The number of saccades that participants performed per second while providing the pain rating. Saccades are ballistic motions during which the eyes rapidly move between fixations, periods in which information is being processed, and the eyes remain fairly still [15]. (c) *Pupil size (no.)*: Average number of camera pixels occluded by the pupil while the participant provided the pain rating.

Paper-and-pencil Numerical Pain Rating Scale (NPRS): The NPRS (length = 10 cm) was presented on an A4 paper. It was identical to the $NPRS_{ETI}$ (e.g., pain scale length, instructions) except for the use of a paper-and-pencil format. Participants marked using a pen their currently experienced pain on a scale ranging from 0 ("no pain at all") and 10 ("unbearable pain").

Self-report questionnaires: The following self-report questionnaires were used: (a) Brief Pain Inventory (BPI): A commonly used questionnaire that assesses the severity of pain and its impact on daily functioning [35, 36]. It includes a screening question, inquiring about the presence of pain and a body chart that is used to indicate locations of experienced pain. The next six items are NPRS scales that are scored from 0 to 10, with higher scores indicating worse pain or more substantial functional impact. The BPI also includes an item rating the pain relief that the patient experienced by medications or other treatments. (b) Patient Health Questionnaire (PHQ-9): A nine-item self-report questionnaire of depressive symptoms [37, 38]. Each response range was from 0 ("not at all") to 3 ("nearly every day"). (c) General Anxiety Disorder-7 (GAD-7): A seven-item questionnaire of anxiety [39]. Responses range was 0 ("not at all") to 3 ("nearly every day"), with the participants rating their anxiety levels during 2 weeks preceding the study. (d) Debriefing survey: A survey assessing participants' motivation to undergo the experiment. It used a 1–7 Likert scale, with higher scores indicating stronger motivation.

Wechsler Adult Intelligence Scale-III (WAIS-III) digit span task: A short task derived from the WAIS-III which assesses attention and other cognitive functions such as working memory and executive functions [40]. As part of the task, the participant repeats increasingly longer strings of numbers that are read aloud by the examiner, in forward and reverse order. This continues until two consecutive strings of the same length are missed, or the longest sequences are successfully repeated.

2.3 Procedure

All participants were given a general description of the study and signed a written informed consent form. They then filled out a demographic-medical questionnaire, the BPI, PHQ-9, and GAD-7. Next, they reported their currently experienced pain using the $NPRS_{ETI}$ and pencil-and-paper NPRS and with their order pseudo-randomized. The participant underwent a nine-point calibration procedure before performing the $NPRS_{ETI}$ (five-point calibration was performed when encountering difficulties calibrating the participant). Participants then completed the WAIS-III digit-span task and filled out the debriefing survey. As in earlier studies (e.g., [41]), the participants were not permitted to compare their second ratings with those of the first one as this may influence patients' ratings.

3. Results

The participation of five participants was discontinued due to either inability to calibrate the eye tracker ($n = 3$) or complaints regarding pain and discomfort ($n = 2$). The final sample included 25 participants, seven of which had learning disabilities or suspected they had such a disability, three were previously diagnosed with attention-deficit/hyperactivity disorder (ADHD), and one participant had a CNS neuropathology that did not impact neuropsychological functioning. Besides comorbid affective depression and anxiety, psychiatric comorbidity included personality disorder ($n = 1$) and adjustment disorder ($n = 1$). Nineteen (76%) patients rated their current pain in the BPI (6th item) as of at least moderate severity using a ≥ 4 cut-off that was chosen in accordance with earlier studies [32, 42]. All participants reported adequate motivation to follow the experimental procedures, scoring $\geq$4 on a 7-point Likert scale in which higher scores indicated stronger motivation (as used in [43]). See **Table 1** for demographic and clinical data.

A comparison of the first and second pain assessments, regardless of the utilized method, revealed that four participants rated their pain one point lower in the second assessment compared to the first. Intra Class Correlation, ICC, calculated according to procedures described by Shrout and Fleiss [44], was 0.99 (95% CI: 0.98–0.99). This indicates excellent agreement based on the interpretative categorization of Koo and Li [45]. Next, we evaluated the match between the $NPRS_{ETI}$ and paper-and-pencil NPRS, with two participants rating their pain as more severe in the former than the latter and two participants showing an opposite pattern (i.e., rated their pain as lower in the $NPRS_{ETI}$). In all cases, the deviations in absolute numbers were one NPRS point. In other words, the scores of 16% of the sample deviated by one point between the two NPRS methods without a trend to these deviations. The match between the $NPRS_{ETI}$ and paper-and-pencil NPRS was additionally assessed using the following methods: (a) Group comparisons: Assumptions for parametric analyses for the pain ratings in each measurement ($NPRS_{ETI}$, NPRS, and BPI 6th item) were checked using Shapiro-Wilk test. This analysis revealed the pain ratings distributions deviated from the normal distribution ($ps < 0.05$) for the $NPRS_{ETI}$ ($W = 0.91$), NPRS ($W = 0.91$), and BPI 6th item ($W = 0.91$). Correspondingly, skewness and kurtosis indicated that

Variable		Participants (n = 25)
Parametric data		**Mean (SD)**
Age (years)		46.92 (11.12)
Education (years)		12.92 (2.13)
Motivation level (1–7)		6.68 (0.80)
PHQ total score (no.)		15.0 (7.29)
GAD score (no.)		10.12 (6.92)
WAIS-III digit span (SS)		8 (2.36)
$NPRS_{ETI}$ pain rating (0–10)		6.4 (2.62)
BPI- 6th item pain rating (0–10)		5.88 (3.07)
Paper-and-pencil NPRS pain rating (0–10)		6.4 (2.66)
Relative Dwell Time (%)	$NPRS_{ETI}$ AOI	81.83 (29.04)
	Instructions AOI	7.15 (19.29)
	Anchors AOI	2.19 (6.15)
Saccade rate (no. per sec.)		1.77 (0.99)
Pupil size (no.)		393.42 (92.97)
Nonparametric data		**Number of cases**
Gender (female / male)		10 / 15
Marital status (married / other)		19 / 6
Birth country (Israel / other)		22 / 3
Medical Cannabis license (yes / no)		11 / 14
Methamphetamine medication (yes / no)		2 / 23

Notes: Area of interest = AOI; Brief Pain Inventory = BPI; Eye tracker-integrated Numerical Pain Rating Scale = $NPRS_{ETI}$; General Anxiety Disorder Questionnaire 7-item = GAD-7; Patient Health Questionnaire-9 = PHQ-9, Scaled Score = SS.

Table 1.
Demographic and clinical data.

the distributions of NPRS, $NPRS_{ETI}$, and BPI 6th item were asymmetrical (S = −0.84, K = 0.37; S = −0.94, K = .43; S = −0.68, K = −0.41; respectively). These findings were expected considering the participants' high pain ratings, as reported earlier. We, therefore, performed a Wilcoxon signed-rank test which indicated no significant difference in the reported pain severity using $NPRS_{ETI}$ (Mdn = 7) and paper-and-pencil NPRS (Mdn = 7), $T = 5, p = 1$. (b) Correlation between NPRS methods: There was a very strong correlation [46] between the $NPRS_{ETI}$ and paper-and-pencil NPRS (ICC = 0.99, 95% CI: 0.98–0.99). Pain severity as evaluated using the $NPRS_{ETI}$ was also strongly correlated with participants' pain rating using the BPI (6th item; ICC = 0.93, 95% CI: 0.84–0.97). The correlation matrix can be found in **Table 2.**

Bland-Altman analysis is an efficient approach for quantifying the limits of agreement between two measurements [47]. However, it could not be used in this study as the differences between the two NPRS scales were not normally distributed [48]. More specifically, assumptions for parametric analyses for the differences between the two measurements ($NPRS_{ETI}$ minus paper-and-pencil NPRS chosen pain ratings) were checked using the Shapiro-Wilk test ($W = 0.57$, $p < 0.001$) and histogram and

DOI: http://dx.doi.org/10.5772/intechopen.111897

	1.	2.	3.	4.	5.	6.	7.	8.	9.
1. Age (years)	____	____	____	____	____	____	____	____	____
2. Education (years)	0.11	____	____	____	____	____	____	____	____
3. PHQ-9 (no.)	−0.14	−0.06	____	____	____	____	____	____	____
4. GAD-7 (no.)	−0.09	−0.23	0.84**	____	____	____	____	____	____
5. Pain rating (BPI 6th item; no.)	0.20	−0.09	0.18	0.05	____	____	____	____	____
6. Pain rating (paper-and-pencil NPRS; no.)	0.33	−0.02	0.04	−0.04	0.89**	____	____	____	____
7. Pain rating ($NPRS_{ETI}$; no.)	0.36	−0.02	0.07	−0.01	0.89**	0.99**	____	____	____
8. Average pupil size (no.)	0.05	−0.06	0.22	0.13	0.02	−0.01	0.01	____	____
9. Saccade rate (no. per second)	0.002	−0.01	−0.24	−0.09	−0.27	−0.10	−0.12	−0.02	____
10. WAIS-III digit span (SS)	0.15	−0.03	−0.51**	−0.39	−0.13	−0.05	−0.08	−0.35	0.25

Note: * $p < 0.05$, ** $p < 0.01$.
Brief Pain Inventory = BPI; Eye-tracker integrated Numerical Pain Rating Scale = $NPRS_{ETI}$; General Anxiety Disorder Questionnaire = GAD-7; Patient Health Questionnaire = PHQ-9; Scaled score = SS.

Table 2.
Pearson product-moment correlations among demographic, clinical, and pain ratings of patients (n = 25).

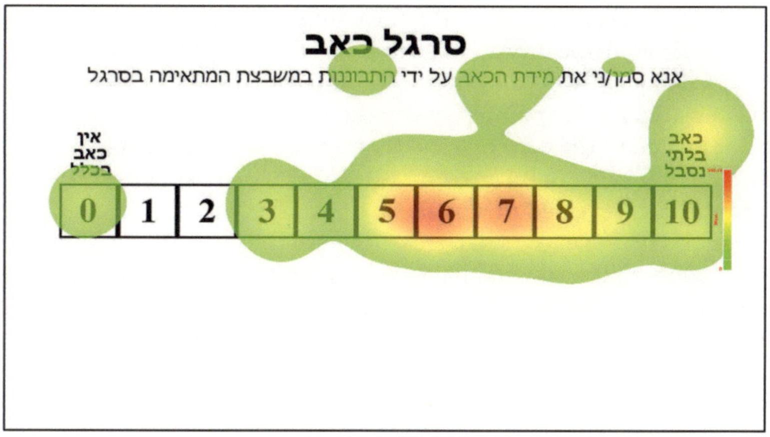
סרגל כאב
אנא סמן/ני את מידת הכאב על ידי התבוננות במשבצת המתאימה בסרגל
אין כאב בכלל
כאב בלתי נסבל
0
1
2
3
4
5
6
7
8
9
10

Figure 4.
Relative gaze duration heatmap; visualizing the proportion of accumulated gaze durations relative to the total duration for rating pain using the $NPRS_{ETI}$ (i.e., time until providing the pain rating).

quantile-quantile (Q-Q) plots. These indicated deviations from the normal distribution, an expected finding considering that the differences between the $NPRS_{ETI}$ and paper-and-pencil NPRS data were expected to be minimal (based on [49]). Correspondingly, kurtosis revealed a heavy-tailed distribution that deviated from the customarily used +1.96 and − 1.96 z-score range, though skewness did not indicate a deviation from a symmetrical distribution (K = 4.29, S = 0).

Additional analysis and general remarks: While most participants noted that $NPRS_{ETI}$ gaze-directed response that was chosen corresponded to their intended rating (n = 17), six participants requested to alter their response, while two additional participants revised their selected response twice. **Figure 4** presents a relative gaze duration heat map that visualizes the proportion of accumulated gaze duration at each AOI. Analyses were performed using IBM SPSS Statistics version 29.

4. Discussion

Earlier studies by our research team indicated the feasibility and utility of integrating an eye tracker with commonly used neuropsychological tests [23, 25–27]. These studies, as well as additional efforts in recent years by other researchers [50, 51], highlighted the potential of this novel technology to enhance daily clinical practice and was the impetus for the current project. We, therefore, set to integrate an eye tracker (i.e., Portable Duo eye-tracker by SR Research Ltd.) with an NPRS. This self-report pain intensity scale is well-established and commonly used in pain clinics [2, 4, 32]. The eye tracker-integrated scale, $NPRS_{ETI}$, is unique as it allows the patient to provide pain ratings without manual manipulation (i.e., use of hands). It thus paves the way for incorporating eye tracker-integrated pain scales in clinical settings (e.g., when evaluating ALS patients with severe physical limitations). The integrated system then underwent an initial validation study in a pain outpatient clinic in which participants filled both the $NPRS_{ETI}$ and conventional paper-and-pencil NPRS in a pseudo-randomized order (N = 25).

The study's findings provide initial validation for the use of the $NPRS_{ETI}$. Overall, excellent agreement was evident between pain ratings made using the $NPRS_{ETI}$ and the gold standard selected for this study, the conventional paper-and-pencil NPRS (ICC = 0.99). A closer inspection reveals that 21 of the participants (84%) rated their pain identically using $NPRS_{ETI}$ and the paper-and-pencil NPRS. The scoring of four participants deviated by one point between the two scales. Significantly, these deviations were not related to the type of scale that was used; two participants rated their pain as weaker, while two others rated it as stronger when using the $NPRS_{ETI}$. A closer inspection of the data revealed that in all cases, the second pain assessment's rating was lower than the first (i.e., two participants were first evaluated using the $NPRS_{ETI}$, and two others were first evaluated using the paper-and-pencil NPRS). Order rather than method, therefore, seemed to have impacted the pain ratings, with a minority of participants decreasing their pain ratings when undergoing temporally close consecutive pain assessments. Though the small number of participants that showed this trend limits speculations regarding its source, a similar decrease was found in other studies in which ratings of pain were performed with a short time interval between them. For example, a similar decline was evident in Bergh, Sjostrom [41] when geriatric patients rated their pain twice (5-minute interval) using the VAS and Graphic Rating Scale (GRS), though not when filling the NRS. As patients' experience of pain likely does change during such short periods [41], any change likely stems from other factors. More specifically, pain is a multidimensional subjective phenomenon [52] that is influenced by environmental factors. These include boredom and loneliness, which patients may experience and consequently view experiments and being attended by the research team as a pleasant experience [41]. This may consequently translate to a decrease in pain ratings, speculation that necessitates further research. Next, we evaluated the match between the $NPRS_{ETI}$ and paper-and-pencil NPRS by both group comparisons and by correlating pain scores obtained using the two NPRS types. The first method revealed that that $NPRS_{ETI}$ did not significantly differ from that of the paper-and-pencil NPRS, while the correlation matrix indicated a very strong correlation between the two methods (ICC = 0.99). Similarly, pain severity as rated using the $NPRS_{ETI}$ was strongly correlated with those made using the BPI (6th item; r ICC = 0.93). Overall, pain ratings using the $NPRS_{ETI}$ and conventional unidimensional scales using the NPRS format were almost identical with deviations likely stemming for momentary changes in experienced pain or other factors (e.g., fluctuating anxiety levels). This corresponds to recent studies, which found similar equivalence between conventional unidimensional pain rating scales and their digital equivalents. For example, Escalona-Marfil, Coda [49] electronic VAS was operated using a tablet and found it to be both highly reliable and interchangeable with the paper-and-pencil VAS (for additional examples, see [53, 54]). Overall, we can conclude that the $NPRS_{ETI}$'s reliability is adequate.

We also performed an initial inspection of eye movement patterns rating their pain using the $NPRS_{ETI}$. First, we produced a relative gaze duration heatmap. Heatmaps visualize the proportion of accumulated fixations—periods in which the eye is relatively still and information is extracted from the scene—at each AOI [55]. Heatmaps, therefore, allow easy visualization of the information that the participant pays attention to. The heatmap reflecting participants' eye movements while rating their pain using the $NPRS_{ETI}$ indicated most fixations were made on the pain scale itself and were concentrated on pain ratings ranging from 5 to 7. Participants' gaze was also directed toward the rightward anchor ("unbearable pain") and keywords in the instructions that were presented above the scale (i.e., "mark", "pain severity", and "gaze"). In other words, participants mostly gazed at pain ratings that corresponded to the pain ratings their later chose (i.e., Median pain rating was 7) and to critical elements in the instructions. Regarding the latter, visual attention tends to be maintained on pain cues that signal potential personal discomfort [56]. It would therefore be of interest to assess in future studies whether patients tended to gaze more at verbal stimuli due to their content (e.g., "unbearable pain," which constitutes the rightward anchor) and whether this correlates with their pain ratings. In addition to analyzing spatial attention based on gaze direction, we analyzed general eye movement measures, saccade rate, and pupil size (see correlation matrix in **Table 2**). The first provides an estimate of periods in which information is being processed [15], while the latter is impacted by various relevant factors; the pupil dilates in response to painful stimuli as well as the effort exerted in a task and other cognitive processes [57]. Both saccade rate and pupil size were not significantly correlated with pain ratings using the unidimensional pain scales used in the study, including the $NPRS_{ETI}$ (see **Table 2**). However, the variability of the pain ratings and the relatively small sample size of this study may have masked associations of interest. Further research is therefore called for.

Several limitations of this study can be mentioned, notably its modest sample size. Repeated measurements using the $NPRS_{ETI}$'s and paper-and-pencil NPRS would have enabled the evaluation of both intermethod and intramethod reliabilities, as research design which would have been preferable in hindsight (as performed by [49, 54]). The median pain ratings (*Mdn* = 7) of the patients in this study may also be in the higher range of patients treated at an outpatient clinic based on our impression of earlier studies (e.g., [5]). This stresses the need to further validate the $NPRS_{ETI}$ using larger samples. This will enable comparisons of different pain etiologies (e.g., neuropathic vs. musculoskeletal) and thereby clarify the generalizability of the findings, as well as evaluating the contribution of factors such as pain medications and sleep quality [58, 59] on $NPRS_{ETI}$ pain ratings. More strongly powered studies will also allow as well a more thorough assessment of the clinical utility, reliability, and validity of the $NPRS_{ETI}$ [1, 60]. Assessing $NPRS_{ETI}$'s usability is also of utmost importance. The comfort and usability of medical devices, with their increasing human-machine interface, have been a focus of increasing research attention [30, 61]. This is especially important as eye tracker-integrated pain scales necessitate calibration and additional components (e.g., gaze-directed pain rating may be incorporated in the scale) and are, therefore, more cognitively demanding than conventional unidimensional pain scales. It is also more challenging for those with visual impairment, which may not be assessed reliably. As part of this study, the participation of three participants was discontinued due to the inability to calibrate the eye tracker. Eight participants requested to alter their response at least once, suggesting that that gaze-directed pain rating may not have been user-friendly. This is disconcerting as these factors already limit the usability of conventional scales. For example, visual and hearing impairment, as well as physical restrictions, led to an inability of about a third of orthopedic post-surgery patients to undergo the VAS [62]. Eye-tracking technology has considerably advanced in recent years with increasingly affordable, precise, and faster eye trackers [63]. Hopefully, this will offset any usability issues that may plague eye trackers such as the one used in this study.

Beyond the earlier mentioned suggestions, several lines of research may be proposed based on the findings of the current study. First, comparisons with other pain scales is of importance, including digital versions that are similar in design to the $NPRS_{ETI}$ (e.g., [64]), and validated pain scales that use a different format (McGill Pain Questionnaire, MPQ; [65]), and more uniquely designed paper-and-pencil scales (e.g., [66]). Second, eye movement analysis can explore cognitive and affective factors associated with rating pain using unidimensional pain scales. Eye movements are sensitive to the effects of cognitive load [67–69], with gaze aversion interpreted in an earlier study performed in our laboratory as an attempt to lessen the cognitive load stemming for attempting to simulate cognitive impairment [23]. Simulators in this study also tended to gaze significantly more at the instructions of the task, which were speculated to serve as “attentional hooks” due to the automatic processing of language and its ability to involuntary draw attention (for a more thorough discussion, see [23]). This is somewhat reminiscent of the pattern evident in this study, with participants gazing toward the marking on the scale’s right anchor (“unbearable pain”) and keywords in the instructions, as noted earlier. Eye movements may therefore be used to explore the association between experienced pain, cognitive load, and likely other cognitive processes involved in rating pain. Eye movements are also impacted by anxiety and other negative affective states [70, 71], as well as stress levels (e.g., stress leads to shorter fixation durations [33]). Regarding the latter, pain is associated with the activation of a stress response—at least in its acute stages—and involves those related to heart rate, respiration, sweating, and muscle tension [1]. Overall, analysis of eye movements constitutes a window through which researchers can explore this various pain-related cognitive and affective factors. Eye movements are only under partial volitional control and were there studies as measures of deception and malingering [23, 26, 72]. Studying participants attempting to feign pain is scales such as the $NPRS_{ETI}$ is therefore also of value, and the interested reader is encouraged to further read about relevant research designs [73]. Finally, researchers are encouraged to integrate other unidimensional pain scales with eye trackers. For example, it was noted in a recent review of adult postoperative patients [7] that older adults and children who have less abstract thinking ability might prefer a categorical scale (e.g., verbal rating scale, VRS), which are easier use for them. This may prove useful as recent research tentatively suggests that the NPRS may have lowered utility in populations of individuals from developing countries with low literacy rates [2]. We hope that researchers can draw ideas from the above-mentioned suggestions, devising comprehensive research plans which may promote the integration of the $NPRS_{ETI}$ or similar eye tracker-integrated pain scales in clinical practice. Recent publications may be useful in devising a comprehensive research plan [15, 74–76].

5. Conclusions

Technological advancements in recent years have enabled clinicians to incorporate increasingly affordable and progressively convenient psychophysiological biomarkers, as also evident in pain research (e.g., [77, 78]). Eye movement analysis provides a window to cognitive and affective processes [75, 76], and as with other biomarkers, there are initial explorations of their utility for evaluating pain (e.g., [79–81]). This study is part of these recent efforts, indicating that the integration of an eye-tracker integrated unidimensional pain rating scale, the $NPRS_{ETI}$, in a hospital-based pain clinic is both feasible and can be used with a relatively diverse adult chronic pain patient population. The study’s findings also provide initial validation of the $NPRS_{ETI}$. More specifically, participants’ pain ratings were very similar to those performed by the conventional NPRS, with no bias in pain ratings associated with the NPRS method that was used. The participants’ gaze indicated that their visual attention was directed toward the relevant range of pain ratings in the scale, as well as the $NPRS_{ETI}$’s anchors and keywords in its instructions. These findings should, however, be considered as preliminary and await further validation using larger samples. These studies can further assess the validity, reliability, and additional key attributes that are mandated from pain scales [1, 60]. Analysis of eye movement also opens a myriad of other research opportunities, ranging from assessing its usability to the exploration of feigning based on the fact that eye movements are under lessened volitional control. The former is particularly important considering the possible deleterious impact of visual and cognitive impairment on utilizing a more complex device such as the $NPRS_{ETI}$. The reduced costs of eye trackers and enhanced usability evident in recent years [21] will hopefully encourage such research. Pending further validation, the NPRS $NPRS_{ETI}$ may find a place among the more established pain assessment tools. The path toward this goal, however, will necessitate a concerted effort by researchers and clinicians.

Acknowledgements

We thank Mr. Lior Golan, Miss Anastasya Garnik, and Miss Astar Lev for assisting in patient recruitment and performing the experimental procedures. We also thank Mrs. Oria Appel for helping with statistical analyses. The project would not have been possible without their aid.

Conflict of interest

The authors declare no conflict of interest.

Author details

Yoram Braw[1*], Motti Ratmansky[2,3] and Itay Goor-Aryeh[2,3]

1 Department of Psychology, Ariel University, Ariel, Israel

2 Pain Clinic, Sheba Medical Center, Ramat Gan, Israel

3 Sackler Faculty of Medicine, Tel Aviv University, Tel Aviv, Israel

*Address all correspondence to: yoramb@ariel.ac.il

References

[1] Strong J, Van Griensven H. Assessing pain (ch. 7). In: Van Griensven H, Strong J, Unruh AM, editors. Pain: A Textbook for Health Professionals. 2nd ed. Edinburgh, Scotland: Churchill Livingstone; 2014. pp. 91-113

[2] Patel KV, Amtmann D, Jensen MP, Smith SM, Veasley C, Turk DC. Clinical outcome assessment in clinical trials of chronic pain treatments. Pain Reports. 2021;**6**(1):e784, 1-e714

[3] Swieboda P, Filip R, Prystupa A, Drozd M. Assessment of pain: Types, mechanism and treatment. Annals of Agricultural and Environmental Medicine. 2013;**1**(1):2-7

[4] Safikhani S, Gries KS, Trudeau JJ, Reasner D, Rudell K, Coons SJ, et al. Response scale selection in adult pain measures: Results from a literature review. Journal of Patient-Reported Outcomes. 2018;**2**(40):1-9

[5] Euasobhon P, Atisook R, Bumrungchatudom K, Zinboonyahgoon N, Saisavoey N, Jensen MP. Reliability and responsivity of pain intensity scales in individuals with chronic pain. Pain. 2022;**163**(12):E1184-E1E91

[6] Modarresi S, Lukacs MJ, Ghodrati M, Salim S, MacDermid JC, Walton DM, et al. A systematic review and synthesis of psychometric properties of the numeric pain rating scale and the visual Analog scale for use in people with neck pain. Clinical Journal of Pain. 2022;**38**(2):132-148

[7] Baamer RM, Iqbal A, Lobo DN, Knaggs RD, Levy NA, Toh LS. Utility of unidimensional and functional pain assessment tools in adult postoperative patients: A systematic review. British Journal of Anaesthesia. 2022;**128**(5):874-888

[8] Trottier ED, Ali S, Dore-Bergeron MJ, Chauvin-Kimoff L. Best practices in pain assessment and management for children. Paediatrics & Child Health. 2022;**27**(7):429-437

[9] Herr KA, Booker SQ, Nakad L, Derrico DJ. Geriatric pain management. In: Benzon HT, Rathmell JP, Wu CL, Turk DC, Argoff CE, Hurley RW, et al., editors. Practical Management of Pain (Ch 44). 6th ed. Philadelphia, PA: Elsevier; 2022. pp. 637-646

[10] Husebo BS, Strand LI, Moe-Nilssen R, Husebo SB, Snow AL, Ljunggren AE. Mobilization-observation-behavior-intensity-dementia pain scale (MOBID): Development and validation of a nurse administered pain assessment tool for use in dementia. Journal of Pain and Symptom Management. 2007;**34**(1):67-80

[11] Hurwitz N, Radakovic R, Boyce E, Peryer G. Prevalence of pain in amyotrophic lateral sclerosis: A systematic review and meta-analysis. Amyotroph Lateral Scler Frontotemporal Degener. 2021;**22**(7-8):449-458

[12] Beswick E, Forbes D, Hassan Z, Wong C, Newton J, Carson A, et al. A systematic review of non-motor symptom evaluation in clinical trials for amyotrophic lateral sclerosis. Journal of Neurology. 2022;**269**(1):411-426

[13] Barzanji A, Zareiyan A, Nezamzadeh M, Mazhari MS. Evaluation of observational and behavioural pain assessment tools in nonverbal intubated critically adult patients after open - heart

surgery: A systematic review. Open Access Macedonian Journal of Medical Sciences. 2019;**7**(3):446-457

[14] Fletcher A, Dunne S, Butler J. A brief history of eye movement research (ch. 2). In: Stuart S, editor. Eye Tracking: Background, Methods, and Applications. New York, NY: Springer; 2022. pp. 15-29

[15] Duchowski AT. Eye Tracking Methodology: Theory and Practice. 3rd ed. Cham, Switzerland: Springer; 2017

[16] Cortese S, Solmi M, Michelini G, Bellato A, Blanner C, Canozzi A, et al. Candidate diagnostic biomarkers for neurodevelopmental disorders in children and adolescents: A systematic review. World Psychiatry. 2023;**22**(1):129-149

[17] Hampel H, Gao P, Cummings J, Toschi N, Thompson PM, Hu Y, et al. The foundation and architecture of precision medicine in neurology and psychiatry. Trends in Neurosciences. 2023;**46**(3):176-198

[18] Ull C, Weckwerth C, Schildhauer TA, Hamsen U, Gaschler R, Waydhas C, et al. First experiences of communication with mechanically ventilated patients in the intensive care unit using eye-tracking technology. Disability and Rehabilitation: Assistive Technology. 2023;**18**(1):44-49

[19] Wang J, Xu S, Dai Y, Gao S. An eye tracking and brain-computer Interface based human-environment interactive system for amyotrophic lateral sclerosis patients. IEEE Sensors Journal. 2022:1-12

[20] Pouget P. Introduction to the study of eye movements (ch. 1). In: Klein C, Ettinger U, editors. Eye Movement Research: An Introduction to its Scientific Foundations and Applications. Switzerland: Springer; 2019. pp. 3-10

[21] Graham L, Das J, Moore J, Godfrey A, Stuart S. The eyes as a window to the brain and mind (ch. 1). In: Stuart S, editor. Eye Tracking: Background, Methods, and Applications. New York, NY: Springer, Humana Press; 2022. pp. 1-14

[22] Young WR, Ellmers TJ. Translating attentional control theory to applied psychological eye tracking research (ch. 8). In: Stuart S, editor. Eye Tracking: Background, Methods, and Applications. New York, NY: Springer; 2022. pp. 131-149

[23] Tomer E, Lupu T, Golan L, Wagner M, Braw Y. Eye tracking as a mean to detect feigned cognitive impairment in the word memory test. Applied Neuropsychology: Adult. 2020;**27**(1):49-61

[24] Schroeder RW, Martin PK. Forced-choice performance validity tests (ch. 3). In: Boone KB, editor. Assessment of Feigned Cognitive Impairment: A Neuropsychological Perspective. 2nd ed. New York, NY: Guilford Press; 2021. pp. 34-63

[25] Lev A, Braw Y, Elbaum T, Wagner M, Rassovsky Y. Eye tracking during a continuous performance test: Utility for assessing ADHD patients. Journal of Attention Disorders. 2022;**26**(2):245-255

[26] Elbaum T, Braw Y, Lev A, Rassovsky Y. Attention-deficit/hyperactivity disorder (ADHD): Integrating the MOXO-dCPT with an eye tracker enhances diagnostic precision. Sensors (Basel). 2020;**20**(21):6386

[27] Lev A, Elbaum T, Berger C, Braw Y. Feigned ADHD associated cognitive impairment: Utility of integrating an eye-tracker and the MOXO-dCPT. Journal of Attention Disorders. 2022;**26**(9):1212-1222

[28] Libon DJ, Baliga G, Swenson R, Au R. Digital neuropsychological assessment: New Technology for Measuring Subtle Neuropsychological Behavior. Journal of Alzheimers Disease. 2021;**82**(1):1-4

[29] Diaz-Orueta U, Blanco-Campal A, Lamar M, Libon DJ, Burke T. Marrying past and present neuropsychology: Is the future of the process-based approach technology-based? Frontiers in Psychology. 2020;**11**:361

[30] McLean E, Cornwell MA, Bender HA, Sacks-Zimmerman A, Mandelbaum S, Koay JM, et al. Innovations in neuropsychology: Future applications in neurosurgical patient care. World Neurosurgery. 2023;**170**:286-295

[31] Treede RD, Rief W, Barke A, Aziz Q, Bennett MI, Benoliel R, et al. Chronic pain as a symptom or a disease: The IASP classification of chronic pain for the international classification of diseases (ICD-11). Pain. 2019;**160**(1):19-27

[32] Karcioglu O, Topacoglu H, Dikme O, Dikme O. A systematic review of the pain scales in adults: Which to use? The American Journal of Emergency Medicine. 2018;**36**(4):707-714

[33] Holmqvist K, Nyström M, Andersson R, Dewhurst R, Jarodzka H, Van de Weijer J. Eye Tracking: A Comprehensive Guide to Methods and Measures. Oxford, UK: Oxford University Press; 2011

[34] SR_Research. Eyelink 1000 user's Manual, Version 1.5.2. Mississauga, Ontario: SR Research Ltd.; 2010

[35] Stanhope J. Brief pain inventory review. Occupational medicine (Oxford, England). 2016;**66**(6):496-497

[36] Cleeland CS. The Brief Pain Inventory User Guide2009 September/15/2022. Available from: https://www.mdanderson.org/research/departments-labs-institutes/departments-divisions/symptom-research/symptom-assessment-tools.html

[37] Kroenke K, Spitzer RL, Williams JB. The PHQ-9: Validity of a brief depression severity measure. Journal of General Internal Medicine. 2001;**16**(9):606-613

[38] Miller RM, Kaiser RS. Psychological characteristics of chronic pain: A review of current evidence and assessment tools to enhance treatment. Current Pain and Headache Reports. 2018;**22**(3):1-6

[39] Spitzer RL, Kroenke K, Williams JB, Lowe B. A brief measure for assessing generalized anxiety disorder: The GAD-7. Archives of Internal Medicine. 2006;**166**(10):1092-1097

[40] Wechsler D. Wechsler Adult Intelligence Scale. 3rd ed. San Antonio, TX: The Psychological Corporation; 1997

[41] Bergh I, Sjostrom B, Oden A, Steen B. An application of pain rating scales in geriatric patients. Aging Clinical and Experimental Research. 2000;**12**(5):380-387

[42] Gerbershagen HJ, Rothaug J, Kalkman CJ, Meissner W. Determination of moderate-to-severe postoperative pain on the numeric rating scale: A cut-off point analysis applying four different methods. British Journal of Anaesthesia. 2011;**107**(4):619-626

[43] Berger C, Astar L, Braw Y, Elbaum T, Wagner M, Rassovsky Y. Detection of feigned ADHD using the MOXO-d-CPT. Journal of Attention Disorders. 2021;**25**(7):1032-1047

[44] Shrout PE, Fleiss JL. Intraclass correlations: Uses in assessing rater

reliability. Psychological Bulletin. 1979;**86**(2):420-428

[45] Koo TK, Li MY. A guideline of selecting and reporting Intraclass correlation coefficients for reliability research. Journal of Chiropractic Medicine. 2016;**15**(2):155-163

[46] Cohen J. A power primer. Psychological Bulletin. 1992;**112**(1):155-159

[47] Bland JM, Altman DG. Agreement between methods of measurement with multiple observations per individual. Journal of Biopharmaceutical Statistics. 2007;**17**(4):571-582

[48] Haghayegh S, Kang HA, Khoshnevis S, Smolensky MH, Diller KR. A comprehensive guideline for Bland-Altman and intra class correlation calculations to properly compare two methods of measurement and interpret findings. Physiological Measurement. 2020;**41**(5):055012

[49] Escalona-Marfil C, Coda A, Ruiz-Moreno J, Riu-Gispert LM, Girones X. Validation of an electronic visual Analog scale mHealth tool for acute pain assessment: Prospective cross-sectional study. Journal of Medical Internet Research. 2020;**22**(2):e13468

[50] Brunye TT, Drew T, Weaver DL, Elmore JG. A review of eye tracking for understanding and improving diagnostic interpretation. Cognitive Research: Principles and Implications. 2019;**4**(1):7

[51] Spering M. Eye movements as a window into decision-making. Annual Review of Vision Science. 2022;**8**:427-448

[52] Unruh AMSJ, Van Griensven H. Introduction to pain (ch. 1). In: Van Griensven H, Strong J, Unruh AM, editors. Pain: A Textbook for Health Professionals. 2nd ed. Edinburgh, Scotland: Churchill Livingstone; 2014. p. 1-7

[53] Delgado DA, Lambert BS, Boutris N, McCulloch PC, Robbins AB, Moreno MR, et al. Validation of digital visual Analog scale pain scoring with a traditional paper-based visual Analog scale in adults. JAAOS Global Research & Reviews. 2018;**2**(3):e088

[54] Turnbull A, Sculley D, Escalona-Marfil C, Riu-Gispert L, Ruiz-Moreno J, Girones X, et al. Comparison of a Mobile health electronic visual Analog scale app with a traditional paper visual Analog scale for pain evaluation: Cross-sectional observational study. Journal of Medical Internet Research. 2020;**22**(9):e18284

[55] Bischof WF, Anderson NC, Kingstone A. Temporal methods for eye movement analysis (ch. 10). In: Klein C, Ettinger U, editors. Eye Movement Research: An Introduction to its Scientific Foundations and Applications. Cham, Switzerland: Springer; 2019. pp. 407-448

[56] Zuo X, Ling Y, Jackson T. Testing links between pain-related biases in visual attention and recognition memory: An eye-tracking study based on an impending pain paradigm. Quarterly Journal of Experimental Psychology. 2023;**76**(5):1057-1071

[57] Laeng B, Alnaes D. Pupillometry (ch. 11). In: Klein C, Ettinger U, editors. Eye Movement Research: An Introduction to its Scientific Foundations and Applications. Cham, Switzerland: Springer; 2019. pp. 449-502

[58] Babiloni AH, De Koninck BP, Beetz G, De Beaumont L, Martel MO, Lavigne GJ. Sleep and pain: Recent

insights, mechanisms, and future directions in the investigation of this relationship. Journal of Neural Transmission. 2020;**127**(4):647-660

[59] D'Souza RS, Langford B, Wilson RE, Her YF, Schappell J, Eller JS, et al. The state-of-the-art pharmacotherapeutic options for the treatment of chronic non-cancer pain. Expert Opinion on Pharmacotherapy. 2022;**23**(7):775-789

[60] Dworkin RH, Burke LB, Gewandter JS, Smith SM. Reliability is necessary but far from sufficient how might the validity of pain ratings be improved? Clinical Journal of Pain. 2015;**31**(7):599-602

[61] Singh HP, Kumar P. Developments in the human machine interface technologies and their applications: A review. Journal of Medical Engineering & Technology. 2021;**45**(7):552-573

[62] Briggs M, Closs JS. A descriptive study of the use of visual analogue scales and verbal rating scales for the assessment of postoperative pain in orthopedic patients. Journal of Pain and Symptom Management. 1999;**18**(6):438-446

[63] Kasprowski P. Eye tracking hardware: Past to present, and beyond (ch. 3). In: Stuart S, editor. Eye Tracking: Background, Methods, and Applications. New York, NY: Springer; 2022. pp. 31-48

[64] Byrom B, Elash CA, Eremenco S, Bodart S, Muehlhausen W, Platko JV, et al. Measurement comparability of electronic and paper Administration of Visual Analogue Scales: A review of published studies. Therapeutic Innovation & Regulatory Science. 2022;**56**(3):394-404

[65] Main CJ. Pain assessment in context: A state of the science review of the McGill pain questionnaire 40 years on. Pain. 2016;**157**(7):1387-1399

[66] He SH, Renne A, Argandykov D, Convissar D, Lee J. Comparison of an emoji-based visual Analog scale with a numeric rating scale for pain assessment. The Journal of the American Medical Association. 2022;**328**(2):208-209

[67] Majumdar D, Mondal K, Sahrawat TR. Eye movement metrics as Indicator of cognitive loading: A systematic review. Research Aspects in Biological Science. 2022;**2**:1-17

[68] Skaramagkas V, Giannakakis G, Ktistakis E, Manousos D, Karatzanis I, Tachos N, et al. Review of eye tracking metrics involved in emotional and cognitive processes. Vol. 16. IEEE Reviews in Biomedical Engineering. 2021

[69] Tao D, Tan H, Wang H, Zhang X, Qu X, Zhang T. A systematic review of physiological measures of mental workload. International Journal of Environmental Research and Public Health. 2019;**16**(15):2716

[70] Rommelse NNJ, Van der Stigchel S, Sergeant JA. A review on eye movement studies in childhood and adolescent psychiatry. Brain and Cognition. 2008;**68**(3):391-414

[71] Clauss K, Gorday JY, Bardeen JR. Eye tracking evidence of threat-related attentional bias in anxiety- and fear-related disorders: A systematic review and meta-analysis. Clinical Psychology Review. 2022;**93**:9

[72] Lancry-Dayan OC, Ben-Shakhar G, Pertzov Y. The promise of eye-tracking in the detection of concealed memories. Trends in Cognitive Sciences. 2023;**27**(1):13-16

[73] Rogers R. Researching response styles (Ch. 30). In: Rogers R, Bender SD, editors. Clinical Assessment of Malingering and Deception. 4th ed.

New York, NY: Guilford Press; 2018. pp. 592-614

[74] Carter BT, Luke SG. Best practices in eye tracking research. International Journal of Psychophysiology. 2020;**155**:49-62

[75] Klein C, Ettinger U, editors. Eye Movement Research: An Introduction to its Scientific Foundations and Applications. Cham: Switzerland: Springer; 2019

[76] Stuart S, editor. Eye Tracking: Background, Methods, and Applications. New York, NY: Humana Press; 2022

[77] Zhang Z, Gewandter JS, Geha P. Brain imaging biomarkers for chronic pain. Frontiers in Neurology. 2021;**12**:734821

[78] Mussigmann T, Bardel B, Lefaucheur JP. Resting-state electroencephalography (EEG) biomarkers of chronic neuropathic pain. A systematic review. NeuroImage. 2022;**258**:119351

[79] Soltani S, van Ryckeghem DML, Vervoort T, Heathcote LC, Yeates KO, Sears C, et al. Clinical relevance of attentional biases in pediatric chronic pain: An eye-tracking study. Pain. 2022;**163**(2):E261-EE73

[80] Alrefaei D, Sankar G, Norouzi NJ, Djamasbi S, Strong D. Examining the Impact of Chronic Pain on Information Processing Behavior: An Exploratory Eye-Tracking Study. Augmented Cognition: 16th International Conference, AC 2022, Held as Part of the 24th HCI International Conference, HCII 2022, Virtual Event, June 26–July 1, 2022, Proceedings. Cham, Switzerland: Springer International Publishing; 2022

[81] Rosker ZM, Vodicar M, Kristjansson E. Oculomotor performance in patients with neck pain: Does it matter which angle of neck torsion is used in smooth pursuit eye movement test and is the agreement between angles dependent on target movement amplitude and velocity? Musculoskeletal Science & Practice. 2022;**59**:59

Chapter 17

Combining Modern Pharmacology with Integrative Medicine: A Biopsychosocial Model for Comprehensive Pain Care

Agnes Mazic De Sonis

Abstract

The medical community recognized last decennia the multidimensional nature of pain and proposed multimodal biopsychosocial management. The most compelling reason to embrace integrative pain strategies is to mitigate patient risk. For patients with chronic pain and pain refractory to conservative medicine, it is essential to assess all factors involved with the chronicity. With significant themes, nutrition and microbiome, neuroplasticity, homeostasis, and the side effects of medication, acupuncture has progressively gained a place in this multimodal evaluation. Therapeutic multimodality approaches the perspective of physiological rehabilitation and chronobiological improvement of the quality of life. Illustrated by various clinical situations, the objective of management is to seek a synergy in the mechanisms of action of treatments to improve quality of life and reduce the need for xenobiotics and, consequently, the side effects. The mechanism of action of integrative medicine, and acupuncture improved with a better understanding of genetics, and epigenetics. As opposed to sham and placebo, acupuncture activates other brain regions. In controlled trials, the strict inclusion and exclusion criteria result in the treatment of a "selected" patient population, which is not always comparable to the patients seen in daily practice. The integrative approach is better illustrated by case reports.

Keywords: acupuncture, nutrition, microbiome, p4medicine, personalized medicine, integrative

1. Introduction

Even for modern medicine, chronic pain remains a complex, multi-faceted problem of nociception, inflammation, and abnormal physiology in the nervous system. Thanks to the knowledge of epigenetics, it becomes clear that environmental factors such as nutrition and chronobiology can modify the parameters involved in all sensitization mechanisms in chronic pain diseases. The deranged sensitization mechanisms suggest restoring the hypersensitive structures to their normal status besides the analgesic treatment.

While more research is needed to understand the progression from acute to chronic pain, the limited pain management strategies have not addressed the scope of pain.

Increased costs and lack of evidence of efficacy are not, according to the physicians (ACP) Clinical Practice Guideline, evidence-informed, comprehensive pain care while conceding that past strategies generally, and the use of opioid medications specifically, have not remedied but rather exacerbated chronic pain, abuse, addiction, illness behavior, and disability [1].

Awareness of serious adverse effects of medications is growing, including the escalating rates of accidental overdoses of prescription opioids and the development of opioid tolerance and hyperalgesia [2].

IASP 2023 global defines integrative pain care as temporally coordinated, mechanism-guided, individualized, and evidence-based integration of multiple pain treatment interventions. Considering the ever-growing burden of chronic pain, current pain management models frequently do not address the clinical problem. The complexity of chronic pain justifies a bio-psycho-social framework, integrating different management and treatment approaches is preferred.

2. Pain chronobiology and epigenetic regulation

A total of 30% genetic and 70% epigenetic factors, such as nutrition and intestinal flora, social, psychological, and affective define the status of an individual [3]. The sensibility for pain is affected by 20 genes. These are also responsible for the variation in reaction to pharmacologic treatment (see **Figure 1**) [5].

The ignition or blocking of specific genes is epigenetically regulated. It is also sensitive to environmental factors [5].

Intra and extracellular homeostasis regulates the peripheral sensitization of the primary nociceptors. Inflammation activates the bidirectional signaling that it modulates. Even though there is no immunological response, certain bacterial infections could be accompanied by a hyperalgesic state (see **Figure 2**) [6].

Pharmacological treatment of chronic pain has dose-dependent side effects, including opioid tolerance, addiction, and even death. Chronic pain involves neuroplastic changes, and neuroinflammation becomes a key question in central sensitization (**Figure 3**).

Pain induces arousal and triggers other neurobiological stress sequels, thus disturbing sleep and enhancing pain sensitivity. Disturbed sleep or pain may induce a cycle whereby both components stabilize or augment each other. Therefore, management of sleep disturbance may alleviate pain, whereas pain relief may restore sleep and enhance long-term pain relief.

Treatment should target the different mechanisms of pain and may require a combination of treatment options. Combining therapies, such as acupuncture, with traditional pharmacology is still in its infancy.

Acupuncture influences the opioid and cannabinoid system by releasing endogenous receptor ligands. Low-dose naltrexone also acts on both systems and upregulates the opioid and cannabinoid receptors.

Dietary choices and drug use (proton pump inhibitors, NSAIDs, steroids, antibiotics, and hormones) can influence inflammation by altering the microbiome and gut permeability. The balance of microorganisms can affect the absorption of nutrients, drugs, and the function of the immune system leading to low-grade inflammation.

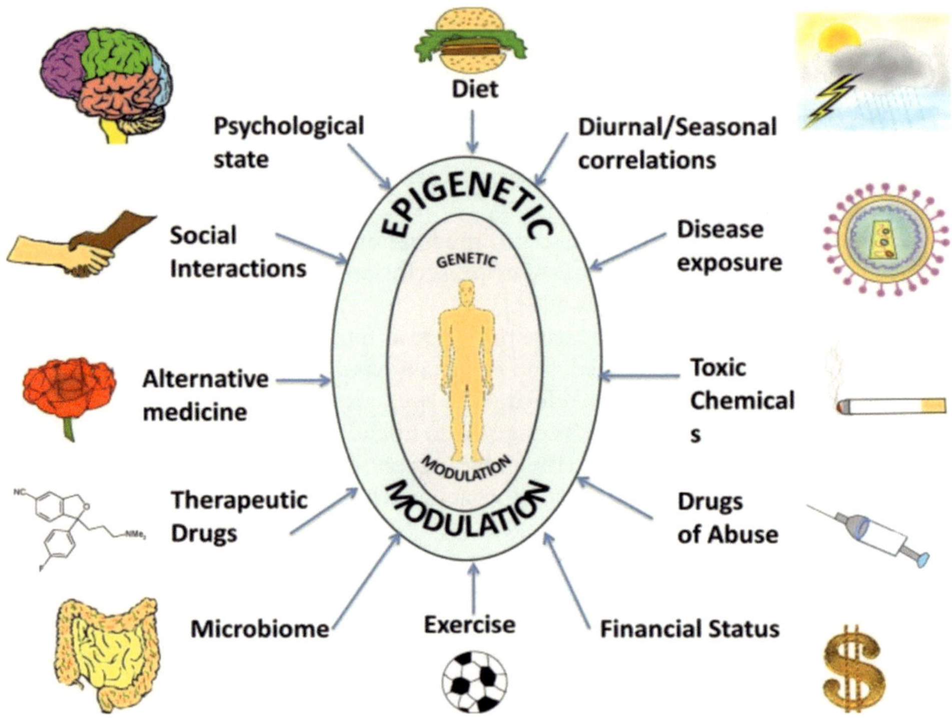

Figure 1.
Influences of the epigenetic modulation system. From Ref. [4].

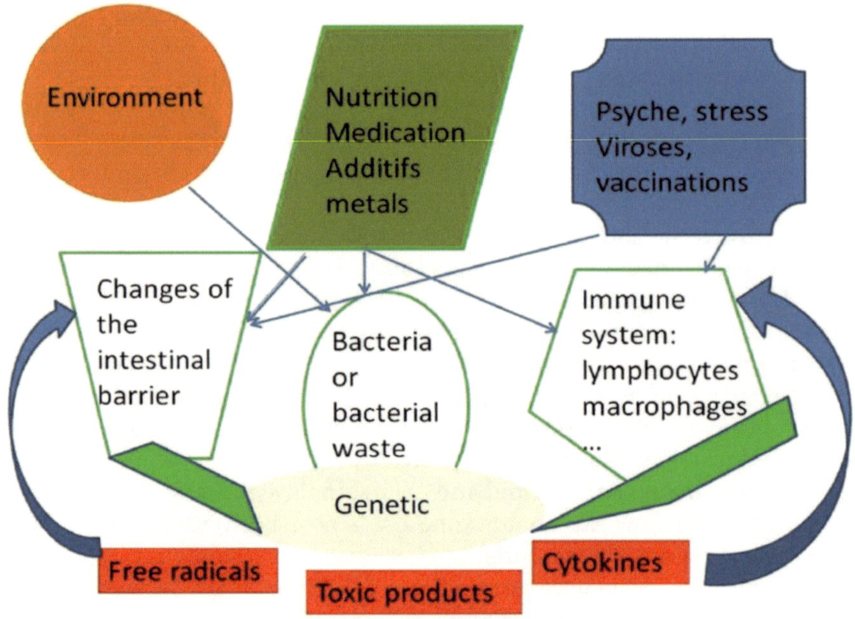

Figure 2.
Interactions leading to vulnerability for pain.

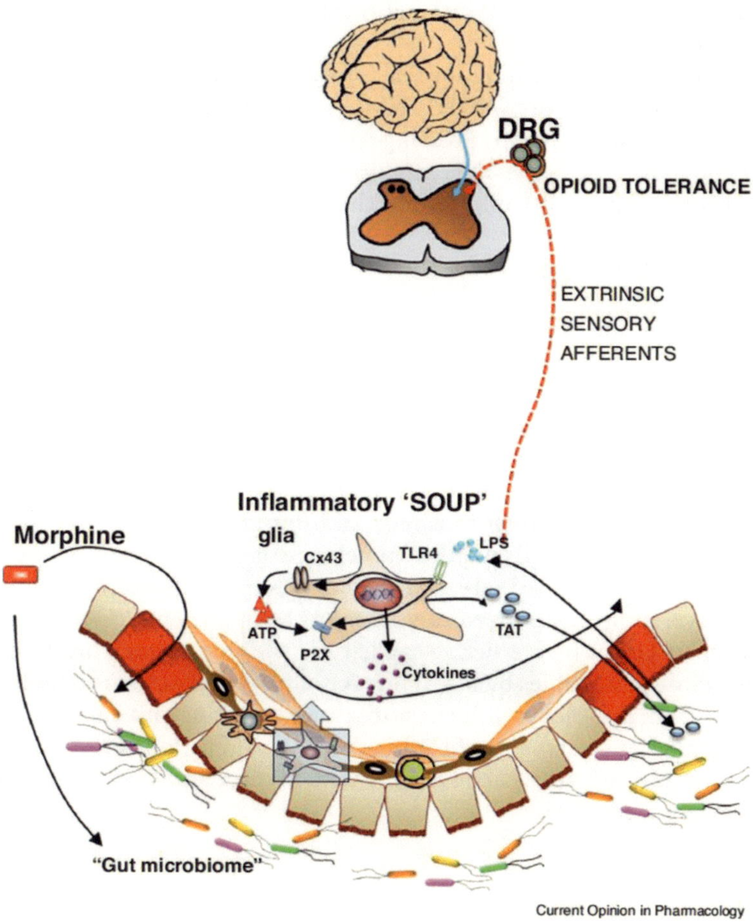

Figure 3.
Schema of gut-brain interaction from [7].

One day after morphine treatment, there is a significant shift in the gut microbiome and metabolome. Morphine-induced gut microbial dysbiosis exhibited distinct characteristic signatures. Drug-microbiota dynamics could help to identify drug-drug interactions and explain inter-individual variation in drug efficacy and adverse effects. The gut microbiome can affect all classes of drugs.

The gastrointestinal microbiome plays a significant role in responses to opioids, including the development of tolerance.

The neuro-immune interactions induced by morphine have direct intestinal functional consequences. Morphine disrupts gut barrier function in a toll-like receptor (TLR)-dependent manner [8]. Low-dose naltrexone (LDN) acts on various gut mechanisms.

Analgesic tolerance to opioids induced by the gut-brain interaction suggests that peripheral mechanisms from the gut can profoundly affect the central control of opioid function. The answer to treatment can be modulated by genetic variations and the inter-individual differences in the bacterial flora of the human digestive tract. The pharmacokinetics of drug metabolism was redefined by the progress in understanding the host-microbial interaction and has improved the management of drug (ab)users.

Acupuncture influences different molecules and receptors, such as GABA, glutamate, and its other receptors (AMPA, NMDA), serotonin (5HT), and the opioid system. The treatment objective is addressing pain and preventing chronicity, focusing on drug and non-drug strategies. Therapeutics directed at maintaining microbiome homeostasis during opioid use may reduce the associated comorbidities.

2.1 Integrative pain medicine and mitigation of risk

The overlap with conventional care is growing as the scientific basis for these therapies expands. Integration across the lifespan to include personal, predictive, preventive, and participatory care.

Personalization of treatment usually means targeting a smaller subset of patients who share a particular phenotype. The economic or financial viability of stratified medicine versus empiric medicine (a medicine prescribed to all patients with a specific condition) was evaluated by Trusheim and Berndt [9] and Ozdemir et al. [10].

Personalized medicine goals require knowledge of which treatment is best for each individual, and promises increased efficiencies for health care systems. Much emphasis in developing customized therapies has been on genetic polymorphisms and blood biomarkers [10]. The predictive capacity of the data pattern must be defined. Determining clinical variables by interview remains the most helpful tool available to a treating physician for selecting the best treatment options on a case-by-case basis. Several recent studies note the need for new models and frameworks that can consistently provide professionals and consumers with helpful knowledge that physicians can meaningfully apply [11].

2.1.1 Acupuncture

Under the premise of selecting acupoints along the meridians and adopting reinforcement and reduction manipulations, acupuncture will bidirectionally regulate the clinical symptoms and signs.

The same stimulation parameters applied to the same acupoint or nerve may result in opposite regulation (restoring homeostatic balance or normalizing function), the so-called "bidirectional regulation".

The peripheral lesions around the needle trigger physiological reactions and initiate a cascade of survival reactions. Via the reflex of the axon due to the increased blood flow in the muscle, Calcitonin Gene-Related Peptide (CGRP) and nitrous oxide (NO) are released after manual acupuncture and contribute to tissue healing [12, 13].

Acupuncture induces a brain response to the stimulation of sensory nerves, making it a physiological therapy. Acupuncture normalizes physiological homeostasis and promotes self-healing. The primary nociceptors are complex in the ligand expression of neurotransmitters and receptors, enabling autocrine and paracrine interactions.

Primary nociceptors generate bidirectional efferent messages toward the innervated tissues, and can modify (facilitate or inhibit) sensory information even before transmission to the central nervous system.

Nociceptors seem to have a mind of their own (see **Figures 4** and **5**) [13].

Pain control might be influenced by the modulation of different molecules and receptors such as GABA, glutamate, and its other receptors (AMPA, NMDA, etc.),

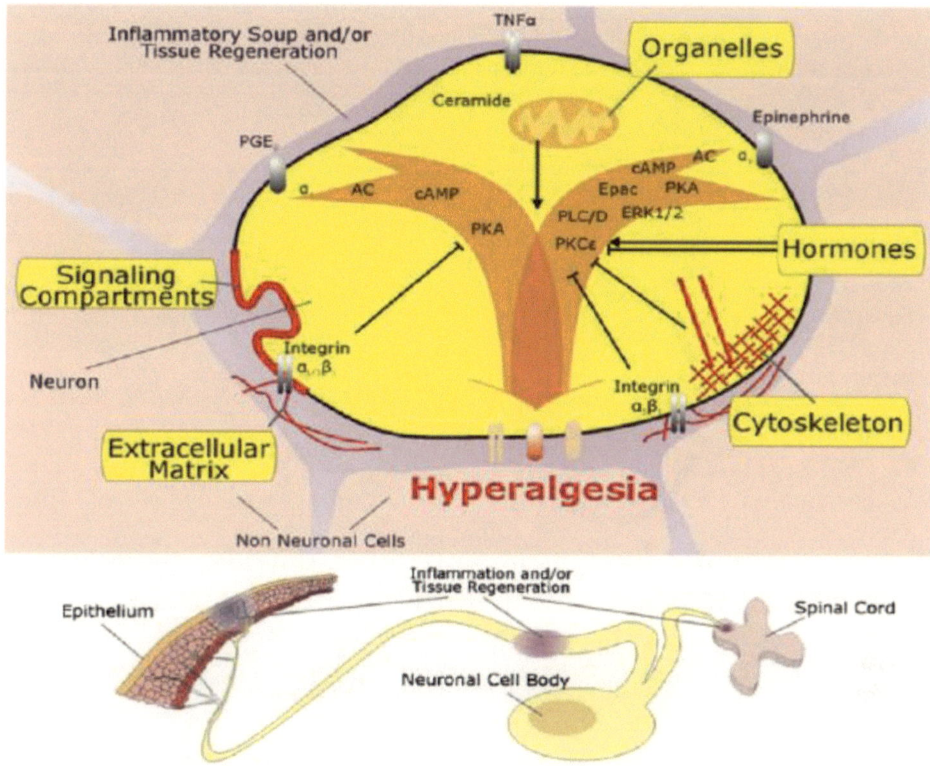

Figure 4.
Hyperalgesia at a cellular level.

the serotonin (5HT) system, the opioid system, norepinephrine (NE), cholinergic receptors, etc. Low-frequency electroacupuncture (EA) has a better effect than a high frequency (100 Hz).

Bidirectional regulation is a unique phenomenon of acupuncture therapy, seen in multiple systemic, cellular, and molecular functional systems. Not all acupoints unconditionally produce the bidirectional regulatory effect, and the corresponding factors remain to be investigated. The body's homeostatic regulation can achieve bidirectional regulation by acupuncture or peripheral stimulation in different functional states. It is not a simple physiological response but a complex pathophysiological process [15, 16].

Acupuncture stimulates brain responses in cortical and subcortical regions, associated with modulation of the pain sensation and perception, including activation in the sensorimotor cortical and deactivation in the limbic-para limbic-neocortical network as demonstrated with functional neuroimaging studies [17]. It is postulated that the therapeutic response to acupuncture, such as down-regulation of inflammation and autonomic nervous system-mediated pain relief, is provided by a mechanistic pathway of the autonomic nervous system.

Event-related (er)-fMRI is used to evaluate the brain correlates of acupuncture stimulation, it seems to be associated with different autonomic nervous system outflow responses to needle stimuli and may result from other sensations elicited by stimuli at different bodily locations [18]. In vivo μ-opioid receptor (MOR) binding effects of traditional Chinese acupuncture versus sham acupuncture were found in chronic pain patients diagnosed with fibromyalgia [17].

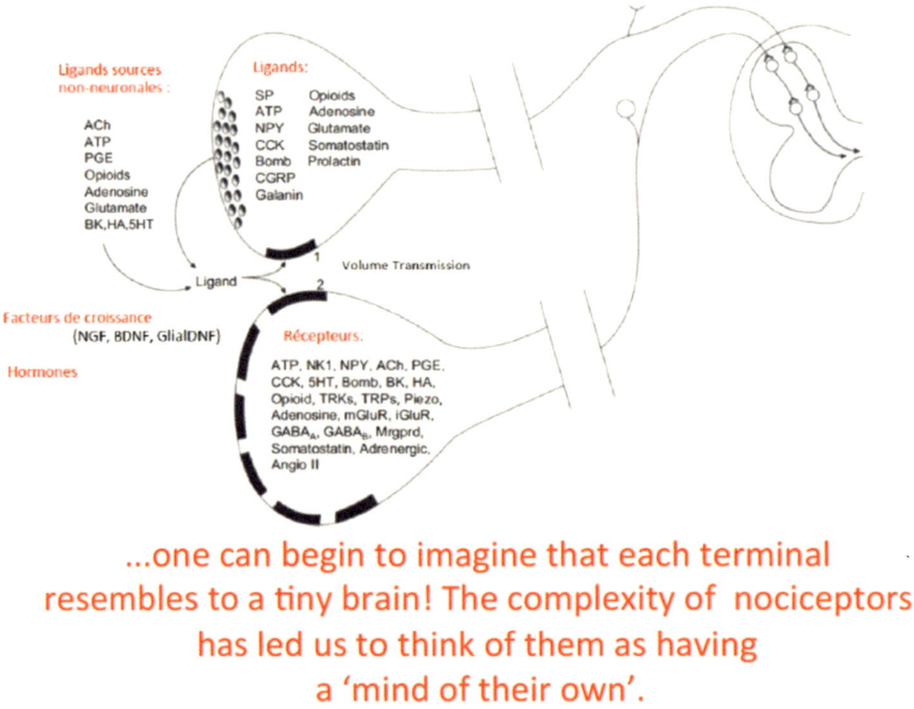

Figure 5.
Interactions at the nerve endings [14].

2.1.2 Nutrition and microbiome

In addition to the severity of the underlying condition, interindividual variability in chronic pain depends on many factors, including its sociocultural context, patients' genetic backgrounds, psychological factors, and pathophysiology, that can be modulated and monitored by altering nutritional habits [19]. Specific nutritional deficiencies can be associated with pain states. A study discovered that patients with pain with insufficient vitamin D levels needed twice the dose of opioids for twice as long as patients without a deficiency.

Many different types of elimination diets can be useful for patients to try.

Food and nutrition are foundational tools in treating painful and inflammatory conditions. Compelling evidence shows the benefits of a healthy diet composed mainly of unprocessed, plant-based foods.

Sugars and facts may feed into many anabolic and catabolic pathways, the handling of the body of nutrients depends on strategically positioned metabolic sensors that link the intrinsic nutritional value of a meal with intermediary metabolism.

Assessing the nutritional status is a cornerstone of integrative pain medicine. Dietary choices increase or decrease inflammation. Free-radical damage of tissues, induced by inflammation, impedes healing mechanisms, and reduces pH to levels where normal enzymatic reactions are no longer optimized. Inflammation can be reduced by an anti-inflammatory diet, such as the Mediterranean diet—which is high in vegetables, fruits, whole grains, fish, and healthy oils but low in meat (**Figure 6**) [21].

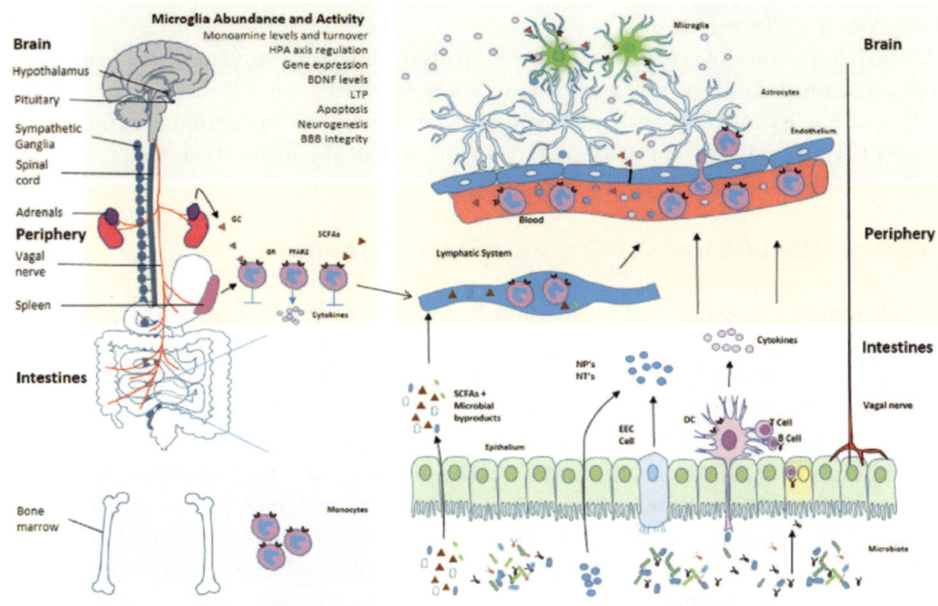

Figure 6.
Schema of microbiota regulation [20].

2.1.3 The effects of drug therapy on the gut microbiome

The individual diversity of the gut microbiome promotes inter-individual variations with pharmacotherapy, drug-induced toxicity, and efficacy.

The gut microbiome is affected by drug effects and the GI tract environment can be altered (e.g., pH and transit time), mucosa integrity, host and bacterial metabolic aqctivity, and the production of microbial metabolites. These changes can have secondary effects on the microbiome and cause drug-drug interactions. Drugs may also challenge both the integrity and permeability of the intestinal mucosa.

2.1.3.1 Drugs and polypharmacy

The combined use of non-steroidal anti-inflammatory drugs (NSAIDs) and PPIs differentially influenced the relative abundance of Bacteroides spp. and Erysipelotrichaceae spp. Compared to NSAIDs alone, the co-administration of drugs may precipitate shifts in the composition of the microbiota to favor the abundance of microbial taxa that have a metabolizing capacity for those drugs [22].

2.1.3.2 Effect of diet-induced changes on the gut microbiome and drug pharmacokinetics

Drug pharmacokinetics may be modulated by probiotics by changing the composition or metabolic activity of the gut microbiota. Probiotic treatment was shown to increase the microbiota-mediated degradation of the antipyretic and analgesic paracetamol, which may be mediated by probiotic-induced modulation of gut microbial enzyme activity.

Some patients are more at risk for food-drug interaction, such as chronic disease, elderly, malnourished, infant, and pregnant women.

Meanwhile, examining and explaining how gut microbiota regulates drug metabolism and toxicity will assist personalized medicine and facilitate strategies for creating new drugs with desired functionality.

2.2 Towards circuit-based tVNS: translational approaches

It is important to estimate the independent effects of the disease or drug treatment in animal and human studies, as both the CNS-related disease itself and the pharmacological treatment of the disease can alter the composition of the microbiota.

This microbiome impacts the properties and function of microglia involved in pain sensitization. To maintain homeostasis, the vagal nerve (VN) actively participates in bidirectional interactions between the gut microbiome and the brain. VN electroacupuncture promotes the expression and localization of junction proteins, decreasing intestinal permeability and protecting the intestinal epithelial barrier. Complex reflexes, such as the autonomic reflex, can be used to explain some therapeutic effects of acupuncture.

Administration of pre/probiotics to modify vagal nerve function could be a promising strategy for treating central nervous system disorders (**Figure 7**).

In human studies, the vital role of the VN in modulating food intake, energy metabolism, and glycemic control has been demonstrated more recently [23–27]. Across disciplines the pathophysiology of several disorders is attributed to the VN on a behavioral and psychological level; VN stimulation, remarkably non-invasive VN stimulation, has been studied, allowing a better understanding of the mechanisms by which VN stimulation exerts psychological and physiological effects. A more important pathway for acupuncture stimuli is via the autonomic center in the brain that works to up or down-regulate the sympathetic or para-sympathetic output. Neuroendocrine and neuroimmune pathways are also crucial for maintaining the stability of various functional systems in the body, and they can be affected by acupuncture stimulation.

2.2.1 Nutraceuticals and others

The purified products derived from plants, animals, microorganisms (e.g., essential fatty acids and enzymes), and marine sources (e.g., glucosamine, chitosan, fish oils) are called nutraceuticals. They are sold in medicinal forms e.g., tablets, capsules, and powders. The bioactive agents the nutraceuticals deliver may also be obtained through a healthy diet. They provide, however, the advantages of a formulation that promotes the absorption and the physiological effect [19].

2.2.1.1 Curcumin

Hu et al. [28] recently determined that curcumin attenuates opioid-induced hyperalgesia by inhibiting Ca^{2+}/calmodulin-dependent protein kinase II α activity and found that a nano-formulation of poly(lactic-co-glycolide)-curcumin-curcumin may reverse opioid-induced hyperalgesia by inhibiting caMKIIa and downstream signaling.

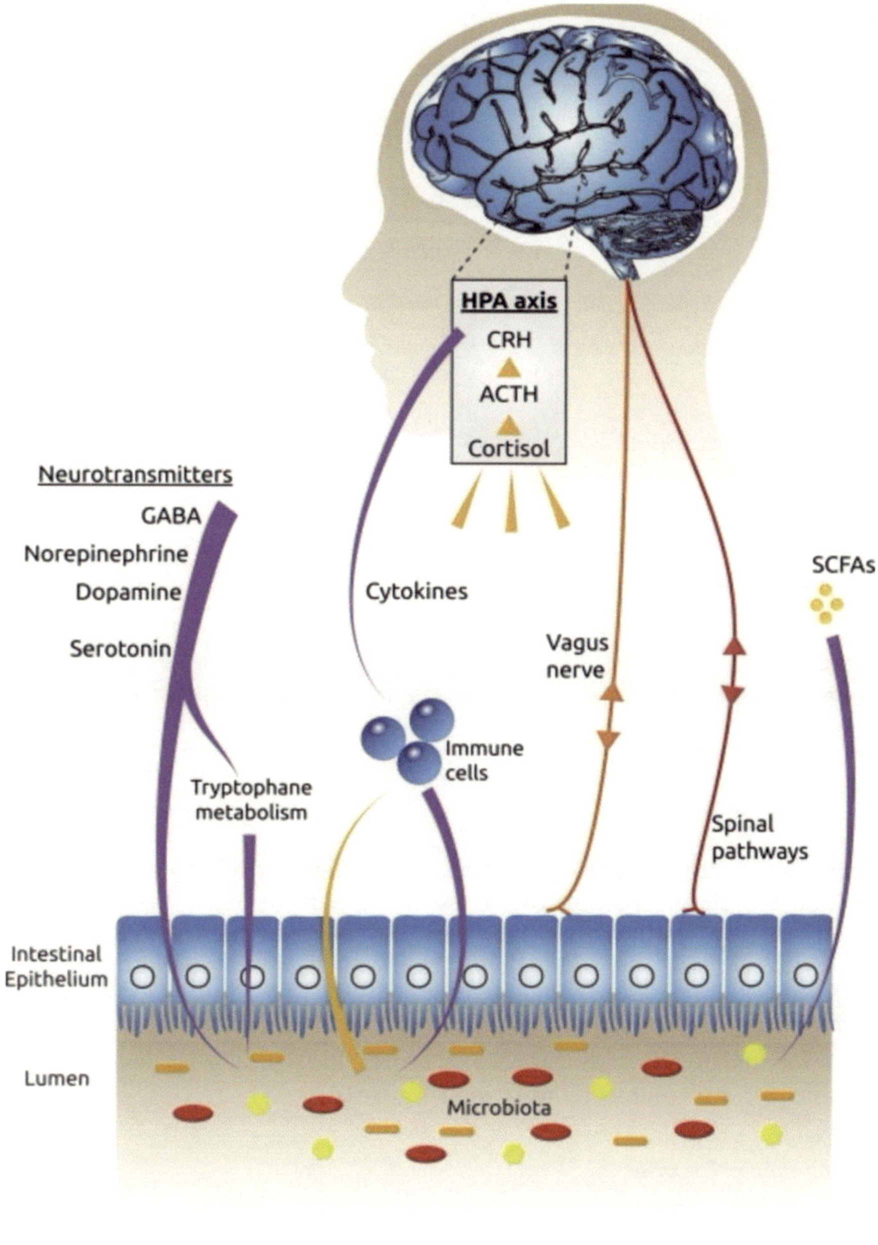

Figure 7.
The multiple bidirectional communication routes between the brain and the gut microbiota. These routes include the vagal nerve, the hypothalamic-pituitary-adrenal axis (HPA), cytokines produced by the immune system, tryptophan metabolism, and short-chain fatty acid production. Adopted from [16].

Curcumin induces mitochondrial biogenesis, and has a direct activity on reactive oxygen species, and induction of NRF2. It regulates the epigenetic patterns and has a synergistic activity on drugs used to treat different painful conditions. The low bioavailability of curcumin can be improved by bio-optimization techniques, thus increasing the therapeutic and preventive potentials of the natural substance [29, 30].

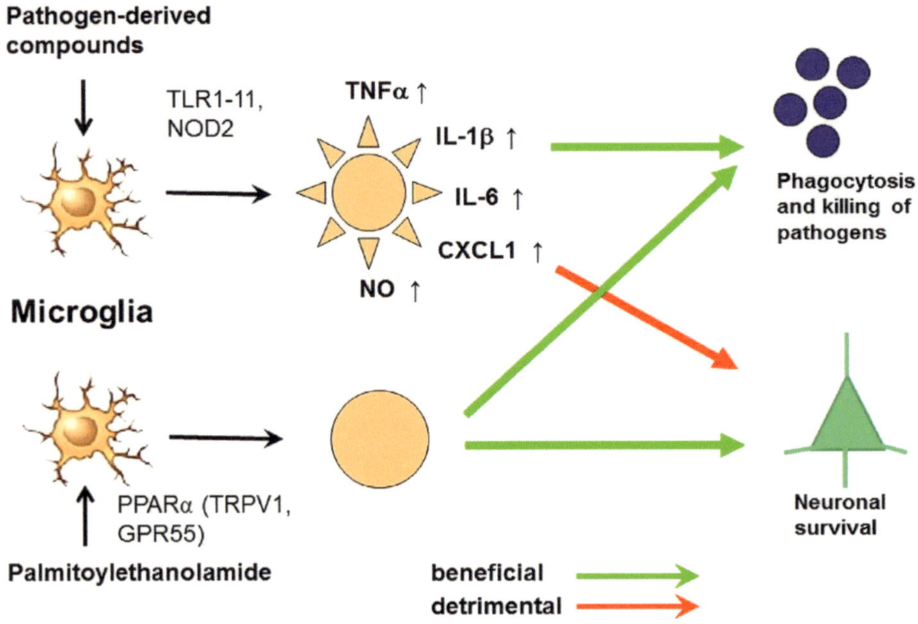

Figure 8.
Activation of microglia by toll-like receptor (TLR) agonists and by palmitoylethanolamide (PEA). Adopted from [31].

2.2.1.2 PEA palmitoylethanolamide

Glia may produce their own endogenous "painkillers" and anti-inflammatory agents through their own modulators. These modulators decrease the winding-up mechanisms in neuropathic pain. Anandamide and its sister molecule PEA are such modulators, and induce a "winding down" in chronic and neuropathic pain and neuroinflammation. Both molecules are classical autacoids, fulfilling the three criteria required for autacoids of lipid transmitters.

PEA is a modulator that reduces pain by decreasing winding-up mechanisms in neuropathic pain and neuroinflammation (**Figure 8**).

2.2.1.3 Low-dose naltrexone

Within a specific dosage window, opioid antagonists such as naltrexone can exert a "paradoxical" analgesic effect. Low-dose naltrexone (LDN) produces the modulation of neuro-inflammation, and stimulates the glial cells to release inflammatory chemicals in the central nervous system. The dosage producing these effects is low compared to the dosage approved for all alcohol and opioid dependency. The pharmacological actions enhance the analgesic effects of endogenous opioids and cannabinoids. Naltrexone modulates the toll-like receptor 4, NO, and filamin A. LDN is safe, with very few side effects, and recent clinical pilot trials in fibromyalgia and multiple sclerosis showed pain reduction and quality of life enhancing impact [32]. It also improved pain tolerance in cold pressor tests and the ability of post-detoxification patients to relate interpersonally with other participants in human relationships (**Tables 1** and **2**).

Synchrome/ model	Type of study (number of subjects)	Notable outcomes	References
Cholestasis pruritis	Case report (1)	Reduction of pruritis and improved mental status despite concurrent opioid therapy	Zylics et al. [34]
Osteoarthritis	Phase II randomized controlled trial (362)	Adding two mcg naltrexone to concurrent opioid therapy provides more significant analgesia. High dropout rate due to opioid side effects.	Chandalore et al. [35]
Low back pain	Phase III randomized controlled trial (712)	Adding two mcg of naltrexone to opioid therapy provides a more favorable response and reduces side effects. A high dropout rate precluded further application.	Webster et al. [36]
Axillary brachial plexus blockade	Randomized controlled trial (112)	Onset of time for motor and sensory blockade was longer with additional 100 ng of naloxone. Added naloxone prolongs motor blockade and analgesia.	Movafegh et al. [37]
Buprenorphine antinociception in healthy subjects	Double-blind crossover trial (10)	Applying buprenorphine with naloxone in 166:1 ratio boost tolerance to cold pressor test	Hay et al. [38]
Postoperative pain control following colorectal surgery	Randomized controlled trial (72)	Adding 0.25 mcg/kg/h of naloxone during surgery and postoperative period lowered opioid consumption shortened length of stay, and hastened bowel function recovery.	Xiao et al. [39]
Postoperative pain control following lumbar discectomy	Randomized controlled trial. (80)	Adding 0.25 mcg/kg/h of naloxone during first 24 h postoperative period reduced opioid consumption and side effects	Firouzian et al. [40]

Table 1.
Summary of clinical experience with low-dose naloxone/naltrexone. Adopted from [33].

3. Observational studies to evaluate the effectiveness of healthcare

The fundamentals of neurophysiology learn that the revalidation of the main chronobiological rhythm results in regulating sleep, food, and the vicious circle involved in pain sensitization.

Although randomized controlled trials are considered the most valuable method for proving the efficacy of a treatment. This method cannot be applied to every treatment. Black [46] discusses the advantages and disadvantages of strictly

Disease classification	Type of study (number of subjects)	Notable outcomes	Reference
Primary progressive multiple sclerosis	Open-label uncontrolled phase II (40)	Safe and tolerable (primary outcome) Significantly reduced spasticity	Gironi et al. [41]
Multiple sclerosis	Randomized placebo-controlled trial (60)	Significant benefits for mental health per quality-of-life indices	Cree et al. [42]
Relapsing-remitting and secondary progressive multiple sclerosis	Retrospective cohort (215)	Majority reported improvement in quality of life and reduced fatigue. Well-tolerated treatment with insomnia and nightmares as adverse effects in a minority of cases	Turel et al. [43]
Relapsing-remitting multiple sclerosis	Retrospective cohort (54)	LDN, as a single therapy, did not result in disease exacerbation.	Ludwig et al. [44]
Multiple sclerosis	Quasi-experimental pharmacoepidemiological cohort (341)	Exposure to LDN did not reduce the amount of disease-modifying therapies used	Raknes and Småkbrekke [45]

Table 2.
Clinical experience on LDN in multiple sclerosis. Adopted from [33].

regulated randomized controlled trials (RCTs). Measuring treatment outcomes of one intervention in patients with complex diseases for whom it would be unethical to drop most ongoing treatments. The numbers to be included in RCTs for demonstrating superiority in effect are too small to identify sometimes rare side effects. The blinding in RCTs cannot be maintained sufficiently long to assess the long-term impact. Building evidence is often a step-wise process, where an effect is noted and reported in a case report. These findings can be confirmed in retrospective and prospective studies, and if possible, the effect can be compared to a placebo or another treatment in an RCT.

The debate regarding these research design issues within conventional medicine has risen in parallel with the growing emphasis on team-based medicine and integrative medical teams for "evidence" of effectiveness and efficacy to meet the standards of "evidence-based medicine."

These standards are predominantly set out for pharmacological treatment, but the EBM model does not evaluate all parts of acupuncture efficacy and strategies in researching complex interventions.

The «whole system» methodology opens the research on Integrative Medicine efficacy with enhanced EBM validation.

Internal and external validity address the usefulness and effectiveness of a treatment. They are complementary and must be addressed separately in different studies. The results must be seen together. The hierarchy of evidence is one of the internal efficacies, not of evidence in general. Other research methodologies must be used and validated.

The results of observational studies help to target treatments and provide information for future research. The mechanisms of action could be elucidated by basic research, and meta-regression could better explain variability in response. Combining the evidence from different sources in a decision-analytical modeling can be used for economic evaluations [47].

4. Conclusions

Pain management is shifting from a model of highly specialized pain care to multimodal evidence-informed options fitted to a patient's whole experience of pain and therapeutic goals. Ideas changed due to the emerging science about the impact on pain states by the microbiome, mitochondria, fascia, glia and neuroplasticity, and movement disorders. Evidence-informed practice is based on evaluating and disseminating current research, including biological, medical, and behavioral science, secondary to pain for future pain treatments.

Emerging epigenetic data show that NPIs are valid approaches in chronic disease treatments on par with allopathic therapies regarding goals and risks. These approaches have proven superior to some conventional treatments because they tend not to cause such severe side effects.

It might be interesting to look at the quantitative and qualitative changes resulting from single interventions or combining non-pharmacological interventions to further test their efficacy and safety, as well as to improvise on existing therapeutic strategies to prevent or cure disease and disability.

Illustrated by various clinical situations, the objective of management is to seek synergy in the mechanisms of action of treatments to improve quality of life, reduce the need for xenobiotics, and consequently the side effects participating in vicious circles chronicity.

The current imperative is to determine what works best under what conditions.

Multiple medical problems often face limited treatment options, the increased risk of adverse effects, complex drug interactions, and the concurrent use of multiple medications.

From our current perspective, the potential benefit of including nutrition in personalizing pain medicine is formidable and highly promising. The role of personalized nutrition and nutraceuticals, by considering how they might be helpful in managing chronic pain, as well as their physiological features (such as body mass and microbiome) and pathological ones.

The need for a multidisciplinary evaluation and treatment focusing on drug metabolism and chronobiology is highlighted. This multimodal approach influences pain via synergistic non-drug associations like pharmaco-nutritional, acupuncture, neuro-acupuncture, and PEA. Acupuncture in this multidisciplinary model is a multimodal pain regulator. The therapeutic and post-effect are augmented by cellular physiological rehabilitation.

Conflict of interest

No conflict of interest to declare.

Abbreviations

5HT	5 hydroxy tryptamine
ACP	association of clinical practice guidelines
AMPA	ampa receptors glutamate receptor
ATP	adenosine triphosphate
Cx43	connexin 43

DRG	dorsal root ganglion
EA	electro acupuncture
er-fMRI	event-related functional magnetic resonance imaging
fMRI	functional magnetic resonance imaging
GABA	gammma aminobutyric acid
IASP	international association for the study of pain
LDN	low dose naltrexone
LPS	lipopolysaccharide binding protein
MOR	mu opioid receptor
NE	norepinephrine
NMDA	n methyl D asparatate receptors
NO	nitrous oxyde
NSAID	non-steroidal anti-inflammatory drug
P2X	recepteurs purinergiques
pH	degree of acidity
TLR4	toll like receptor 4
tVNS	transcutaneous vagus nerve stimulation
VN	vagal nerve

Appendix

The philosophy behind the score sheets states that individuals or groups define a standard for the quality of their performance. Then, they describe the standard in terms of a set of requirements. This set is the score sheet. It allows for peer evaluation and self-evaluation of an activity. Grading proceeds by determining the fraction of requirements fulfilled and is objective and reproducible. The score sheet exists prior to the execution of any activity and thus induces iteration until the performance becomes satisfactory. Any individual or group can adapt the method to any professional activity by selecting the pertinent requirements to fulfill their standard of excellence.

Author details

Agnes Mazic De Sonis
Pain Medicine Pole Neuroscience, Chirec Delta Hospital, Brussels, Belgium

*Address all correspondence to: a_mazic@yahoo.com

References

[1] Tick H et al. Evidence-based nonpharmacologic strategies for comprehensive pain care: The consortium pain task force white paper. Explore (New York, N.Y.). 2018;**14**(3):177-211

[2] Hay JL et al. Hyperalgesia in opioid-managed chronic pain and opioid-dependent patients. The Journal of Pain. 2009;**10**(3):316-322

[3] Junien C. Early determinants of health and disease: Epigenetics and environment. Bulletin de L'academie Nationale de Medecine. Mar 2011; **195**(3):511-526; discussion 526-527. DOI: 10.1016/s0001-4079(19)32060-6. PMID: 22292301

[4] Kanherkar RR, Bhatia-Dey N, Csoka AB. Epigenetics across the human lifespan. Frontiers in Cell and Development Biology. 2014;**2**:49

[5] Mazic-de Sonis A. Multimodal management of chronic pain: Litterature on the basic research and clinical expertise. In: 14 Congrès National de la SFETD. Lyon, France: La Société Française d'Études et de Traitement de la Douleur; 2014

[6] Plaghki L. Update on nociceptors. In: Quarterly Meeting October. Liège: GRID; 2014

[7] Akbarali HI, Dewey WL. The gut-brain interaction in opioid tolerance. Current Opinion in Pharmacology. 2017;**37**:126-130

[8] Meng J et al. Morphine induces bacterial translocation in mice by compromising intestinal barrier function in a TLR-dependent manner. PLoS One. 2013;**8**(1):e54040

[9] Trusheim MR, Berndt ER. Economic challenges and possible policy actions to advance stratified medicine. Personalized Medicine. 2012;**9**(4):413-427

[10] Ozdemir V et al. Mapping translational research in personalized therapeutics: From molecular markers to health policy. Pharmacogenomics. 2007;**8**(2):177-185

[11] Arar N et al. The genome-based knowledge management in cycles model: A complex adaptive systems framework for implementation of genomic applications. Personalized Medicine. 2011;**8**(2):191-205

[12] Sandberg M et al. Different patterns of blood flow response in the trapezius muscle following needle stimulation (acupuncture) between healthy subjects and patients with fibromyalgia and work-related trapezius myalgia. European Journal of Pain. 2005;**9**(5):497-510

[13] Shinbara H et al. Participation of calcitonin gene related peptide released via axon reflex in the local increase in muscle blood flow following manual acupuncture. Acupuncture in Medicine. 2013;**31**(1):81-87

[14] Carlton SM. Nociceptive primary afferents: They have a mind of their own. The Journal of Physiology. 2014;**592**(16):3403-3411

[15] Pan WX. Bidirectional regulation of acupuncture and its plausible mechanisms. Zhen Ci Yan Jiu. 2019;**44**(11):843-853

[16] Dinan TG et al. Collective unconscious: How gut microbes shape human behavior. Journal of Psychiatric Research. 2015;**63**:1-9

[17] Harris RE et al. Traditional Chinese acupuncture and placebo (sham) acupuncture are differentiated by their effects on mu-opioid receptors (MORs). NeuroImage. 2009;**47**(3):1077-1085

[18] Napadow V et al. Brain correlates of phasic autonomic response to acupuncture stimulation: An event-related fMRI study. Human Brain Mapping. 2013;**34**(10):2592-2606

[19] De Gregori M et al. Combining pain therapy with lifestyle: The role of personalized nutrition and nutritional supplements according to the SIMPAR Feed Your Destiny approach. Journal of Pain Research. 2016;**9**:1179-1189

[20] Rea K, Dinan TG, Cryan JF. The microbiome: A key regulator of stress and neuroinflammation. Neurobiol Stress. 2016;**4**:23-33

[21] IASP. Integrative pain medicine: A holistic model of care. IASP: Pain Clinical Update. 2014;**22**:1-6

[22] Ticinesi A et al. Gut microbiota composition is associated with polypharmacy in elderly hospitalized patients. Scientific Reports. 2017;**7**(1):11102

[23] Burneo JG et al. Weight loss associated with vagus nerve stimulation. Neurology. 2002;**59**(3):463-464

[24] Cork SC et al. Extracellular pH monitoring for use in closed-loop vagus nerve stimulation. Journal of Neural Engineering. 2018;**15**(1):016001

[25] Ikramuddin S et al. Effect of reversible intermittent intra-abdominal vagal nerve blockade on morbid obesity: the ReCharge randomized clinical trial. JAMA. 2014;**312**(9):915-922

[26] Shikora S et al. Vagal blocking improves glycemic control and elevated blood pressure in obese subjects with type 2 diabetes mellitus. Journal of Obesity. 2013;**2013**:245683

[27] Pardo JV et al. Weight loss during chronic, cervical vagus nerve stimulation in depressed patients with obesity: An observation. International Journal of Obesity. 2007;**31**(11):1756-1759

[28] Hu X et al. PLGA-curcumin attenuates opioid-induced hyperalgesia and inhibits spinal CaMKIIα. PLoS One. 2016;**11**(1):e0146393

[29] Teiten MH, Dicato M, Diederich M. Curcumin as a regulator of epigenetic events. Molecular Nutrition & Food Research. 2013;**57**(9):1619-1629

[30] Anand P et al. Bioavailability of curcumin: Problems and promises. Molecular Pharmaceutics. 2007;**4**(6):807-818

[31] Nau R et al. Strategies to increase the activity of microglia as efficient protectors of the brain against infections. Frontiers in Cellular Neuroscience. 2014;**8**:138

[32] Hesselink JM, Kopsky DJ. Enhancing acupuncture by low dose naltrexone. Acupuncture in Medicine. 2011;**29**(2):127-130

[33] Toljan K, Vrooman B. Low-dose naltrexone (LDN)-review of therapeutic utilization. Medical Sciences. 2018;**6**(4):82

[34] Zylicz Z, Stork N, Krajnik M. Severe pruritus of cholestasis in disseminated cancer: Developing a rational treatment strategy. A case report. Journal of Pain and Symptom Management. 2005;**29**(1):100-103

[35] Chindalore VL et al. Adding ultralow-dose naltrexone to oxycodone

enhances and prolongs analgesia: A randomized, controlled trial of Oxytrex. The Journal of Pain. 2005;**6**(6):392-399

[36] Webster LR et al. Oxytrex minimizes physical dependence while providing effective analgesia: A randomized controlled trial in low back pain. The Journal of Pain. 2006;**7**(12):937-946

[37] Movafegh A et al. An ultra-low dose of naloxone added to lidocaine or lidocaine-fentanyl mixture prolongs axillary brachial plexus blockade. Anesthesia and Analgesia. 2009;**109**(5):1679-1683

[38] Hay JL et al. Potentiation of buprenorphine antinociception with ultra-low dose naltrexone in healthy subjects. European Journal of Pain. 2011;**15**(3):293-298

[39] Xiao Y et al. A randomized clinical trial of the effects of ultra-low-dose naloxone infusion on postoperative opioid requirements and recovery. Acta Anaesthesiologica Scandinavica. 2015;**59**(9):1194-1203

[40] Firouzian A et al. Ultra-low-dose naloxone as an adjuvant to patient controlled analgesia (PCA) with morphine for postoperative pain relief following lumber discectomy: A double-blind, randomized, placebo-controlled trial. Journal of Neurosurgical Anesthesiology. 2018;**30**(1):26-31

[41] Gironi M et al. A pilot trial of low-dose naltrexone in primary progressive multiple sclerosis. Multiple Sclerosis. 2008;**14**(8):1076-1083

[42] Cree BA, Kornyeyeva E, Goodin DS. Pilot trial of low-dose naltrexone and quality of life in multiple sclerosis. Annals of Neurology. 2010;**68**(2):145-150

[43] Turel AP et al. Low dose naltrexone for treatment of multiple sclerosis: A retrospective chart review of safety and tolerability. Journal of Clinical Psychopharmacology. 2015;**35**(5):609-611

[44] Ludwig MD et al. Long-term treatment with low dose naltrexone maintains stable health in patients with multiple sclerosis. Multiple Sclerosis Journal—Experimental, Translational and Clinical. 2016;**2**:2055217316672242

[45] Raknes G, Småbrekke L. Low dose naltrexone in multiple sclerosis: Effects on medication use. A quasi-experimental study. PLoS One. 2017;**12**(11):e0187423

[46] Black N. Why we need observational studies to evaluate the effectiveness of health care. BMJ. 1996;**312**(7040):1215-1218

[47] Philips Z et al. Review of guidelines for good practice in decision-analytic modelling in health technology assessment. Health Technology Assessment. 2004;**8**(36):iii-iv, ix-xi, 1-158